Diagnosis and Psychopharmacology
of Childhood and Adolescent Disorders

WILEY SERIES IN CHILD AND ADOLESCENT MENTAL HEALTH

Joseph D. Noshpitz, Editor

FATHERLESS CHILDREN

by Paul L. Adams, Judith R. Milner and Nancy A. Schrepf

DIAGNOSIS AND PSYCHOPHARMACOLOGY OF CHILDHOOD AND ADOLESCENT DISORDERS

by Jerry M. Wiener

DIAGNOSIS AND PSYCHOPHARMACOLOGY OF CHILDHOOD AND ADOLESCENT DISORDERS

Edited by

JERRY M. WIENER

George Washington University School of Medicine

A Wiley-Interscience Publication

JOHN WILEY & SONS

New York / Chichester / Brisbane / Toronto / Singapore

This publication is designed to provide accurate and
authoritative information in regard to the subject
matter covered. It is sold with the understanding that
the publisher is not engaged in rendering legal, accounting,
or other professional service. If legal advice or other
expert assistance is required, the services of a competent
professional person should be sought. *From a Declaration
of Principles jointly adopted by a Committee of the
American Bar Association and a Committee of Publishers.*

Library of Congress Cataloging in Publication Data:

Main entry under title:

Diagnosis and psychopharmacology of childhood and
  adolescent disorders.

  (Wiley series in child and adolescent mental health)
  "A Wiley-Interscience publication."
  Includes indexes.
  1. Child psychopathology.   2. Adolescent psychopathology.   3. Psychopharmacology.   4. Pediatric pharmacology.
I. Wiener, Jerry M., 1933–   .   II. Series. [DNLM:
1. Mental Disorders—in adolescence.   2. Mental Disorders
—in infancy & childhood.   3. Psychopharmacology—in
adolescence   4. Psychopharmacology—in infancy & childhood.   WS 350 D536]

RJ499.D49   1985   618.92′89′18   84-25797
ISBN 0-471-80071-6

Printed in the United States of America

10 9 8 7 6 5 4 3

To Louise,
and to
Matthew, Ethan, Ross, and Aaron

List of Contributors

Paul J. Ambrosini, M.D., *Assistant Professor of Psychiatry, College of Physicians and Surgeons, Columbia University, New York, New York*

Magda Campbell, M.D., *Professor of Psychiatry, New York University Medical Center, New York, New York*

Donald J. Cohen, M.D., *Professor of Pediatrics, Psychiatry and Psychology, Child Study Center, Yale University, New Haven, Connecticut*

C. Keith Conners, Ph.D., *Professor of Psychiatry and Behavioral Sciences and Child Health and Development, George Washington University Medical School, and Director of Research, Department of Psychiatry, Children's Hospital National Medical Center, Washington, DC*

Maureen Donnelly, M.D., *Section on Child Psychiatry, National Institute of Mental Health, Bethesda, Maryland*

Robert L. Hendren, D.O., *Assistant Professor of Psychiatry and Behavioral Sciences, Co-Director, Eating Disorders Program, George Washington University Medical School, Washington, DC*

Steven L. Jaffe, M.D., *Associate Professor of Psychiatry (Child), Emory Univer-*

sity, and Director, Adolescent Psychiatry Program, Parkwood Hospital, Atlanta, Georgia

Peter J. Knott, Ph.D., *Associate Professor of Psychiatry and Pharmacology, Mount Sinai School of Medicine, New York, New York*

James F. Leckman, M.D., *Associate Professor of Pediatrics and Psychiatry, Child Study Center, Yale University, New Haven, Connecticut*

Leonard I. Leven, M.D., *Research Fellow in Child and Adolescent Psychiatry, Mount Sinai School of Medicine, New York, New York*

J. Vernon Magnuson, M.D., *Assistant Professor of Psychiatry (Child), Emory University, and Director, Division of Child and Adolescent Psychiatry, Grady Memorial Hospital, Atlanta, Georgia*

Daniel J. O'Donnell, M.D., *Assistant Professor of Psychiatry and Behavioral Science and Child Health and Development, George Washington University Medical School, and Director, Inpatient Psychiatric Service, Children's Hospital National Medical Center, Washington, DC*

Joaquim Puig-Antich, M.D., *Professor of Psychiatry, University of Pittsburgh School of Medicine, and Chief, Child and Adolescent Psychiatry, Western Psychiatric Institute and Clinic, Pittsburgh, Pennsylvania*

Harris Rabinovich, M.D., *Instructor of Clinical Psychiatry and Research Psychiatrist, College of Physicians and Surgeons, Columbia University, New York, New York*

Judith L. Rapoport, M.D., *Chief, Section of Child Psychiatry, National Institute of Mental Health, Bethesda, Maryland, and Clinical Professor of Psychiatry, George Washington University School of Medicine, Washington, DC*

Neal D. Ryan, M.D., *Instructor of Clinical Psychiatry, College of Physicians and Surgeons, Columbia University, New York, New York*

David Shaffer, M.R.C.P., F.R.C. Psych., *Chief, Division of Child Psychiatry, New York State Psychiatric Institute, and Professor of Clinical Psychiatry and Pediatrics, College of Physicians and Surgeons, Columbia University, New York, New York*

Theodore Shapiro, M.D., *Professor of Psychiatry and Pediatrics, and Director of Child Psychiatry, New York Hospital-Cornell Medical College, New York, New York.*

Jerry M. Wiener, M.D., *Leon Yochelson Professor and Chairman, Department of Psychiatry and Behavioral Sciences, George Washington University School of Medicine, Washington, DC*

J. Gerald Young, M.D., *Professor of Psychiatry and Pediatrics, Mount Sinai School of Medicine, New York, New York*

Preface

A precursor of this book appeared in 1977. Although this was only seven years ago, the field of psychopharmacology in childhood disorders is changed in significant ways from its status in the mid-1970s, more than justifying a new volume. I stated in the preface to the earlier work that the time seemed overdue for such a book; of this edition I can say the time seems just about right. Why so?

First, and perhaps foremost, major advances occurred during the mid-to-late 1970s in the development of reliable, operationally defined, and generally accepted diagnostic classifications. This culminated in the 1980 publication of the *Diagnostic and Statistical Manual* (DSM-III) by the American Psychiatric Association. This has made possible the study of homogenous groups of children and comparisons among different studies in different centers. Accordingly, the clinical section of this book is organized by DMS-III categories.

Second, both the methodology of drug studies, and the reliability and validity of standardized assessment instruments, are significantly improved and more widely used. These issues are fully explored and explicated in Chapter 3.

Third, and related to the above two points, the number of child psychiatrists and others doing creditable psychopharmacology research has increased, and accordingly, the number of high quality research findings on the indications, pharmacodynamics, efficacy, and adverse effects of psychoactive drug use in children.

The contributors to this volume represent a combination of outstanding research scientists and experienced senior clinicians and teachers. Together they present the current state of the science of psychopharmacology in childhood disorders, and the art of their use in clinical practice. Working as editor with this outstanding group of authors has been again, as it was before, "stimulating, at times frustrating, but always greatly rewarding." The real reward for me, as I hope it will be for the reader, is in what I have learned from this volume, not in what I have done for it.

I have had much help, and in particular must thank Herb Reich of Wiley for shepherding this book to publication, and Steve Jaffe who always was helpful when I asked.

JERRY M. WIENER, M.D.

May 1985
Washington, D.C.

Contents

**2. *Developmental Considerations in Psychopharmacology:
The Interaction of Drugs and Development***   *51*

Theodore Shapiro, M.D.

Central Nervous System Untoward Effects 137
Behavioral and Other Withdrawal Effects 140
Supersensitivity Psychosis 140
Abnormal Laboratory Findings 140
Miscellaneous 141
Effects on Height and Weight 141
Patient Sample, Design, and Assessment 142

7. *Anxiety Disorders* 199

Steven L. Jaffe, M.D.
J. Vernon Magnuson, M.D.

J. Gerald Young, M.D.
Leonard I. Leven, M.D.
Peter J. Knott, Ph.D.
James F. Leckman, M.D.
Donald J. Cohen, M.D.

SECTION III: CONCLUSION

*Diagnosis and Psychopharmacology
of Childhood and Adolescent Disorders*

Basic Issues

Historical Overview of Childhood and Adolescent Psychopharmacology

JERRY M. WIENER, M.D. and STEVEN L. JAFFE, M.D.

Parts of this chapter, reviewing the period up to 1970, have appeared previously in J. Wiener (Ed.), *Psychopharmacology in Childhood and Adolescence*, published in 1977 by Basic Books.

A scientific psychopharmacology for childhood and adolescent disorders essentially did not exist before the 1930s. Reflecting the state of the science at that time, Kanner (1935) commented in the first edition of his textbook: "Pharmacological aids are indicated in demonstrable endocrine disorders, in lues, in the epilepsies, in migrane and other severe headaches, and in a number of other conditions. The indiscriminate use of toxics and sedatives as placebos cannot be discourged emphatically enough" (p. 133). Progress in the field remained minimal until the later 1950s, as illustrated by the second edition of Kanner's textbook (1957), which included only two pages of discussion and sixteen references on drug therapy.

During the 1930s and 1940s the entire emphasis was on the use of Benzedrine sulfate and Dilantin sodium with hyperactive, "brain-damaged," and behavior-disordered children. After the introduction of the "tranquilizers" in the 1950s, the number of studies on the use of drugs for the emotional and behavioral disorders of childhood and adolescence increased, at first slowly, and then dramatically. By 1958, Freedman (1958) listed 63 references from the literature, covering 14 different "tranquilizer" drugs and three "stimulant" drugs. Subsequently Eveloff (1966) published an excellent review of the literature on pharmacology in child psychiatry, citing 63 articles for the preceding five-year period. He offered a clinical classification that included the major tranquilizers, minor tranquilizers, stimulants (dextroamphetamine sulfate and methylphenidate) and the antidepressants (MAO inhibitors and tricyclic compounds).

In 1956 the National Institute of Mental Health established the Psychopharmacology Service Center to serve as the focal source of support for research in psychopharmacology (Psychopharmacology Bulletin, 1973). Following a Center-sponsored Conference on Child Research in Psychopharmacology, the first NIMH grant to study childhood pharmacotherapy was awarded in 1958 to Dr. Leon Eisenberg of the Johns Hopkins University. This grant was for the study of two major tranquilizers and meprobamate. A second grant for childhood pharmacotherapy was awarded in 1961, a third grant was not awarded until 1968. Although blame for this minimal support has been placed on the unsophisticated state of methodology in the field (Lipman, 1973), nevertheless, a low level of priority seems to have been assigned to research in childhood pharmacotherapy.

As a measure of both progress and the lack of it, and echoing an observation made 12 years earlier by Freedman (1958), Di Mascio stated in 1970 that, "The majority of these articles [in childhood psychopharmacology] show a marked lack of application of sophisticated research

4

techniques required for the appropriate assessment of a drug's actions" (p. 479). He referred by that time, however, to almost 500 articles in the American literature.

It is indeed true that most studies in childhood pharmacotherapy have serious methodological flaws, including absent or inadequate control groups; nonstandardized dosage schedules; insufficient attention to the placebo effect; absent or inadequate attention to standardized observation techniques, rating scales, and other measurements; poorly defined study groups; and an inadequate basis for diagnostic classification of psychiatric disorders in childhood.

At the same time, significant progress can be noted. A wealth of clinical experience with psychoactive medication has accumulated. Studies published in the past few years have been increasingly sophisticated in their attention to considerations of methodology. The field of childhood psychopharmacology is vigorous and expanding. This chapter will trace the history by decades of this growth and expansion. The first two decades (1930–1950) dealt almost exclusively with stimulants (and anticonvulsants) in hyperactive and brain-damaged children. The decade of the fifties marked the beginning of the so-called modern era in psychopharmacology with the introduction of the major tranquilizers. During the 1960s the antidepressants and new classes of major tranquilizers were introduced, and there was a revival of studies on the stimulant drugs in the hyperkinetic syndrome. This decade was also marked by an increasing concern for methodology and more refined approaches to diagnostic classification.

The decade of the seventies was marked by increasingly sophisticated verification and comparison studies, an expanding base of knowledge about the biological aspects of normal and deviant child development, and a concomitant interest in the kinetics and mechanisms of action of psychoactive drugs in children.

THE 1930s

All psychopharmacological agents for the treatment of behavioral and emotional problems in children were first studied in adult populations. In 1936 a series of studies (Sargant & Blackburn, 1936; Myerson et al., 1936) described Benzedrine (a combination of the dextro and levo forms of amphetamine) as a central nervous system stimulant affecting mood and behavior and possibly increasing intelligence. In the next year, Bradley (1937) reported the effects of Benzedrine on behavior problem children in residential treatment at the Emma Pendleton Bradley Home.

This report marked the beginning of a clinical psychopharmacology in children. Because of its historical significance and because most of its results were subsequently confirmed in studies with more sophisticated methodology 30 years later, this first report is presented in some detail. Thirty children, ages 5 to 14 years and of normal intelligence, received an average morning dose of 20 mg of Benzedrine during the middle week of a three-week observation period. Diagnostically, the children varied from "specific educational disabilities, with secondarily disturbed school behavior, to the retiring schizoid child on one hand and the aggressive, egocentric, epileptic child on the other" (p. 578). Effects of Benzedrine were rapid and, in many children, remarkable. Fourteen of the 30 improved "spectacularly" in school performance with increased interest, speed of comprehension, and accuracy. This effect appeared on the first day Benzedrine was given and disappeared on the first day it was discontinued. Eight children demonstrated temporary school improvement, five showed no change in school performance but had an "emotional response," and two had no response at all. Under the category of emotional response, 15 of the 30 became "subdued," which meant that they became placid, easygoing, and had decreased mood swings yielding improvement in social relationships. Seven of the children with the subdued-improved emotional response also demonstrated the "spectacular" increase in school performance. Negative responses included three who cried more easily, two who became more anxious, and one who became more hyperactive, aggressive and defiant. Side effects were delay in falling asleep, malaise, nausea, and epigastric distress. Twenty children were given EEGs and over half of these were definitely abnormal. Thus, in a small study using careful clinical observation and each child as his own control, Bradley described remarkable changes in school performance and improvement in emotional response level in about half of the children after administration of Benzedrine. Despite these markedly positive findings, Bradley was cautious as to the use of medication affecting behavior and emotions. He stated, "Any indiscriminate use of Benzedrine to produce symptomatic relief might well mask reactions of etiological significance that should in every case receive adequate attention" (p. 584). This approach is as pertinent now as it was in 1937.

In the same year as Bradley's first report, Molitch et al. (Molitch & Sullivan, 1937; Molitch & Eccles, 1937) studied the effects of Benzedrine on preadolescent and adolescent boys who were committed to the New Jersey State Home for Boys. Using a comparison group that received placebo, but without statistical analysis, they reported greater improvement with the drug on the New Stanford Achievement Test and on verbal intelligence scores. In a third study (Molitch & Poliakoff, 1937) eight of the 22 most severe enuretics at the Home improved with placebo, while increasing doses of Benzedrine led to continence in 12 of the remaining 14.

Cutts and Jasper (1939), also at the Bradley Home, were the first to describe the reverse effects of phenobarbital in certain behavior-disordered children. Twelve children aged 7 to 10 who had abnormal EEGs and behavior characterized by hyperactivity, impulsivity, and marked variations in personality unrelated to environmental changes were administered Benzedrine and phenobarbital. Seven improved with Benzedrine, while phenobarbital caused an increase of irritability, impulsivity, destructiveness, and temper tantrums in nine.

THE 1940s

Bradley continued to study the effects of Benzedrine at the Bradley Home in Rhode Island while Bender and her co-workers concomitantly studied the effects of Benzedrine on children hospitalized at Bellevue Hospital in New York. Bradley and his group (Bradley & Bowen, 1940; Bradley & Green, 1940) reported that children administered Benzedrine who showed marked improvement in school performance especially improved in arithmetic, but that Benzedrine did not significantly affect performance on the revised Stanford Binet scale. They concluded that the improved intellectual performance following Benzedrine administration represented primarily an improved attitude by the subject toward the intellectual task.

Bradley and Bowen (1941) summarized their studies on Benzedrine from the previous three-year period. Administered to 100 children with a variety of behavior disorders, 72 improved, of whom 54 were "subdued" from a hyperactive labile impulsive state, 12 were stimulated from a previously abnormally underactive or preoccupied condition, and six improved in school performance without other behavioral change. Twenty-one were unaffected, and seven had negative effects described as excessive activity or irritability. These results were related to clinical diagnosis but no definite correlation was found. Bradley commented at that time on the chaos in child psychiatric diagnostic classification.

Bender and Cottington (1942) reported the effects of Benzedrine on 40 hospitalized children who were not otherwise accessible to treatment. Dosage at 10–20 mg were administered, and results grouped according to a diagnostic classification. In the psychoneurosis group, which included hysterical, depressed, phobic, obsessive-compulsive, and anxiety states, eight improved and four became more tense and irritable. An immediate and dramatic effect was noted in the "neurotic" or "usual" behavior disorder group in the direction of decreased hyperactivity, increased attention span, improved integration and more constructive activity. Children with schizophrenia, organic brain disease, or psychopathic personalities either did not respond or worsened. One girl with persistent masturbation and sexual preoccupations responded with relief of "sexual tension." Two of four children with severe reading disabilities had a definite increase in attention span and improved motivation for learning. This was the first report of the effects of stimulant medication on children with a specific learning disability. Bender, like Bradley, put into perspective the possible roles and uses of medication. She commented: "The successful use of this drug in the behavior problems in children depends on a clear understanding of the causes of the child's problems, the proper choice of children to receive the drug, and the use of the drug only as an adjunct to adequate personal psychotherapy, tutoring, and social adjustment" (p. 12).

THE 1950s

Stimulants

At the beginning of this decade, Bradley (1950) summarized the results of 12 years of study during which Benzedrine and dextroamphetamine were administered to over 350 children under the age of 13 years. Of the 275 children who received Benzedrine, 60–75 percent improved with 50–60 percent subdued from a previous hyperactive, impulsive state; 20 percent stimulated from a shy, regressing state; 5 percent improved in school performance with no behavioral changes; and no effect was produced in 15–20 percent of the cases. Unfavorable responses occured in 10–15 percent in which excessive stimulation predominated, and a few were excessively subdued. These results were very similar to Bradley's previous report on 100 children in 1941. The effects of dextroamphetamine were compared with those of Benzedrine in 82 children; about a third did better with dextroamphetamine and a third did better with Benzedrine.

Bender and Nichtern summarized their clinical psychopharmacological studies in 1956. Drugs were given to children with a variety of symptoms. If improvement occurred, this drug was then given to other children with the same symptom complex. At least four to five drugs were used on the ward at the same time, with ward personnel generally being unaware of which drug was given. They reported that neurotic behavior patterns responded best to amphetamines with most children becoming quieter, more cheerful, and relaxed with decreased mood swings and relief of tension. In comparing Benzedrine with Dexedrine, they reported that Dexedrine was equally effective at half the dose.

Laufer et al. (1957) defined the hyperkinetic impulse disorder as characterized by hyperactivity, short attention span, impulsivity, low frustration tolerance, poor school work, visual motor problems, writing and reading reversals, and poor handwriting. "Although each of these symptoms or any combintion may also have a purely emotional origin, this total symptom complex, at the time of its origin at least, does not seem to be related to any particular psychological precipitant, though it may have concomitant psychological effects and sequelae" (p. 38). Laufer stated that the positive effects of amphetamines on behavior disordered children, as described by Bradley, were observed primarily in children presenting the hyperkinetic impulse disorder Thus Laufer, also working at the Bradley Home, set the stage for the later numerous studies of the effects of stimulants on the diagnostic grouping of hyperactive children. He further demonstrated that children with the hyperkinetic impulse disorder had a photometrazol threshold significantly lower than did children of comparable age without the syndrome. In addition, 13 of the children with the hyperkinetic impulse disorder who were administered amphetamines demonstrated a rise in the mean photometrazol threshold up to the level previously noted as characteristic for children who are hypokinetic. Laufer hypothesized that the hyperkinetic impulse disorder was due to a dysfunction of the diencephalon causing unusual sensitivity to stimuli from both peripheral receptors and viscera.

Methylphenidate (Ritalin) was first synthesized in 1954. Although it was hoped that this drug would be a central nervous system stimulant free of the side effects and abuse potential of the amphetamines, double-blind studies in adults did not bear this out (Fisher & Wilson, 1971). Zimmerman and Burgemeister (1958) reported results in a mixed-age (i.e., 4–33 years) outpatient population with a variety of emotional problems. Sixty-five percent of those treated with methylphenidate improved, while 60 percent of a matched group improved with Reserpine. Verbal intelligence retest quotients following six months of treatment with either drug were not significantly affected, but results of the motor test favored the methylphenidate group.

The "Tranquilizer" Medications

The synthesis of chlorpromazine (R.P. 4560, Largactil) in 1950 by Charpentier in France initiated the modern era of psychopharmacology

(Dundee, 1954). Because of its sedative and hypothermic effects, the drug's original use was as an adjunct and supplement to anesthesia.

Delay and Deniker (1952) were the first to report on the value of chlorpromazine in psychiatric patients, and the first clinical report of its use as the sole treatment drug for psychiatric conditions appeared in July 1952 (Delay et al.).

The first report on the use of chlorpromazine in children appeared in 1953, describing its value in cases of "psychomotor excitement," with favorable results as long as the medication was maintained (Heuyer et al., 1953).

Lehman and Hanrahan (1954) published the first report in the English literature on the use of chloropromazine in adult psychiatric patients, concluding that "the drug is of unique value in the symptomatic control of almost any kind of severe excitement" (p. 232).

Several studies were published in 1955 on the use of chlorpromazine in three types of children, the "emotionally disturbed," "mentally retarded", and cerebral palsied. Except for one study by Freedman et al. (1955a), all the reports in this first round of experience were essentially impressionistic clinical trials. Silver (1955) reported anecdotally on the use of chlorpromazine for the control of restless behavior and "autonomic imbalance." Gatski (1955) and Flaherty (1955) reported on the use of chlorpromazine for emotionally disturbed boys in residential treatment centers, with dramatic improvement in behavior, tractability, and social relatedness. The age range in these latter two studies was from 6–15 years, dosage ranged from 40–100 mg/day, administration and/or observation were nonblind, and there were no control groups.

Bair and Herold (1955) and Rettig (1955) reported on the use of chlorpromazine in very heterogeneous populations of behaviorally disturbed, mentally retarded children and adolescents. Dosages ranged from 75–200 mg/day, with an impressive improvement in behavior reported in both studies. Rettig commented that the greater the "actual brain damage, the less the effectiveness of the drug" (p. 194). Neither of these studies included control groups or standardized observations and ratings.

Denhoff and Holden (1955) gave chlorpromazine to children with cerebral palsy. Although the anticipated muscle relaxant effect did not occur, they reported an improvement in overall behavior in half of the 18 children studied, allowing for better rehabilitation and ratings.

Freedman et al. (1955a) presented the results up to that time of a three-year psychopharmacology study on the Children's Service of the Psychiatric Division of Bellevue Hospital in New York City. This was a multidrug comparison study involving 105 boys between 7 and 12 years, selected randomly from admissions to the inpatient service. A well-defined methodology is described, including the use of placebo control, rating scales, and a single-blind drug administration. Comparing six drugs (Benadryl, Tolserol, Artane, Ambodryl, Thorazine hydrochloride, and Serpasil) with one another, the authors concluded that Benadryl (diphenhydramine) had the best overall effect, particularly in children with the diagnosis of primary behavior disorder displaying anxiety. Chlorpromazine in doses from 30–100 mg/day was most beneficial for children with a diagnosis of schizophrenia who were "hyperactive." Artane, Ambodryl, and Serpasil were not superior in effect to placebo.

Contributions during 1956 included papers by Heuyer et al., Freed & Peifer, Hunt et al., and Miksztal et al. Freed & Peifer reported the first study on the use of chlorpromazine with outpatient children who were "overactive and emotionally disturbed," having a diagnosis of "primary behavior disorder." Twenty-five children ages 7–15 years were treated in doses ranging from 10–250 mg/day, including a comparison period on placebo therapy. A decrease in hyperactivity, greater calmness, facilitated learning, and better interpersonal relationships were recorded at a level of "marked improvement" in 70 percent of the cases.

Hunt et al. (1956) reported the most ambitious and carefully controlled study of chlorpromazine use in children to that time. They employed a blind chlorpromazine-placebo crossover study in two groups matched for age and, most important, for diagnosis. Diagnostic groups included schizophrenic reactions classified as chronic, "sub-acute and borderline," and acute; primary behavior disorder; adolescent delinquent behavior; and severely brain-damaged children. Although the number in each group was too small for statistical significance, hyperactivity and social relatedness were consistently improved. Side effects were minimal and mild as dosage levels increased to the point of drowsiness and sedation.

Two reports appeared in 1957 (Carter & Maley, Tarjan et al.). The latter reported the use of chlorpromazine in a nonblind, nonrandom, uncontrolled study with 178 defective adults and children (141) of 19 years old or below with a subjective conclusion of improvement in 70 percent.

Reviewing the field in 1958, Freedman stated: "one is appalled at the number of drugs recommended and the conflicting claims both as to efficacy and absence of toxicity" (p. 573). He criticized the common shortcomings of faulty methodology, lack of adequate controls, and uncertainty of diagnosis. Freedman listed 154 "tranquilizer" drugs and three "stimulant" drugs for which there was some report or experience in the literature. The tranquilizers were divided into (1) phenothiazine derivatives, (2) reserpine, (3) diphenylmethane derivatives, and (4) the propanediol derivatives, maphanesin (Tolserol), and meprobamate. The stimulants listed were Benzedrine, Dexedrine, and marsilid. Freedman concluded that chlorpromazine was particularly useful in the treatment of hyperkinetic children, particularly when associated with schizophrenia. On the other phenothiazine drugs—promazine (Sparine), prochlorperazine (Compazine), perphenazine (Trifalon), triflupromazine (Vesprin), and promethazine (Phenergan)—either there were no published reports of experience with children or only subjectively substantiated or unconfirmed impressions.

Of the diphenylmethane compounds, diphenylhydramine (Benadryl) was reported as particularly helpful and superior to placebo at a statistically significant level in "primary behavior disorders displaying anxiety." This conclusion was based on a preliminary report (Effron & Freedman, 1953) and a later single controlled study (Freedman et al, 1955b). Otherwise, the remainder of this group of compounds—azacyclonol (Frenquel), hydroxyzine (Atarax), benactyzine (Suavitil), captodiamine (Suvren)—were all reported of positive or variable usefulness in the treatment of impulsivity, diffuse anxiety, overactivity, behavior disorders, and brain-injured children. However, none of these drugs had been studied with any adequate methodology up to that time, and no subsequent reports of such studies appeared in the literature. It is of some historical interest that Freedman (1958) cited a study by Bayart presented at a meeting in July 1956, which reported dramatic improvement in 90 percent of children with tics treated with 30 mg/day of hydroxyzine (Atarax). A published report of this presentation cannot be found and, despite this extremely impressive result with a symptom so often refractory to any treatment, no subsequent reports appeared on the use of hydroxyzine for the treatment of children with tics.

For the propanediol derivatives, Freedman cited his earlier experience with myanesin (Tolserol) (Freedman et al., 1955b), and also reported his impression of meprobamate as useful in children with "organic behavior disorders" characterized by symptoms of hyperactivity, restlessness, distractibility, and short attention span.

Between 1957 and 1961 several articles appeared on the use of meprobamate in children with behavioral and/or emotional disturbance (Littchfield, 1957; Kraft et al, 1959; Zier, 1959; Breger 1961). By and large these studies included heterogeneous groups of children by age, symptomatology, and diagnosis. Dosage ranged from 50–1200 mg/day in the various studies, and methodology ranged from absent to minimally adequate except for the study by Breger, which was methodologically sound and concluded that placebo was as effective as meprobamate for the treatment of childhood enuresis. The other studies reported positive to enthusiastic results for meprobamate in the treatment of everything from petit mal epilepsy to schizophrenia, from enuresis to stuttering, and for various behavioral problems. No further studies of meprobamate in children appeared in the literature to either refute or further validate these results.

THE 1960s

The decade of the 1960s is characterized by several developments:

1. An almost quantum leap forward in the study of stimulants in children with the hyperkinetic syndrome.

2. The introduction into childhood pharmacotherapy of two additional classes of phenothiazine compounds, (1) the piperazines: trifluoperazine (Stelazine), fluphenazine (Prolixin), perphenazine (Trilafon), prochlorperazine (Compazine), and (2) the piperidine compound thioridazine (Mellaril).

3. The first use in children of two additional categories of major tranquilizing drugs: the thioxanthenes and butyrophenones.

4. Use of the antidepressant drugs—MAO inhibitors and the tricyclic compounds—in various categories of childhood disorders.

5. An increasing concern with the methodology required to yield either reliable or valid results, along with attention to the related issue of adequate diagnostic classification.

Stimulants

Fish (1960a) reported the results of treatment with 85 outpatient children under age 12 in whom various medications were used as a part of overall treatment programs. In response to amphetamines nine of 12 children with school phobia had rapid relief of their sexual and hypochondriacal preoccupations.

Knobel (1962) in an uncontrolled study treated 150 children with the hyperactivity syndrome with 20–40 mg/day of methylphenidate (Ritalin) for eight months. He reported that 40 percent showed "good" improvement, 50 percent "moderate" improvement, and 10 percent "no" improvement.

Eisenberg and co-workers, after reporting negative results with tranquilizers (Cytryn et al., 1960), began to study the effects of the stimulants on hyperkinetic children. Eisenberg et al. (1963) first studied the effects of dextroamphetamine on the 21 most troublesome male adolescents at a state training school. A double-blind, placebo controlled design was used in three groups matched on the basis of symptom scores from behavioral ratings done by cottage parents, teachers, and peers. The three groups were indistinguishable by the pretreatment ratings. At the end of the seven weeks of treatment, the amphetamine group rated significantly superior to the placebo and control groups. Then Conners and Eisenberg (1963) reported a study of 81 disturbed children aged 7–15 years in residential care who were randomly assigned to drug and placebo groups. The drug group received 30–60 mg/day of methylphenidate over a 10-day period. This was a double-blind placebo controlled study with symptomatology ratings by house parents and child care workers. A statistically significant improvement occurred in the drug group on total symptom score, a paired association learning test, and the Porteus Maze test. These two studies established the short-term efficacy of the stimulant in reducing hyperactivity, distractibility, and impulsivity.

Except for the grants to Eisenberg's group and to Fish's group, there was a hiatus of funding support between 1961 and 1968 from the Psychopharmacology Service Center of the National Institute of Mental Health. Lipman (1973) described the few grants reviewed and not approved as reflecting the unsophisticated state of methodology in pediatric psychopharmacology. Funding support began again in 1968. Conners was given a personal service contract to develop a reliable and sensitive standardized rating system. The Conners Teacher Rating Scale (Conners, 1969) and the Conners Parent Symptom Questionnaire (Conners, 1970), became standard rating scales in most subsequnt studies.

Research on the effects of stimulants in the late 1960s was characterized by improved research design and more emphasis on cognitive functioning. Conners et al. (1967) reported on a double-blind placebo controlled, crossover design study involving one month of 10 mg/day of Dexedrine and one month of placebo administered to fifth and sixth graders referred by the school because of significant academic and/or school behavior difficulties. Significant improvement occurred by teacher ratings for the active drug group, including a reliable increase on that rating scale factor thought to reflect assertiveness and drive.

Millichap et al. (1968) reported on a double-blind placebo controlled crossover design study in which methylphenidate at 1.5 mg/kg for a three-week period was administered to 30 school-age children of normal I.Q. with hyperactivity and school underachievement. Significant and specific beneficial effects attributable to the drug occurred only on the

Draw-A-Man and Frostig figure-ground perception test. Conners et al. (1969) then reported on a placebo controlled, double-blind randomized study of dextroamphetamine in dosages up to 25 mg/day administered to outpatient children referred for problems in learning. Significant improvement attributable to the drug occurred as measured by the Porteus Maze test, some visual perception, auditory synthesis, rote learning, and reduction of the hyperkinetic factor on parent symptom ratings.

While the milder side effects, such as anorexia, irritability, insomnia, and abdominal pain had been repeatedly described since 1937, it was not until the late 1960s that toxic psychosis (Ney, 1967) and dyskinesia were reported (Mattson & Calverley, 1968).

Major Tranquilizers

Fish published two companion papers in 1960 (a and b), which introduced most of the important issues that were to occupy the field of childhood psychopharmacology for the next several years. In those studies the use and comparative effects of Benadryl, chlorpromazine (Thorazine), prochlorperazine (Compazine), trifluoperazine (Stelazine), and perphenazine (Trilafon) were reported in a group of 85 children under 12 drawn from a private practice population. These papers reported what were probably the first clinical trials with prochlorperazine, perphenazine, and trifluoperazine in children. The conditions of the studies included a total treatment program, an attempt at more precise diagnostic classification, a definition of average dosage in mg/kg of body weight, the utilization of a variety of assessment techniques to rate different aspects of ego functioning, and the introduction of a developmental approach that defined age as an important variable in drug effect. Fish provided a good discussion of the philosophy and pragmatics of drug administration in children as well as a description of qualitative differences in potency among the drugs, related more to differences in overall severity of impairment and type of developmental disturbance than to either diagnosis alone or to isolated symptoms.

In a study already mentioned as supported by the first NIMH grant awarded for childhood pharmacotherapy (Psychopharmacology Bulletin, 1973), Cytryn et al. (1960) reported the first effort at a methodologically sound clinical study on outpatient children that compared the efficacy of two major and one minor tranquilizers to placebo in children undergoing psychotherapy. Four diagnostic categories were identified: neurotic, hyperkinetic (both constitutional and secondary to anxiety), defective with behavior disorder, and antisocial. None of the active drugs studied—prochlorperazine, perphenazine (Eisenberg et al. 1961), or meprobamate—was superior to placebo for any of the diagnostic groups.

As methodology of drug studies improved, earlier enthusiastic reports of efficacy underwent modification. Rosenblum et al. (1960) found no advantage for prochlorperazine (Compazine) over either placebo or no drug in affecting behavior disturbance in a group of borderline retarded children. La Veck et al. (1960) reported the first use of fluphenazine (Prolixin) in a double-blind placebo cntrolled study of behaviorally disturbed retarded children, finding no statistically significant advantage for the drug over placebo.

In a study mentioned previously, Fish (1960a) reported a beneficial stimulating effect for trifluoperazine (Stelazine) on withdrawn, hypoactive, schizophrenic children. Another study in the same year (Beaudry & Gibson, 1960) proposed that trifluoperazine would provide a calming effect in a hyperactive group and a stimulating effect in a hypoactive group of a population of children hospitalized for "behavioral disorders . . . with malignant emotional disturbances." Changes occurred in the direction of the hypothesis.

Clinical reports began to appear in the early 1960s on the use of thioridazine (Mellaril), from the piperidine subclass of phenothiazine compounds. Similar to initial enthusiastic reports in uncontrolled studies with earlier "new" compounds, thioridazine was introduced with claims for significant advantages in efficacy and many fewer side effects than the previously used aliphatic and piperazine subclasses of phenothiazines. Le Vann (1961), for example, reported 90 percent "complete or great improvement" with virtually no side effects in children ranging from institutionalized severely retarded to seriously emotionally disturbed at dosages ranging from 40–800 mg/day. In a study of outpatient children, Oettinger and Simonds (1962) reported about equally significant improvement (60.6% overall) in groupings of children that included the hyperkinetic behavior syndrome and behavior problems associated with retardation or with seizures. Administration of the drug was by a modified single-blind procedure, no suitable control was defined, and the ratings were largely subjective.

However, the reports of fewer side effects with thioridazine than the aliphatic and piperazine phenothiazines encouraged further studies. Shaw et al. (1963) compared thioridazine with trifluoperazine, trifluopromazine (Vesprin), and fluphenazine (Prolixin) in a well-controlled study, but with a very heterogeneous group of emotionally disturbed children. They reported no significant differences in efficacy among these four drugs when compared either by diagnosis or by degree of improvement. Alderton and Hoddinott (1964) reported a statistically significant superiority for thiordazine over amphetamine and placebo on the hyperactive and distubed behavior of mentally retarded children, but with no significant effect on cognitive functioning (Alexandris & Lundell, 1968). Two further studies compared thioridazine with the butyrophenone compound, haloperidol (Haldol); one in an inpatient population of "emotionally disturbed retarded children" (Ucer & Kreger, 1969), and another very heterogeneous population of outpatient children being seen in a mental health clinic (Claghorn, 1972). Both were double-blind comparison studies; the first found a statistically significant advantage in efficacy but significantly greater side effects for haloperidol; the second found no significant difference for efficacy between the two drugs.

In addition, experience with chlorpromazine and various of the piperazine class of phenothiazines continued to accumulate through the 1960s. Garfield et al. (1962) compared chlorpromazine and placebo in a well-controlled, double-blind study on children aged 6–13 in a university residential treatment progam. At doses of 75–450 mg/day, chlorpromazine resulted in "depressing" and inhibiting certain behaviors; but in the setting of an active treatment program, actual differences in results between the active drug and placebo were quite small. This study, as much as any, underscored the importance of the total treatment approach in giving medication, consistent with the results of previous studies of drug effect on children in outpatient psychotherapy (Cytryn et al., 1960; Eisenberg et al., 1961).

In the study mentioned earlier by Shaw et al. (1963), four phenothiazines—trifluoperazine (Stelazine) and fluphenazine (Prolixin) from the piperazine class, trifluopromazine (Vesprin) from the aliphatic class, and thioridazine (Mellaril) from the piperadine class—were all reported effective in relieving symptoms of anxiety, excitability, aggressiveness, and impulsivity in a heterogeneous group of children in residential treatment, but no drug was superior to the others. This study also reported reserpine, meprobamate, deanol and benactyzine (Suavitil) as ineffective on the basis of screening trials.

One of the more significant papers in childhood psychopharmacology was published by Fish and Shapiro in 1965. Following up on Fish's earlier work (1960a, 1960b), the authors compared chlorpromazine with diphenylhydramine (Benadryl) and placebo in four groups of young inpatient children. To do so, they introduced a concept of classification according to severity and patterns of impairment and deviation in ego function. Their "types" I and II included severely impaired children with low-level functioning; Types III and IV children were more intact and integrated and of higher I.Q., with behavior disorder and/or paranoid thinking. Sixty percent improved with chlorpromazine, 43 percent with placebo, and none with diphenylhydramine (Benadryl). Clearly chlorpromazine was a potent, active, and effective drug, especially with the more severely impaired children for whom the milieu and placebo were ineffective. Moreover, the classification by severity and type of impairment, along with the methodology used in this study, were introduced in the first of a series of valuable studies on severely disturbed young children from the Children's Psychopharmacology Research Unit of the New York University Medical Center and Bellevue Hospital (Fish et al., 1966; Fish et al., 1969a; Campbell et al., 1970; Campbell et al., 1972a; Campbell et al., 1972b; Campbell et al., 1972c).

Fish et al. (1966) next reported their results using trifluoperazine (Stelazine) with severely disturbed inpatient preschool children. Utilizing a carefully matched control group, a placebo comparison, ratings by a "blind" psychiatrist, and doses ranging from .11–1.60 mg/kg/day (6–20 mg/day), they found the drug significantly effective for, and only for, the most severely impaired group of children, in particular those with no language function. Trifluoperazine offered no advantages over placebo for the children with language function and with lesser functional impairment (all the children were diagnosed autistic or schizophrenic). These latter children responded most to the ward treatment program. These findings supported an earlier suggestion that the piperazine phenothiazines with stimulating effects increased the responsiveness of severely impaired children (Fish, 1960b) and underlined the usefulness of the typology classification.

In the mid-1960s, reports began to appear on the effect of the phenothiazines in children with the hyperactivity or minimal brain dysfunction syndrome. Werry and co-workers (Werry et al., 1966; Weiss et al., 1968) compared chlorpromazine (a more sedating phenothiazine) with dextroamphetamine and placebo in groups of children carefully selected for normal I.Q. and free of overt neurological disease, so as to be relatively homogeneous for characteristics of the hyperactivity or minimal brain dysfunction syndrome. Their studies showed both chlorpromazine and dextroamphetamine to be superior to placebo to a statistically significant degree in the reduction of hyperactivity and without impairment of cognitive functions. Chlorpromazine was more consistent in its effect, but for that group of children who did benefit from dextroamphetamine, the improvement "seems to be superior to that of chlorpromazine," especially in reduction of distractibility. Jumping ahead somewhat, Greenberg et al. (1972) compared the effects of chlorpromazine, dextroamphetamine, hydroxyzine (Atarax), and placebo in a well-designed study on 61 boys with the hyperkinetic syndrome, characterized by hyperactivity, impulsivity, poor attention span, and poor academic performance. Consistent with the previous finding, they found both chlorpromazine and dextroamphetamine significantly better than placebo in affecting the behavior of these children, that hydroxyzine was generally ineffective, and that dextroamphetamine produced either strongly favorable or strongly unfavorable reactions, with fewer of the latter.

The remaining major work on the "tranquilizing" antipsychotic drugs during the 1960s and into the 1970s was with two new classes of compounds: the thioxanthenes, chlorprothixene (Taractan) and thiothixene (Navane), and the butyrophenones, haloperidol (Haldol) and trifluperidol (or triperidol). Both of these new classes were introduced first for use in adults in 1959. According to Di Mascio (De Mascio & Shader, 1970), the thioxanthenes are characterized by less toxicity but a higher incidence of extrapyramidal side effects than the phenothiazine compounds, to which they are structurally very similar. The butyrophenones have a different chemical structure than the phenothiazines with the advantage of greater potency, calming without sedating, and some stimulant-like activity, but were reported to have the highest potential for inducing extrapyramidal side effects.

An early report on the use of chlorprothixene (Taractan) in children compared it to previous results with thioridazine for symptoms of hyperactivity and habit and conduct disorders (Oettinger, 1962). At an average dose of 2.2 mg/kg/day (range 60–200 mg/day), chlorprothixene compared favorably with thioridazine, having a less sedative and a more stimulating effect, but the ratings were not controlled and there was no comparison to placebo.

The first report on the use of thiothixene (Navane) in children appeared in 1966 (Wolpert et al.) and was followed by two further studies (Wolpert et al., 1967, 1968). The latter studies compared thiothixene with chlorprothixene in 20 matched male inpatients ages 9–13 years with a diagnosis of primary behavior disorder. Double-blind ratings of improvement consistently favored thiothixene (Navane).

The first report in the English literature on the use of haloperidol (Haldol) in children (except in the treatment of Gilles de la Tourette Syndrome, reported below) appeared in 1965 (Rogers), describing improvement in destructive, aggressive behavior. Two following studies with groups of children hospitalized for severe behavior disorder without psychosis found haloperidol somewhat but not strikingly superior to placebo in affecting aggressive behavior (Cunningham et al., 1968; Barker & Fraser, 1968). Le Vann (1969) then reported on the use of haloperidol in 100 children and adolescents, both retarded and nonretarded with behavioral disturbances within a wide range of diagnoses. This was a noncontrolled nonblind study that reported striking improvement in hyperactive, assaultive self-injurious, and other disturbed or disturbing behavior, more so in the nonretarded subjects. Ucer and Kreger (1969) compared haloperidol with thioridazine in mentally retarded children, finding haloperidol significantly superior for control of disturbed behavior but also with a significantly greater incidence of extrapyramidal reactions, ataxia, and agitation. This was a reasonably well-designed study except for the heterogeniety of the study and control groups and the rather low mean daily dosage of thioridazine (53 mg/day), which casts some doubt on the validity of the comparison.

This decade fittingly closed with a report by Fish et al. (1969) on the use of another butyrophenone, trifluperidol (or triperidol).

The Antidepressants

The antidepressant medications (MAO inhibitors and tricyclics) were introduced for use in adults in the late 1950s. The first reports on the effects of antidepressants in children was in 1960, when MacLean reported relief of enuresis by administration of 25–50 mg of imipramine (Tofranil) each evening. Munster et al., (1961) and Salgado et al. (1963) described three unusual reactions to imipramine, which included allergic rash, relief of sleepwalking, and cessation of chronic headbanging. Poussaint and Ditman (1965) reported the first controlled study of imipramine in enuresis with a crossover design on 47 enuretic children. In doses of 25 mg for children under 12 years and 50 mg for those over age 12, imprimine was markedly superior to placebo, both clinically and statistically, in decreasing the frequency of enuretic nights.

In 1968 placebo controlled, double-blind studies (Bindelglass et al.) with crossover (Shaffer et al.) further demonstrated the significant effect of imipramine in decresing enuresis.

Reports on the use of antidepressants for the treatment of depression in children and for hyperkinetic children appeared in 1965. Lucas et al. (1965) administered amitriptyline (Elavil) in dosages of 30–50 mg/day to 10 hospitalized children with mixed diagnoses (including psychosis), whose presenting symptom was depression. A placebo controlled, double-blind, crossover study was done for a 12-week period, yielding equivocal results.

Rapoport (1965) reported a high improvement rate using imipramine in hyperkinetic children, but this was an uncontrolled study. Krakowski (1965) reported on 50 hyperkinetic children given amitriptyline (Elavil) in doses of 20–75 mg/day in a double-blind placebo controlled study.

The nonresponders to placebo and the initial drug group were given amitriptyline and follwed for one month to one year, with a good response reported in 70 percent. In an uncontrolled study of 123 children of mixed diagnoses, Kraft et al. (1966), reported a 60 percent improvement (by phone follow-up) after treatment with amitriptyline. Kurtis (1966) reported improvement in sixteen hospitalized psychotic children who received nortriptyline (Aventil) in an uncontrolled study. In a double-blind, crossover outpatient study of 31 patients diagnosed as having depressive illness, Frommer (1967) compared combined phenelzine (an MAO inhibitor) and chlordiazepoxide (Librium) with treatment by phenobarbital combined with an inert capsule. About half of these patients had phobic symptomatology and the other half had depressed mood disorder. The combination of phenelzine and chlordiazepoxide was superior to placebo to a statistically significant degree. Foster (1967) reported an uncontrolled study of 27 children aged three to eleven with mixed behavioral and anxiety symptoms. Twenty-one had moderate to marked improvement after treatment with nortriptyline.

1970 TO THE PRESENT

The Stimulants

Psychopharmacological research on the stimulants during the past several years has first of all further supported by better methodological studies the positive effects of dextroamphetamine and methylphenidate for treatment of the symptoms of Attention Deficit Disorder (ADD). DSM-III (American Psychiatric Association, 1980) replaced the diagnosis of Hyperkinetic Reaction with Attention Deficit Disorder (ADD) because the attention span problems were felt to be central to the disorder, and hyperactivity may or may not be present. The validity of this distinction has yet to be demonstrated.

Improved placebo-controlled studies on dextroamphetamine have been done. Huestis et al. (1975) in a placebo crossover study obtained significant improvement for the drug by teachers' and parents' ratings for hyperactivity and distractibility. Gordon et al. (1978) in a placebo controlled crossover study found improved attention and increased task related behavior for 15 hyperactive children when on dextroamphetamine.

In a similar manner, more sophisticated studies on methylphenidate (MPH) continue to demonstrate significant improvement for the symptoms of ADD with hyperactivity. Schain and Reynard (1975) report a double-blind placebo controlled study of 98 hyperactive children in which the code was broken if maximum dose did not produce improvement. MPH was markedly superior to placebo. Gittelman-Klein et al. (1976) demonstrated significant superiority for MPH over placebo for conduct problems, inattentiveness, hyperactivity, and sociability in the classroom by teacher ratings. Numerous studies (Firestone et al., 1978; Conners & Taylor, 1980) show significant drug effect, and Barkley's review (1977) of over 110 studies demonstrated an improvement rate of approximately 75 percent. Gittelman (1980a) points out that studies with more restrictive diagnostic selection criteria yield more significant drug effects. Other factors that affect results are whether high enough stimulant dosage is administered and whether observations for the rating scale are done after the 4–6 hour period of drug effectiveness (i.e., the parent rating scale was made from observations in late afternoon and evening when the last dose administered was at noon).

Since Conners' (1972) study on magnesium pemoline, which demonstrated positive effects for ADD symptoms only after six weeks, a few further studies have been done. A study by Page et al. (1974) demonstrated a significant drug effect beginning at three weeks, while the study by Conners and Taylor (1980) showed a weak but significant effect after eight weeks.

Along with the studies demonstrating significant effect of the stimulants on the symptoms of ADD with hyperactivity, there have been many laboratory studies with hyperactive children demonstrating that stimulants positively effect laboratory measures of learning. Cohen et al. (1971) showed that MPH produces faster and more consistent reaction time in hyperactive childen. MPH improves sustained attention on the Continuous Performance Test (Sykes et al., 1971) lowers error scores on the matching Familiar Figures Test measuring impulsivity (Brown & Sleator, 1979). Swanson et al. (1978) demonstrated that 70 percent of hyperactive children show significant improvement with MPH on a paired association test.

Because of the demonstration that stimulants improve behavior and the cognitive processes of attention and short term memory for ADD children, it was expected that stimulants would enhance academic achievement. Barkley and Cunningham (1978) reviewed 120 studies and concluded that there was little support for the view that stimulants improve academic performance. This has become a major conceptual and therapeutic issue in this decade, with the interpretation by some that the ADD child is not "really" helped by medication but only "slowed down." Aman's review (1980) of seven different follow-up studies similarly indicates no long term educational gains resulting from stimulant medication treatment. There have been a number of possible explanations for this discrepancy. Some relate to research methodological problems such as lack of clearly defined diagnostic criteria for group studied or lack of a good control group. Others propose (Gadow, 1981, 1983) that the samples studied include hyperactive children who are nondrug responders or under or overmedicated (Swanson et al., 1978). Of most importance is the issue of the effect on specific learning disabilities in the "hyperactive" population studies. Although Lerer et al. (1977) demonstrated that MPH improved handwriting, studies on learning disabled (LD) and reading disordered children who do not have behavior problems (LD but no ADD) show no positive effects from treatment with stimulants (Aman & Werry, 1982; Gittelman, 1980b). Since it appears that a significant number of ADD children also have specific learning disabilities (Silver, 1981), then stimulant treatment alone will only treat the attention span–behavior impulsivity symptoms and not the learning disability. The learning disability needs to be remediated by special education. This aspect may account for the poor results on academic achievement and also the relatively poor results of most long term follow-up studies. In contrast to these poor outcome studies, a follow-up study of up to three years indicates that multimodality treatment leads to improvement in a number of areas including decreased antisocial behavior, improved academic performance, and improved adjustment at home and at school (Satterfield et al., 1981). In this study of ADD-hyperactive children, stimulant medication *plus* other therapies (e.g., education therapy, family therapy, parent training, individual or group therapy) were administered according to the child's needs.

During the past decade, the side effects of the stimulants have been further studied and a clear contraindication for use of stimulants has been described. While studies in the early 1970s raised the issue of growth inhibition (Safer et al., 1972), other studies did not substantiate this finding (Gross, 1976). A recent study by Mattes and Gittelman (1983), using revised growth charts, demonstrates a significant decrease in weight and height percentile. After controlling for age and pretreatment height and weight, the MPH dosage accounted for only two percent of the variance in final height, indicating the magnitude of the drug effect is small.

Recently for the first time, a clear contraindication for the use of stimulants has been described. While there is some disagreement (Shapiro & Shapiro, 1981), Lowe et al. (1982) present evidence that stimulant medication may precipitate Tourette's Syndrome. Because of the possible development of this severe syndrome, they recommend that the development of motor tics in a child receiving stimulant medication is a clear indication for immediate discontinuation of the stimulant. Stimulants are contraindicated in a child who has motor tics or who has been diagnosed as having Tourette's Syndrome, and a family history of tics or Tourette's Syndrome indicates that stimulants should be used very cautiously.

A number of studies relate stimulant dosage level to clinical effects. Halliday et al. (1980) studied 15 hyperactive children at three dosage levels. Teacher ratings showed that the group did better at the higher dosage administered, but a few had better results at the lower level. Sprague and Sleator (1977) compared placebo with MPH at dosage of 0.3 mg/kg and 1.0 mg/kg. The effect on a visual memory task was optimal at the lower dosage, but the clinical effect using teacher ratings was best for the higher dosage. Swanson et al. (1978) used a paired association learning task to show that higher than optimal dosage may yield decreased task performance.

In contradistinction to the findings of dosage level relating to clinical effects, studies on plasma levels have not yielded a relationship to clinical effects. Brown et al. (1980) was not able to correlate a specific plasma level of amphetamine to clinical response, and Gualtieri et al. (1982) found a wide range of both inter and intraindividual variations in serum levels on different days. Also MPH serum levels did not differentiate responders from nonresponders.

While previous studies on activity levels of hyperactive children have yielded mixed results, Porrino et al. (1983) studied this issue using a solid state activity monitor worn on a belt. Studying twelve matched 6–12 year olds in their natural environments, they demonstrated that hyperactive children show consistently and substantially higher levels of motor movement in many diverse settings including sleep. Administration of dextroamphetamine decreased the activity level down to, but not below, the activity level of the normal boys. Motor activity was most strikingly decreased during structured classroom activity. As the drug effects diminished, a distinct behavioral rebound occurred.

There is one study on the effects of stimulants on normal children. Rapoport et al. (1978) in a double-blind placebo controlled study of normal prepubertal boys demonstrated that amphetamine had similar effects on normal children as on ADD children. Motor activity and reaction time were decreased, and performance on cognitive tests was increased. Although this study is at variance with the view that stimulants have a "paradoxical effect" on ADD children, Rapoport states that "lack of specificity of a treatment is no argument against its use."

The issue of state dependent learning continues to be studied. A recent study suggests that while stimulants enhance the acquisition of information and its retrieval 24 hours later, there is no evidence of poorer retrieval of information learned in a state different from the retrieval state (Weingartner et al., 1982).

A few studies comparing stimulant treatment with other treatment modalities for ADD-hyperactive children have been done, but further research in this area is sorely needed to further define what treatment methods are best for which children. Gittelman-Klein et al. (1980) compared methylphenidate alone, placebo plus behavior modification, and methylphenidate and behavior modification for an eight-week treatment period. Results demonstrated significant improvement on parent and teacher ratings for all three, but MPH plus behavior modification was the most effective. MPH alone was next, and was better than behavior modification. Firestone et al. (1980) compared parent training in behavior modification plus placebo, MPH alone, and MPH and parent training over a three-month period. All groups showed improved home and school behavior, but only with MPH were there gains in measures of attention and impulse control. There was no evidence of significant benefit from the addition of parent training to the administration of MPH. These studies are only preliminary in an area that needs much more extensive research.

After a backlash against medication use in children in the late 1960s, it appears that a more considered approach has been adopted in the late 1970s. With diminished popularity of the Feingold diet, as well as the increased recognition of severe side effects with major tranquilizers (tardive dyskinesia), we expect an increase in the use and acceptance of stimulants through the 1980s. Future directions include studies on more defined diagnostic groupings, neurochemical studies (Hunt et al., 1982), better follow-up studies, and studies comparing stimulant medication in combination with and as compared to other treatment modalities.

The Antipsychotics

Studies during this period of the indications for use and comparative efficacy of antipsychotics reflect the period before and after the introduction of DSM-III (American Psychiatric Association, 1980). Studies before DSM-III are difficult to evaluate and compare because of diagnostic variability and heterogeneity both within and among the study populations. After DSM-III the diagnostic criteria used to define study groups became more standardized into the categories of schizophrenic disorders, autism, and childhood onset pervasive developmental disorders.

Campbell et al. (1970) compared thiothixene (Navane) to the results obtained in a previous study with trifluperiodol (Fish et al., 1969). In a well-matched population of 10 preschool autistic-schizophrenic children, the two drugs were not significantly different in effectiveness, but thiothixene had a much greater margin of safety with no side effects observed at therapeutic levels.

Waizer et al. (1972) supported this positive impression of thiothixene efficacy on an outpatient population of 18 school-age children diagnosed by the Creak criteria as childhood schizophrenics. This group of children was considered highly homogenous for severe to moderate illness. Ratings were by a single blind observer, with a preceding period of placebo. They reported thiothixene to be highly effective and very safe at a mean daily dose of 17 mg/day. Significant improvement over placebo occurred in motor activity, stereotyped behavior, coordination and affect, with little improvement in language function in short term administration.

In a study measuring both clinical change and neurophysiological correlates, Saletu et al. (1974) compared thiothixene (Navane) with placebo in then hospitalized boys aged five to 15 (mean age 10), diagnosed as psychotic with longstanding illness and severe functional impairment. Compared to placebo, thiothixene produced a significant and persistent improvement, beginning in the second week, in areas of motor activity, speech, social relationships, affect and behavior disturbance. In addition, the drug treatment period was correlated with a trend toward normalization of the visual evoked potential recorded by the EEG, as compared to normal controls.

Three further studies of haloperidol compared its effects with those of thioridazine (Claghorn, 1972) and with fluphenazine (Faretra et al., 1970; Engelhardt et al., 1973). Methodological problems make the results reported by Claghorn difficult to evaluate. The other two studies found haloperidol and fluphenazine to be significantly and about equally effective in producing improvement in the target symptoms of children diagnosed as schizophrenic. Haloperidol tended to be quicker acting and effective at a mean daily dose of 10.4 mg/day (Engelhardt et al., 1973).

By way of some contrast to the above results comparing a butyrophenone with a piperazine phenothiazine, Campbell et al. (1972a) reported a comparison study of trifluperiodol ("prototype of a stimulating neuroleptic") with chlorpromazine (a sedating aliphatic phenothiazine), and placebo. Following the methodology previously established by this research group, 15 preschool severely disturbed children were studied. Trifluperiodol was consistently statistically significantly better than chlorpromazine or placebo in producing improvement in functioning and target symptoms. They found consistent sedative effect and worsening of hyperactivity with chlorpromazine.

Infantile Autism. Campbell (1975) provides a comprehensive review and commentary on pharmacotherapy in "early infantile autism" up to that time.

Campbell et al. (1978) report that haloperidol in doses of .5–4.0 mg/day is significantly superior to placebo in improving withdrawal and stereotypy in young (2.6–7.2 years) autistic children (but not in those below four years of age), and that the combination of haloperidol with behavior therapy was more effective than either alone was in facilitating the acquisition of imitative speech. The beneficial effects of haloperidol on stereotypy and attention in autistic children was replicated by this same group of workers (Cohen et al., 1980). A further report extends the efficacy of haloperidol in doses of .5–3.0 mg/day on decreasing maladaptive behaviors and increasing discriminate learning performance in the classroom (Anderson et al., 1984).

The question of antipsychotic medication dosage, plasma level, and response relationships in children is as yet little studied. One report on haloperidol finds a 15-fold variability between dose and plasma level, with younger patients having lower plasma levels than older patients at equivalent doses, and a plasma level to response relationship in Tourette's disorder but not in psychosis (Morselli et al., 1979).

Pervasive Developmental Disorders, Schizophrenic and Conduct Disorders, and Tourette's Syndrome. Pervasive development disorders are defined in DSM-III as onset after 30 months, but are different from schizophrenia in the absence of hallucinations, delusions, and overt thought disorder. There is remarkably little in the literature that specifically defines this disorder as a subject for drug studies. These children are generally included in studies of children with autism or with older children and adolescents who are diagnosed "psychotic" or "schizophrenic." (See review by Mikkelsen, 1982.)

The same can be said for children with the diagnosis of schizophrenic disorder made by DSM-III criteria, which are the same for children as for adults. Although many children with this diagnosis probably are included in earlier studies of childhood "psychosis," most of these are older children with earlier onset autism. The presumption of DSM-III is that schizophrenic disorder as seen in adults may and does begin in childhood (although Kydd and Werry, 1982 found only six cases in prepubertal children out of 1000 consecutive admissions), and such children should respond similarly to antipsychotic medication. So far, no study is reported of medication efficacy in carefully diagnosed pre-pubertal onset schizophrenic disorder.

Conduct disorders (aggressive/nonaggressive and socialized/un-socialized subtypes) is another DSM-III category extensivly treated with antipsychotics, based on many reports of their antiagressive properties. (For a review, see Campbell et al., 1982.)

To further define this question, Campbell et al. (1984) studied the comparative efficacy of haloperidol, lithium, and placebo in prepubertal hospitalized children diagnosed as conduct disorder, unsocialized aggressive type, without evidence of psychosis and without evidence of overt affective disorder. In this group of impulsive, destructive, explosively aggressive children haloperidol and lithium are both superior to placebo in decreasing the behavioral symptoms. Optimal doses of haloperidol range from 1.0–6.0 mg/day, and more side effects are noted with haloperidol than with lithium (at doses of 500–2000 mg/day).

The other major use of haloperidol has been in the treatment of Gilles de la Tourette Syndrome. The first report of such use was by Seignot (1961). Shapiro et al. (1973) cited an additional 10 studies between 1962 and 1970 reporting haloperidol as the most effective treatment for the syndrome. These authors summarized their experience with haloperidol in the treatment of 34 cases of the Tourette Syndrome with a mean age of onset of seven plus years. They reported strikingly successful results in 21 of 34 cases on whom there was adequate follow-up. These patients required a median daily dose of 4 mg, with a daily maintenance dose ranging from 1.5–44 mg. In a subsequent report, Shapiro and Shapiro (1982) report haloperidol providing an 80 percent decrease in symptoms in upwards of 80 percent of patients followed for up to eight years, but with significant adverse effects on cognition, mood and extrapyramidal symptoms. They also report pimozide at doses of 2–30 mg/day as or more effective than haloperidol and with significantly fewer side effects. Clonidine, a centrally active alpha-adrenergic agonist is also reported effective (Leckman et al., 1982) in up to 50 percent of patients in doses of .5–0.9 mg/day, with relatively few side effects but somewhat unpredictable response.

Side Effects. The study and better understanding of the adverse effects of antipsychotic medication usage in children is a feature primarily of the past five or six years.

Engelhardt and Polizos (1978) reported that symptoms involving the skin (rash and photosensitivity), bone marrow depression, liver function, and the autonomic system are either rare and/or clinically insignificant. However, many authors observe weight gain and sedation as common and potentially serious (Engelhardt & Polizos, 1978; Campbell et al., 1984). Most attention focuses on the extrapyramidal adverse effects: dystonic, Parkinsonlike, akathesic, and dyskinetic reactions.

McAndrew et al. (1972) and Polizos et al. (1973) reported dyskinetic and akathesic symptoms in children after withdrawal from relatively long term administration of chlorpromazine and haloperidol, respectively. This syndrome was described as reversible, usually spontaneously remitting, and was termed the "withdrawal emergent syndrome" (WES) by Engelhardt and Polizos (1978). The relationship of this syndrome to tardive dyskinesia in children is still unsettled. Gualtieri and Hawk (1980) and Campbell et al. (1983) published extensive reviews and their own studies of tardive and withdrawal dyskinestic reactions in neuroleptically treated children, extending the work done previously by Engelhardt and Polizos (1978). Overall, 20–50 percent of children treated with and then withdrawn from antipsychotics will develop dyskinesias ranging from mild to severe, and more likely with high potency/low dose than with low potency/high dose neuroleptics. Symptoms appear within a few days to weeks following withdrawal and in most reported cases spontaneously remit after several weeks to months, or remit on restarting the medication.

Antidepressant Medication

Important research during this period reports on indications and efficacy of the tricyclic antidepressants (TCAs) in separation anxiety disorders (school phobia), affective disorders, anorexia nervosa, hyperactivity, and enuresis. From the mid 1970s onward, studies on the diagnosis and treatment of depression in childhood are the dominant theme around which research is organized.

1. *Separation anxiety disorders.* Gittelman-Klein and Klein (1970) reported on the efficacy of imipramine at doses of 100–200 mg/day in the treatment of children with the school phobia syndrome, considered an expression of separation anxiety. In this controlled study children treated with imipramine and psychotherapy returned to school significantly sooner than children treated with psychotherapy and placebo.

2. *Hyperactivity.* Attention deficit disorder with hyperactivity (ADDH) and without hyperactivity (ADD) are defined as diagnostic categories in DSM-III (1980), replacing the diagnosis of minimal brain dysfunction/disorder and the hyperactive child syndrome. Earlier studies used hyperactivity per se as the major identifying and target symptom for medication efficacy.

Rapoport et al. (1974) studied imipramine in doses up to 80 mg/day in 76 outpatient hyperactive, middle-class grade-school boys. Comparing imipramine to methylphenidate in a double-blind placebo controlled study, both drugs are superior to placebo, but all ratings favor methylphenidate, with a higher incidence of imipramine discontinuance on follow-up (Quinn & Rapoport, 1975). Both drugs were associated with a decreased rate of weight gain, but with no effect on height. Winsberg et al. (1972) also compared imipramine (150 mg/day × one week), and dextroamphetamine (15–30 mg/day × one week) in a double-blind placebo controlled study of 32 children with hyperactivity and aggressiveness (the latter not necessarily a symptom of ADDH). Both drugs decreased target symptoms, but only imipramine affected attention span. Comparing imipramine in doses of 100–200 mg/day to placebo, Waizer et al. (1974) report significant advantage for imipramine in reducing hyperactivity and defiance, and increasing attention span and sociability. Additional studies (Greenberg et al., 1975; Yepes et al., 1977) support the efficacy of imipramine in treating hyperactivity, but see it overall as less useful and with more side effects than the stimulants.

3. *Anorexia nervosa.* Initial open trials and single case studies reported successful treatment with tricyclic antidepressants (Mills, 1976; Needleman & Waber, 1977; White & Schnaulty, 1977). More recent double blind placebo controlled studies fail to demonstrate any significant advantage over placebo or efficacy for antidepressant medication (Lacey & Crisp, 1980; Biederman et al., 1982).

4. *Enuresis.* Clinical efficacy for tricyclics in treating enuresis is well established (see Chapter 11). The major clarifying studies regarding phenomenology, relationship to sleep architecture, associated psychopathology, response to tricyclics, and correlation of response to plasma level appear in two reports from Rapoport and her colleagues at the NIMH (Mikkelson et al., 1980; Rapoport et al., 1980). They report on 40 severely enuretic boys treated with imipramine (75 mg/day), desipramine (75 mg/day), methscopolamine bromide and placebo in a carefully controlled double blind study. Both tricyclics were equally effective and significantly superior to placebo and methscopolamine. Neither enuresis itself or response is related to sleep stage, nor is response related to associated psychopathology or to peripheral anticholinergic or psychotropic effect. There is a weak but significant correlation with plasma level. Both true nonresponders and patients who develop tolerance are identified.

5. *Depression.* Since the 1972 publication and application to children

of the Research Diagnostic Criteria (RDC), a large number of studies (see below and Chapter 5) report on the reliability and validity of adult criteria for the diagnosis of depressive disorder and assessment instruments for use in childhood, on the psychobiological correlates and biological continuity of childhood depressive disorder with the adult condition, and on the efficacy of antidepressant medication. Since its 1980 publication, DSM-III criteria are generally accepted for the diagnosis of affective disorders in childhood as well as in adults, although many research studies continue to use the somewhat more stringent RDC criteria.

Weinberg et al., (1973), and many others since then, accepted and applied the reliability and validity of RDC and the later DSM-III criteria, eliminating from common use the previously held concepts of "masked depression" and "depressive equivalents" (Cytryn et al., 1980; Puig-Antich et al., 1978; Gittelman-Klein, 1977; Carlson & Cantwell, 1979; Carlson & Cantwell, 1980). Several authors suggest specific features related to age and developmental level (Malmquist, 1971; Poznanski et al., 1982), with Poznanski, for example, describing a different sleep pattern in children and less diurnal variation in mood.

Studies on the biological correlates of childhood depression are early in development but support the validity of the diagnosis and its continuity with the adult disorder. Reports in prepubertal depressed children include cortisol hypersecretion in two of four children (Puig-Antich et al., 1981), a reduction in urinary MHPG excretion (McKnew & Cytryn, 1979), a decreased response of growth hormone using the insulin tolerance test (Puig-Antich et al., 1981), and a response similar to that in adults to the dexamethasone suppression test (Poznanski et al., 1982).

Clinical efficacy for tricyclic antidepressants is reported in a number of open or otherwise methodologically limited clinical trials (Kuhn & Kuhn, 1972; Weinberg et al., 1973; Puig-Antich et al., 1978; Frommer, 1972), generally finding improvement in over 50 percent of subjects. A further most recent open study reports very significant efficacy for imipramine in a group of 20 hospitalized prepubertal children carefully diagnosed by DSM-III criteria for a major depressive episode (Weller et al., 1983). In this study all children who responded had a total TCA level between 125–225 ng/ml, without benefit from either lower or higher levels.

Two double blind controlled studies report the superiority of imipramine to placebo in treating hospitalized prepubertal children with a DSM-III or RDC diagnosis of major depressive disorder (Puig-Antich et al., 1979; Petti & Law, 1982). In the Puig-Antich study imipramine in doses up to 5 mg/kg/day strongly supports efficacy for imipramine over placebo when the total TCA plasma level is in the range of 200 ng/ml, with a positive response in many children at or above 150 ng/ml (quite similar to the finding in the above Weller et al. study).

In the Petti and Law study, seven children were randomly administered either placebo or imipramine in doses of 5 mg/kg/day, with significant advantage for improvement in the imipramine treated children. The authors acknowledge the limitations in generalization imposed by the small sample size and some imperfections in the degree of matching between the two groups.

6. Reported side effects include:

   a. Anorexia and weight loss; insomnia; an increase in heart rate, systolic and diastolic blood pressure; stomach aches and tearfulness (Rapoport et al., 1974; Greenberg et al., 1975).

   b. Anticholinergic effects of dry mouth, constipation, and blurring of vision.

   c. Precipitation of seizures (Brown et al., 1973; Petti & Campbell, 1975)

   d. Cardiotoxic effects at doses approaching 5 mg/kg/day are reported by Winsberg et al. (1975), with cases of EKG changes including three with a first degree atrioventricular block. The Federal Drug Administration now recommends EKG monitoring of children on doses of imipramine approaching 5 mg/kg/day. One sudden cardiaclike death is reported in a six-year-old girl receiving imipramine at a dosage of 200 mg/day (14.7 mg/kg/day) (Saraf et al., 1974).

   e. Withdrawal symptoms include abdominal pain, nausea, vomiting, drowsiness, decreased appetite, tearfulness and agitation. Gradual tapering may require several weeks (Law et al., 1981).

Lithium

Large scale studies in the United States demonstrating the efficacy of lithium treatment in adults with affective disorders began in the late 1960s. Case studies of children and adolescents with possible bipolar disorder treated with lithium have been reported throughout the 1970s. Van Krevelen and Van Voorst in 1959 (Campbell et al., 1972b, p. 235) reported on an adolescent retarded boy with alternating depression and hypomanic states who responded to lithium. Annell (1969b) reported on 15 patients ages 10 to 18 with serious emotional disorders of an episodic nature who responded favorably to lithium. Kelly et al. (1976) and Horowitz (1977) reported adolescents with bipolar illness who responded to lithium. Youngerman and Canino (1978) reviewed the literature and analyzed 46 cases, of which approximately two-thirds responded to lithium treatment. A positive family history for affective disorder and a strong affective component as part of presenting symptoms appeared to be related to a positive lithium response.

During the past few years, recognition of bipolar illness in adolescents has increased. Carlson and Strober (1979) described nine adolescents with manic-depressive disorder where the diagnosis was previously missed because of the following: insufficient inquiry into signs and symptoms, irritability and manic lability being interpreted as adolescent turmoil, and depressive or grandiose delusions being interpreted as schizophrenia. Six of the nine responded well to treatment programs, which included lithium.

Although bipolar illness in prepubertal children appears to be quite rare, there are some clinical reports of positive responses to lithium. Brumback and Weinberg (1977) described five such children where adult therapeutic plasma levels yielded positive results, and McKnew et al., (1981) described two latency aged children with bipolar disorder who were part of a double-blind placebo controlled crossover study and responded positively to lithium. Puig-Antich (1980) states that there is enough pilot work accumulated so that properly controlled studies of bipolar disorder in children and adolescents should now be undertaken.

Studies of lithium treatment for severely hyperactive children have been negative (Greenhill et al., 1973). Studies on psychotic children have yielded weak or negative results. Gram and Rafaelsen (1972) described a significant decrease in disturbed activity, mood, and aggressiveness, while Campbell et al., (1972b) in a study of severely disturbed preschool children, did not obtain significant improvement.

During the past few years, lithium's effectiveness in reducing aggressiveness has been studied in various types of patients and in scientifically controlled studies. Clinical reports on mentally retarded aggressive and/or self-mutilating children and adolescents relate a positive response to lithium (Goetzl & Berkowitz, 1977; Dostal & Zvolsky, 1970). Sheard et al. (1976) in a double-blind placebo controlled study of chronically aggressive, antisocial teenagers in a correctional facility demonstrated that lithium treatment reduced the number of reported aggressive incidents and decreased self-reported aggressive affect. In a recent major double-blind placebo controlled study by Campbell et al. (1984), hospitalized children with the diagnosis of undersocialized aggressive conduct disorder were treated with lithium, haloperidol, or placebo. Results demonstrated lithium to be as effective as haloperidol in reducing aggressiveness and temper outbursts. These findings may indicate a major psychopharmacological contribution to treatment programs. There are many retarded and delinquent youth who require residential care because of severe self- and other-directed aggression who have been unresponsive to other drugs and therapeutic modalities. Further studies of lithium in this area are indicated (Campbell et al., 1978).

Other Medications

Triiodothyronine T₃.   A report by Sherwin et al. (1958) noted improvement in two euthyroid autistic boys after receiving triiodothyronine. Campbell et al. (1972c) administered triiodothyronine (T_3) to an inpatient population of 16 euthyroid preschool autistic-schizophrenic children with severe developmental deviations. On a daily dose of 12.5–75 mg of T_3, marked improvement was noted in 11 children consisting of changes in affect, social responsiveness, language production, and self-initiated activity; with decreases in stereotypy, hyperactivity, distractibility, and so on. Blind ratings, using treatment results with dextroamphetamine as the control, indicated statistically significant improvement with T_3 in overall symptomatology. This study has important methodological limitations, and a subsequent placebo controlled double-blind study fails to demonstrate any significant superiority for T_3 over placebo in the treatment of 30 young euthyroid children with autism (Campbell et al., 1978).

LSD.   In two papers published in 1962 and 1963, Bender and co-workers reported on the use of LSD-25 in the treatment of hospitalized, severely disturbed children with diagnoses of schizophrenia and autism. Favorable results reported included mood elevations, spontaneous play with adults and other children, improvement in social relatedness, responsiveness to contact and affection, and reduced rhythmic and whirling behavior. The dosage was 100 mg of LSD-25, with the response lasting over several hours beginning 30–40 minutes after ingestion. The drug was given one to three times per week over a six-week period. The methodology and data were not presented.

Simmons et al. (1966), commenting on the methodological limitations of the earlier studies, administered LSD to a pair of four-year, nine-month-old identical male twins using an intrasubject replication design with LSD interspersed with control and placebo observations and objective behavior records. Both twins satisfied the diagnostic criteria for childhood autism. Changes included an increase in social behaviors with better eye-to-face contact and responsiveness to adults, an increase in smiling and laughing behavior indicating a pleasurable affective state, and a decrease in self-stimulation behavior. They found the drug responses to be consistent with those reported by Bender, and mentioned unpublished data from a population of 18 psychotic children to whom LSD was also administered. In this more heterogeneous population, there was a tendency for the autisticlike children to respond as described, while the less retarded schizophrenic children became more withdrawn and disorganized. The effects of the LSD were transient and required continued administration.

Despite these relatively optimistic findings, there are no further reports or follow-up on these studies.

Anticonvulsants. Merritt and Putnam (1938) reported on the efficacy of diphenylhydantoin in the treatment of convulsive disorders. Since that time, reports of its effect on children with emotional or behavioral problems have intermittently occurred.. Lindsley and Henry (1942) described that diphenylhydantoin improved the behavior scores of 13 behavior problem children, but there was no significant difference in mean scores between diphenylhydantoin and no drug at the conclusion of the study. Brown and Solomon (1942) administered diphenylhydantoin for seven weeks to seven behavior-disordered adolescents with grossly abnormal EEGs at a state training school and described improvement in three of them. Walker and Kirkpatrick (1947) administered diphenylhydantoin to 10 behavior-disordered children with abnormal EEGs and described improvement during the 9–18 month outpatient follow-up. Pasamanick (1951) reported little positive effect of diphenylhydantoin on 21 hospitalized behavior-disordered children aged 6–13 with abnormal EEGs. One improved slightly with diphenylhydantoin; another improved markedly on trimethadione. Gross and Wilson (1964) studied 48 hyperactive children with abnormal EEGs who were treated with medication. Diphenylhydantoin was rarely effective. A child with severe temper tantrums and an EEG with left temporal spikes responded dramatically to Celontin. Looker and Conners (1970) reported three cases of children who responded to diphenylhydantoin following nonresponse to stimulant medication. Because these three children had in common a history of violent temper outbursts, 17 children ages 5½–14½ who had a history of periodic outbursts of violent temper were studied in a nine-week double-blind placebo controlled crossover trial of diphenylhydantoin. The authors reported no statistically significant group changes attributable to drug effect, and concluded that diphenylhydantoin was of little clinical benefit in a group of children characterized by severe temper tantrums. All of these children subsequently improved with dextroamphetamine or methylphenidate. Millichap (1973), in a study of 22 children with learning and behavior disorders reported a significant elevation of the auditory perception quotient following treatment with diphenylhydantoin in a group of children with paroxysmal dysrhythmias. Wender (1971) reported on four children with periodic rather than continuous MBD symptoms who failed to respond to amphetamines, but responded dramatically to diphenylhydantoin. Thus, individual case reports with marked improvement in response to diphenylhydantoin continue to be reported, despite the fact that controlled studies demonstrating positive effects do not exist.

Carbamazepine is established in the treatment of seizure disorders, with apparent special usefulness in temporal lobe seizures and so-called psychomotor epilepsy. There is also an established relationship in some children between epilepsy and learning and behavior disorders (Stores, 1978). Furthermore, carbamazepine is considered to have independent psychotropic properties and is reported effective in the treatment of affective disorders in adults. Based on the above, a number of studies report efficacy for carbamazepine in the treatment of a variety of symptoms occurring both with and without evidence of association with a seizure disorder. These symptoms include hyperactivity, aggressive behaviors, and mood disturbances. These studies vary greatly in the quality of design and methodology and their results are not consistent; so while the use of carbamazepine in childhood disorders is promising it is so far not established. (See review by Remschmidt, 1976.) An extended discussion of this issue is presented in Chapter 9.

SUMMARY

The use of psychoactive medications for the treatment of childhood psychiatric disorders began with Benzedrine during the 1930s. Little was added until the onset of the "biological revolution" in psychiatry beginning in the 1950s. This decade and the next witnessed a steadily progressive increase in reports of efficacy for antipsychotic, antidepressant, "minor tranquilizer," and stimulant medications for a wide variety of chilhood disorders.

Almost without exception the interpretation of the results reported in these studies is compromised by methodological limitations. These included diagnostic heterogeneity, the absence of a standardized diagnostic classification system, inadequate attention to control groups, absence of double-blind procedures, the unavailability of standardized assessment instruments, and variable dosage schedules.

Nonetheless, evidence accumulated for the efficacy of drugs in certain childhood disorders: stimulants for "hyperactive" children, the antidepressant imipramine for enuresis, antipsychotic medication for psychosis and aggressive behaviors in children and adolescents, and early reports on the treatment of depression in children.

During the 1970s several major changes occurred to dramatically affect the field of childhood psychopharmacology:

1. The introduction and gradual acceptance by 1980 of agreed upon diagnostic criteria for psychiatric disorders (RDC and DSM-III).

2. An increasing number of child psychiatry research scientists sophisticated in the application of scientific methodology.

3. The development of a number of reliable assessment instruments.

4. An increasing knowledge about pharmacokinetics of psychoactive medications.

5. A growing attention to and concern about immediate and longer term adverse effects of medications.

6. A considerable broadening of the conditions considered responsive to medication and/or appropriate for drug trials, including depressive disorders, bipolar disorders, Tourette's Syndrome, eating disorders, aggressive conduct disorders, and separation anxiety disorders (school phobia).

So far, almost midway into the 1980s, the field of childhood psychopharmacology is actively exploring the indications, contraindications, efficacy, pharmacokinetics, and adverse effects of several groups of drugs: stimulants, antidepressants, antipsychotics, lithium, anticonvulsants (carbamazepine), and benzodiazepines.

Concurrently studies are underway in refining the reliability and validity of diagnostic criteria, assessment instruments, dosage/plasma level relationships, the genetics of childhood and adolescent disorders and their continuity or discontinuity with adult conditions, and the comparative efficacy of different treatment approaches.

Taken together these studies, often complementary and overlapping, represent a solid, vigorous, and exciting area for continued research.

REFERENCES

Alderton, H. R., & Hoddinott, B.A. (1964). A controlled study of the use of thioridazine in the treatment of hyperactive and aggressive children in a children's psychiatric hospital. *Canad. Psych. J., 9*, 239–247.

Alexandris, A., & Lundell, F. W. (1968). Effect of thioridazine, amphetamine, and placebo on the hyperkinetic syndrome and cognitive area in mentally deficient children. *Canadian Medical Association Journal, 98*, 92–96.

Aman, M. G. (1980). Psychotropic drugs and learning problems, a selective review. *Journal of Learning Disabilities, 13* (2), 87–97.

Aman, M. G., & Weery, J. S. (1982). Methylphenidate and diazepam in severe reading retardation. *Journal of the American Academy of Child Psychiatry, 1*, 31–37.

American Psychiatric Association. (1980). *Diagnostic and statistical manual of mental disorders* (3rd. ed.), Washington, DC: American Psychiatric Association.

Anderson, L. T., Campbell, M., Grega, D. M., Perry, R., Small, A. M., & Green W. H. (1984). Haloperidol in infantile autism: Effects on learning and behavioral symptoms. *American Journal of Psychiatry* (in press).

Annell, Anna-Lisa. (1969b), Manic-depressive illness in children and effects of treatment with lithium carbonate. *Acta Paedopsychiatrica 36*, 282–301.

Bair, H. V., & Herold, W. (1955). Efficacy of chlorpromazine in hyperactive mentally retarded children. *A.M.A. Archives of Neurology and Psychiatry, 74*, 363.

Barker, P., & Fraser, I. A. (1968). A controlled trial of haloperidol in children. *British Journal of Psychiatry, 114*, 855–857.

Barkley, R. A. (1977). A review of stimulant drug research with hyperactive children. *Journal of Child Psychology and Psychiatry, 18*, 137–166.

Barkley, R. A., & Cunningham, C. E. (1978). Do stimulant drugs improve the academic performance of hyperkinetic children? *Clinical Pediatrics, 17*, 85–92.

Beaudry, P., & Gibson, D. (1960). Effect of trifluoperazine on the behavior disorders of children with malignant emotional disturbances. *American Journal of Mental Deficiency, 64*, 823.

Bender, L., & Cottington, F. (1942). The use of amphetamine sulfate (Benzedrine) in child psychiatry. *American Journal of Psychiatry, 99*, 116–121.

Bender, L., Faretra, F., & Cobrink, L. (1963). LSD & UML treatment of hospitalized disturbed children. *Recent Advances in Biological Psychiatry, 5*, 84–92.

Bender, L., Goldschmidt, L., & Siva Shanka, D. V. (1962). Treatment of autistic schizophrenic children with LSD-25 and UML-491. *Recent Advances in Biological Psychiatry, 4*, 170–177.

Bender, L., & Nichtern, S., (1956), Chemotherapy in child psychiatry. *New York State Journal of Medicine, 56*, 2791–1796.

Biederman, J., Herzog, D. B., Rivinus, T., Haber, G., Feber, R., Rosenbaum, J., Harmatz, J. S., Tandorf, R., Orsulak, P., & Schildkraut, J. (1982). Amitriptyline in the treatment of anorexia nervosa: A double blind placebo controlled study. Presented at the annual meeting of the American Academy of Child Psychiatry, October, 1982, Washington, DC.

Bindelglass, P. M., Dec, G. H., & Enos F. A. (1968). Medical and psychosocial factors in enuretic children treated with imipramine hydrochloride. *American Journal of Psychiatry, 124*, (8), 1107–1112.

Bradley, C. (1937). The behavior of children receiving Benzedrine. *American Journal of Psychiatry, 94*, 577–585.

Bradley, C., & Bowen, M. (1940). School performance of children receiving amphetamine (Benzedrine) sulfate. *American Journal of Orthopsychiatry, 10*, 782–788.

Bradley, C., & Green, E. (1940). Psychometric performance of children receiving amphetamine (Benzedrine) sulfate. *American Journal of Psychiatry, 97*, 388–394.

Bradley, C., & Bowen, M. (1941). Amphetamine (Benzedrine) therapy of children's behavior disorders. *American Journal of Orthopsychiatry, 11*, 92–103.

Bradley, C. (1950). Benzedrine and Dexedrine in the treatment of children's behavior disorders. *Pediatrics, 5*, 24–37.

Breger, E. (1961). Meprobamate in the management of enuresis. *Journal of Pediatrics* (October), 571–576.

Brown, D., Winsberg, B. G., Bialer, I., & Press, M. (1973). Imipramine therapy and seizures: Three children treated for hyperkinetic behavior disorders. *American Journal of Psychiatry, 130*, 210–212.

Brown, G. L., Ebert, M. H., Mikkelsen, E. J. & Hunt, R. D. (1980). Behavior and motor activity response in hyperactive children and plasma amphetamine levels following a sustained release preparation. *Journal of the American Academy of Child Psychiatry, 19*, 225–239.

Brown, R. T., & Sleator, E. K. (1979). Methylphenidate in hyperkinetic children: Differences in dose effects on impulsive behavior. *Pediatrics, 64*, 408–411.

Brown, W. T., and Soloman, C. I. (1942). Delinquency and the electroencephalogram. *American Journal of Psychiatry, 98*, 499–503.

Brumback, R. A., & Weinberg, W. A. (1977). Mania in childhood *American Journal of Diseases in Children, 131*, 1122–1126.

Campbell, M. (1975). Pharmacotherapy in early infantile autism. *Biological Psychiatry, 10*(4), 399–423.

Campbell, M., Anderson, L. T. Meier, M., et al. (1978). A comparison of haloperidol and behavior therapy and their interaction in autistic children. *Journal of the American Academy of Child Psychiatry, 17*, 640–655.

Campbell, M., Cohen, I. L., & Small, A. M. (1982). Drugs in aggressive behavior. *Journal of the American Academy of Child Psychiatry, 21*, 107–117.

Campbell, M., Fish, B., Shapiro, T., & Floyd, A. (1970). Thiothixene in young disturbed children. *Archives of General Psychiatry, 23*, 70–72.

Campbell, M., Fish, B., Shapiro, T., & Floyd, A. (1971). Imipramine in preschool autistic and schizophrenic children. *Journal of Autism and Childhood Schizophrenia, 3*, 260–282.

Campbell, M., Fish, B., Shapiro, T., & Floyd, A. (1972a). Acute responses of schizophrenic children to a sedative and a "stimulating" neuroleptic: A pharmacologic yardstick. *Current Therapy Research, 14*, 759.

Campbell M., Fish, B., Korein, J., Shapiro T., Collins, P., & Koh, C. (1972b). Lithium and chlorpromazine: A controlled crossover study of hyperactive severely disturbed young children. *Journal of Autism and Childhood Schizophrenia, 2*, 234–263.

Campbell, M., Fish, B., David, R., Shapiro, T., Collins, P., & Koh, C. (1972c). Response to triiodothyronine and dextroamphetamine: A study of preschool schizophrenic children. *Journal of Autism and Childhood Schizophrenia, 2,* 343–358.

Campbell, M., Grega, D. N., Green, W. H., & Bennett, W. G. (1983). Neuroleptic induced dyskinesias in children. *Clinical Neuropharmacology, 6,* 207–222.

Campbell, M., Perry, R., & Green, W. H. (1984). Use of lithium in children and adolescents. *Psychosomatics, 25, 95–106.*

Campbell, M., Schulman, D., & Rapoport, J. L. (1978). The current status of lithium therapy in child and adolescent psychiatry. *Journal of the American Academy of Child Psychiatry, 17,* 717–720.

Campbell, M., Small, A. M., & Green, W. H. (1982). Lithium and haloperidol in hospitalized aggressive children. *Psychopharmacological Bulletin, 18,* 126–130.

Campbell, M., Small, A. M., Green, W. H., Jennings, S. J., Perry, R., Bennett, W. G., & Anderson, L. (1984). Behavioral efficacy of haloperidol and lithium carbonate. Archives of General Psychiatry, 41,650–656.

Campbell, M., Small, A. M., Hollander, C. S., Korein, J., Cohen, I., Kalmijn, M., & Ferris, S. (1978). A controlled crossover study of triiodothyranine in autistic children. *Journal of Autism and Childhood Schizophrenia, 8*(4), 371–381.

Carlson, G. A., & Strober, M. (1979) Affective disorders in adolescence. *Psychiatric Clinics of North America, 2,* (3), 511–525.

Carlson G. A., & Cantwell D. P. (1979). A survey of depressive symptoms in a child and adolescent psychiatric population. *Journal of the American Academy of Child Psychiatry, 18,* 587–599.

Carlson G. A., & Cantwell D. P. (1980) Unmasking masked depression in children and adolescents. *American Journal of Psychiatry, 137,* 445–449.

Carter, C. H., & Maley, M. C. (1957). Chlorpromazine therapy in children at the Florida Farm Colony, *American Journal of Medical Science, 233,* 131.

Claghorn, J. L. (1972). A double-blind comparison of haloperidol (Haldol) and thioridazine (Mellaril) in outpatient children. *Current Therapy and Research, 14,* 785–789.

Cohen, I. L., Campbell, M., Posner, B. A., Small, A. M., Triebel, D., & Anderson, L. T. (1980). Behavioral effects of haloperidol in young autistic children. *Journal of the American Academy of Child Psychiatry, 19*:655–677.

Cohen, N. J., Douglas, C. I., Weiss, G., & Minde, K. K. (1971). Attention in hyperactive children and the effect of methylphenidate. *Journal of Child Psychology and Psychiatry, 12,* 129–139.

Conners, C. K., & Eisenberg, L. (1963). The effect of of methylphenidate on symptomatology and learning in disturbed children. *American of Journal of Psychiatry, 120,* 458–463.

Conners, C. K., Eisenberg, L., & Barcai, A. (1967). Effect of dextroamphetamine on children. *Archives of General Psychiatry, 17,* 478–485.

Conners, C. K. (1969). The teacher rating scale for use in drug studies with children. *American Journal of Psychiatry, 126,* 884–888.

Conners, C. K., Rothchild, G., Esenberg, L., Schwartz, L. S., & Robinson, E. (1969). Dextroamphetamine sulfate in children with learning disorders. *Archives of General Psychiatry, 21,* 182–190.

Conners, C. K. (1970). Symptom patterns in hyperkinetic neurotic and normal children. *Child Development, 41,* 667–682.

Conners, C. K. (1972). Psychological effects of stimulant drugs in children with minimal brain dysfunction. *Pediatrics, 49,* 702–708.

Conners, C. K., & Taylor E. (1980). Pemoline, methylphenidate and placebo in children with minimal brain dysfunction. *Archives of General Psychiatry, 37,* 922–930.

Cunningham, M. A., Pillai, V., & Rogers, W. J. B. (1968). Haloperidol in the treatment of children with severe behavior disorders. *British Journal of Psychology, 114,* 845–854.

Cutts K. K., & Jasper, H. H. (1939). Effect of benzedrine sulfate and phenobarbital on behavior problem children with abnormal electroencephalograms. *Archives of Neurology and Psychiatry, 41, 1138–1145.*

Cytryn, L., Gilbert, A., & Eisenberg, L. (1960). The effectiveness of tranquilizing drugs plus supportive psychotherapy in treating behavior disorder of children: A double-blind study of eighty outpatients. *American Journal of Orthopsychiatry, 30,* 113–129.

Cytryn L., McKnew D. H., Jr., & Bunney W. E., Jr. (1980). Diagnosis of depression in children: A reassessment. *American Journal of Psychiatry, 137,* 22–25.

Delay, J., & Deniker, P. (1952). Reactions biologiques observées au cours du traitement par le chlorthydrate de dimethylaminopropyl-N-chlorophenothiazine (4560 r.p.), Congrès des psychiatres de langue francaise, Luxembourg, July 22–26.

Delay, J., Deniker, P., & Harl, J. M. (1952). Traitement des états d'excitation et d'agitation par une méthode médicamenteuse derivée de l'hibernotherapie. *Annales Medico-Psychologiques, 110,* 267–273.

Denhoff, E., & Holden, R. H. (1955). The effectiveness of chlorpromomazine (Thorazine) with cerebral palsied children. *Journal of Pediatrics, 47,* 328–332.

Di Mascio, A. (1970). Classification and overview of psychotropic drugs. In A. Di Mascio, and R. I. Shader (Eds.), *Clinical handbook of psychopharmacology* (pp. 3–15). New York: Aronson.

Dostal, T., & Zvolsky, P. (1970). Antiaggressive effects of lithium salts in severely mentally retarded adolescents. *International Pharmacopsychiatry, 5,* 203–207.

Dundee, J. W. (1954). A review of chlorpromazine hydrochloride. *British Journal of Anaesthesia, 26,* 357–379.

Effron. A. S., & Freedman, A. M. (1953). The treatment of behavior disorders in children with Benadryl, A preliminary report. *Journal of Pediatrics, 42,* 261.

Eisenberg, L., Gilbert, A., Cytryn, L., Molling, P. A. (1961). The effectiveness of psychotherapy alone and in conjunction with perphenazine or placebo in the treatment of neurotic and hyperkinetic children. *American Journal of Psychiatry, 117,* 1088–1093.

Eisenberg, L., Lackman R., Molling, P. A., Lockner, A. Mizelle, J. D., & Conners, C. K. (1963). A psychopharmacologic experiment in a training school for delinquent boys: Methods, problems, findings. *Journal of Orthopsychiatry, 33,* 431–447.

Engelhardt, D. M., & Polizos, P. (1978). Adverse effects of pharmacotherapy in childhood psychosis. In M. A. Lipton, A. Di Mascio, and K. F. Killam (Eds.), *Psychopharmacology: A generation of progress.* New York: Raven Press.

Engelhardt, D. M., Polizos, P., Waizer, J., & Hoffman, S. P. (1973). A double-blind comparison of fluphenazine and haloperidol in outpatient schizophrenic children. *Journal of Autistic and Child Schizophrenia, 3,* 128–237.

Eveloff, H. H. (1966). Psychopharmacologic agents in child psychiatry. *Archives of General Psychiatry, 14,* 472–481.

Faretra, G., Dooher, L., & Dowling, J. (1970). Comparison of haloperidol and fluphenazine in disturbed children. *American Journal of Psychiatry, 126,* 1670–1673.

Firestone, P., Davey, J., Goodman, J. T., & Peters, S. (1978). The effects of caffeine and methylphenidate on hyperactive children. *Journal of the American Academy of Child Psychiatry. 17,* 445–456.

Firestone, P., Kelly, M. J., Goodman, J. T., & Davey, J. (1980). Differential effects of parent training and stimulant medication. *Journal of the American Academy of Child Psychiatry, 20,* 135–147.

Fish, B. (1960a). Drug therapy in child psychiatry: Psychological aspects. *Comprehensive Psychiatry, 1,* 55–61.

Fish, B. (1960b). Drug therapy in child psychiatry: Pharmacological aspects. *Comprehensive Psychiatry, 1,* 212–227.

Fish, B., and Shapiro, T. (1965). A typology of children's psychiatric disorders. Its application to a controlled evaluation of treatment. *Journal of the American Academy of Child Psychiatry, 4,* 32–52.

Fish, B., Campbell, M., Shapiro, T., & Floyd, A. (1969a). Comparison of trifluperidol, trifluoperazine, and chlorpromazine in preschool, schizophrenic children: The value of less sedative antipsychotic agents. *Curr. Ther. Res., 11,* 589–595.

Fish, B., Shapiro, T., & Campbell, M., (1966). Long term prognosis and the response of schizophrenic children to drug therapy: A controlled study of trifluoperazine. *American Journal of Psychiatry, 123,* 32–39.

Fisher, K. C., & Wilson, W. P. (1971). Methylphenidate and the hyperkinetic state. *Diseases of the Nervous System,* 695–698.

Flaherty, J. A. (1955). Effect of chlorpromazine medication on children with severe emotional disturbance. *Delaware State Medical Journal, 27,* 180–184.

Foster, P. (1967). Treatment of childhood depression. *Newton Wellsley Medical Bulletin, 19,* 33–36.

Freed, H., & Peifer, C. A. (1956). Treatment of hyperkinetic emotionally disturbed childen with prolonged administration of chlorpromazine. *American Journal of Psychiatry, 113,* 22–26.

Freedman, A. M. (1958). Drug therapy in behavior disorders. *Pediatric Clinics of North America, 5,* 573–594.

Freedman, A. M., Effron, A. S., & Bender, L. (1955a). Pharmacotherapy in children with psychiatric illness. *Journal of Nervous and Medical Diseases, 122,* 479–486.

Freedman, A. M., Kremer, M. W., Robertiello, R. C., & Effron, A. S. (1955b). The treatment of behavior disorders in children with tolserol. *Journal of Pediatrics, 47,* 369–372.

Frommer, E. A. (1967). Treatment of childhood depression with antidepressant drugs. *British Medical Journal, 1,* 729–732.

Frommer, E. A. (1972). Indications for antidepressant treatment with special reference to depressed preschool children. In A. L. Annell (Ed.), *Depressive states in childhood and adolescence.* Stockholm: Almquist & Wiksell.

Gadow, K. D. (1981). Effects of stimulant drugs on attention and cognitive deficits. *Exceptional Education Quarterly, 2* (3), 83–93.

Gadow, K. D. (1983). Effects of stimulant drugs on academic performance in hyperactive and learning disabled children. *Journal of Learning Disabilities, 16,* 290–300.

Garfield, S. L., Helper, M. M., Wilcott, R. C., & Murrly, R. (1962). Effects of chlorpromizine on behavior in emotionally disturbed children. *Journal of Nervous Mental Diseases, 135,* 147–154.

Gatski, R. L. (1955). Chlorpromazine in the treatment of emotionally maladjusted children. *Journal of the American Medical Association, 157,* 1298–1300.

Gittelman-Klein R. (1977). Definitional and methodological issues concerning depressive illness in children. In J. G. Schulterbrandt and A. Raskin (Eds.) *Depression in childhood: Diagnosis, treatment, and conceptual models.* New York: Raven Press.

Gittelman, R. (1980a). Diagnosis and drug treatment of childhood disorders. In D. F. Klein et al. (Eds.), *Diagnosis and drug treatment of psychiatric disorders: Adults and children, (2nd ed.) (pp. 590–776). Baltimore: Williams & Wilkins Company.*

Gittelman, R. (1980b). Indications for the use of stimulant treatment in learning disorders. *Journal of the American Academy of Child Psychiatry, 19,* 623–636.

Gittelman-Klein, R., and Klein, D. F. (1970). Controlled imipramine treatment of school phobia. *Archives of General Psychiatry, 25,* 204–207.

Gittelman-Klein, R., Klein, D. F., Katz, S., Saraf, K., & Pollack, E. (1976). Comparative effects of methylphenidate and thioridazine in hyperkinetic children. *Archives of General Psychiatry, 33,* 1217–1231.

Gittelman-Klein, R., Abikoff, H., Pollack, E., Klein, D., Katz, S. & Mattes, J. (1980). A controlled trial of behavior modification and methylphenidate in hyperactive children. In C. Whalen and B. Henker (Eds.), *Hyperactive children: The social ecology of identification and treatment.* New York: Academic Press.

Gordon, D. A., Forehand, R., & Picklesimer, D. K. (1978). The effects of dextroamphetamine on hyperactive children using multiple outcome measures. *Journal of Clinical Child Psychiaology, 7,* 125–128.

Goetzl, U. & Berkowitz, B. (1977). Lithium carbonate in the management of hyperactive aggressive behavior of the mentally retarded. *Comprehensive Psychaitry, 18,* 599–606.

Gram, L. F., & Rafaelsen, O. J. (1972). Lithium treatment of psychotic children and adolescents. *Acta Psychiatrica Scandinavica, 48* (3), 253–260.

Greenberg, L. M., Deens, M. A., & McMahon, A. (1972). Effects of dextroamphetamine, chlorpromazine, and hydroxyzine on behavior and performance in hyperactive children. *American Journal of Psychiatry, 129,* 532–539.

Greenberg, L., Yellin, A., Spring, C., & Metcalf, M. (1975). Clinical effects of imipramine and methylphenidate in hyperactive children. In R. Gittelman-Klein (Ed.), *Recent advances in child psychopharmacology.* New York: Human Science Press.

Greenberg, L., Yellin, A., Spring, C., & Metcalf, M. (1975). Clinical effect of imipramine and methylphenidate in hyperactive children. *International Journal of Mental Health, 4,* 144–156.

Greenhill, L. L., Rieder, R. O., Wender, P. H., Bucksbaum, M., & Zahn, T. P. (1973). Lithium carbonate in the treatment of hyperactive children. *Archives of General Psychiatry, 28,* 636–640.

Gross, M. D., & Wilson, W. C. (1964). Behavior disorders of children with cerebral dysrhythmias. *Archives of General Psychiatry, 11,* 610–619.

Gross, M. (1976). Growth of hyperkinetic children taking methylphenidate, dextroamphetamine or imipramine/desipramine. *Pediatrics, 58,* 423.

Gualiteri, C. T., & Hawk, B. (1980). Tardive dyskinesia and other drug-induced movement disorders among handicapped children and youth. *Applied Research in Mental Retardation, 1,* 55–69.

Gualtieri, C. T., Wargin, W., Kanoy, R., Patrick, K., Shen, C., Youngblood, W., Mueller, R., & Breese, G. (1982). Clinical studies of methylphenidate serum levels in children and adults. *Journal of the American Academy of Child Psychiatry, 21*, 19–26.

Halliday, R., Gnanck, K., Rosenthal, J. R., McKibben, J. L., & Callaway, E. (1980). The effects of methylphenidate dosage on school and home behaviors of the hyperactive child. In R. M. Knight & D. J. Bakker (Eds.) *Treatment of Learning Disabilities*. University Park Press: Baltimore.

Heuyer, G., Gerard, G., & Galibert, J. (1953). Traitement de l'excitation psychometrics chez l'enfant pare (13456 r.p.) *Archives Francaises de Pediatrie, 9*, 961.

Heuyer, G., Dell, C., & Prinquet, G. (1956). Emploi de la chlorpromazine en neuro-psychiatric infantile. *Encephale, 45*, 576–578.

Horowitz, H. A. (1977). Lithium and the treatment of adolescent manic-depressive illness. *Diseases of the Nervous System, 37*, 90–92.

Huestis, R. D., Arnold, L. E., & Smeltzer, D. J. (1975). Caffeine versus methylphenidate and D-amphetamine in minimal brain dysfunction: A double-blind comparison. *American Journal of Psychiatry, 132*, 868–870.

Hunt, B.R., Frank, T., & Krush, T. P. (1956). Chlorpromazine in the treatment of severe emotional disorders of childhood. *Journal of the Diseases of Children, 9*, 268–277.

Hunt, R D., Cohen, D. J., Shaywitz, S. E., & Shaywitz, B. A. (1982). Strategies for study of neurochemistry of attention deficit disorder in children. *Schizophrenia Bulletin, 8*, 236–252.

Kanner, L. (1935). *Child Psychiatry* (p. 133). Springfield: Charles C. Thomas.

Kanner, L. (1957). *Child Psychiatry*. (2nd ed.). Springfield: Charles C. Thomas.

Kelly, J.T., Koch, M., & Buegel, D. (1976). Lithium carbonate in juvenile manic-depressive illness. *Diseases of the Nervous System, 37*, 90–92.

Knobel, M. (1962). Psychopharmacology for the hyperkinetic child. *Archives of General Psychiatry, 6*, 30–34.

Kraft, I. A., Marcus, I. M., Wilson, W., Swander, D. V., Rumage, N. W., & Schulhoffer, E. (1959). Methodological problems in studying the effect of tranquilizers in children with specific reference to meprobamate. *Southern Medical Journal, 52*, 179–185.

Kraft, I. A., Ardali, C., Duffy, J., Hart, J., & Pearce, P. R. (1966). Use of amitryptyline in childhood behavior disturbances. *International Journal of Neuropsychiatry, 2*, 611–614.

Krakowski, A. J. (1965). Amitryptyline in treatment of hyperkinetic children: A double-blind study. *Psychosomatics, 6*, 355–360.

Kuhn, V., & Kuhn R. (1972). Drug therapy for depression in children. Indications and methods. In A. L. Annell (Eds.), *Depressive states in childhood and adolescents*. Stockholm; Almquist & Wiksell.

Kurtis, L. B. (1966). Clinical study of the response to nortriptyline on autistic children. *International Journal of Neuropsychiatry, 2*, 298–301.

Kydd, R. R., & Werry, J. S. (1982). Schizophrenia in children under 16 years. *Journal of Autism and Development Disorders, 12*(4), 343–356.

Lacey, J. H., & Crisp, A. H., (1980). Hunger, food intake and weight: The impact of clomipramine on a refeeding anorexia nervosa population. *Postgraduate Medical Journal, 56, (supplement 1)*, 79–85.

Laufer, M., Denhoff, E., & Solomons, G. (1957). Hyperkinetic impulse disorder in children's behavior problems. *Psychosomatic Medicine, 19*, 38–49.

La Veck, G. D., De La Crug, F., & Simundson, E. (1960). Fluphenazine in the treatment of mentally retarded children with behavior disorders. *Diseases of the Nervous System, 23,* 82–85.

Leckman, J. F., Cohen, D. J., & Detlor, et al. (1982). Clonidine in the treatment of Tourette Syndrome: A review of the data. In A. J. Friedhoff and T. N. Chase (Eds.), *Gilles de la Tourette Syndrome.* New York: Raven Press.

Lehmann, H. E., & Hanrahan, G. E. (1954). Chlorpromazine, new inhibiting agent for psychomotor excitement and manic states. *Archives of Psychiatry and Neurology, 71,* 227–237.

Lerer, R. J., Lerer, M. P., & Artner, J. (1977). The effects of methylphenidate on the handwriting of children with minimal brain dysfunction. *Journal of Pediatrics, 91,* 127–132.

Le Vann, L. J. (1961). Thioridazine, a psychosedative virtually free of side-effectts. *Alberta Medical Bulletin.*

Le Vann, L. J. (1969). Haloperidol in the treatment of behavioral disorders in children and adolescents. *Canadian Psychiatric Association Journal, 14,* 217–220.

Lindsley, D. B., & Henry, C. E. (1942). The effects of drugs on behavior and the electroencephalograms of children with behavior disorders. *Psychosomatic Medicine, 4,* 140–149.

Lipman, R. S. (1973). NIMH-PRB support of research in minimal brain dysfunction and other disorders of childhood. *Psychopharmacology Bulletin* Special Issue. Pharmacotherapy of children. NIMH. pp. 1–8 DHEW Publication No. (HSM) 73–9002.

Litchfield, H. R. (1957). Clinical evaluation of meprobamate in disturbed and prepsychotic children. *Annals of the New York Academy of Science, 67,* 828–832.

Looker, A., & Conners, C. K. (1970). Diphenylhydantoin in children with severe temper tantrums. *Archives of General Psychiatry, 23,* 80–89.

Lowe, T. L., Cohen, D. J., Detlor, J., Kremenitzer, M. W. & Shaywitz, B. A. (1982). Stimulant medications precipitate Tourette's Syndrome. *JAMA, 247,* 1729–1731.

Lucas, A. P., Lockett, H. J., & Grimm, F. (1965). Amitriptyline in childhood depression. *Diseases of the Nervous System, 28,* 105–113.

MacLean, R. E. G. (1960). Imipramine hydrocholoride (Tofranil) and enuresis. *American Journal of Psychiatry, 117,* 551.

Malmquist C. P. (1971). Depressions in childhood and adolescence. *New England Journal of Medicine, 284,* 887–893.

Mattes, J., & Gittelman, K. (1983). Growth of hyperactive children on a maintenance regimen of methylphenidate. *Archives of General Psychiatry, 40,* 317–321.

Mattson, R. H., & Calverley, J. R. (1968). Dextroamphetamine sulfate induced dyskinesias. *JAMA, 205,* 400–402.

McAndrew, J. B., Case, Q., & Treffert, D. (1972). Effects of prolonged phenothiazine intake on psychotic and other hospitalized children. *Journal of Autistic and Child Schizophrenia, 2,* 75.

McKnew, D. H. Jr., & Cytryn, L. (1979). Urinary metabolities in chronically depressed children. *Journal of the American Academy of Psychiatry, 18,* 608–615.

McKnew, D. H., Cytryn, L, Buschbaum, M. S., et al. (1981). Lithium in children of lithium-responding parents. *Psychiatry Research, 4,* 171–180.

Merritt, H. H., & Putnam, T. J. (1938). Sodium diphenylhydantoinate in treatment of convulsive disorders. *JAMA, 111,* 1068–1073.

Meyerson, A. (1936). Effect of benzedrine sulfate on mood and fatigue in normal and neurotic persons. *Archives of Neurology and Psychiatry, 36,* 816–822.

Meyerson, A., Lomar, J., & Dameshek, W. (1936). Physiological effects of Benzedrine and its relationship to other drugs affecting the autonomic nervous system. *American Journal of Medical Science, 192,* 560–574.

Mikkelsen, E. J. (1982). Efficacy of neuroleptic medication in pervasive development disorders of childhood. *Schizophrenic Bulletin, 8,*(2), 320–332.

Mikkelson, E. J., Rapoport, J., Nee, L., Grunenau, C., Mendelson, W., & Gillin J. C. (1980). Childhood enuresis I. Sleep patterns and psychopathology. *Archives of General Psychiatry, 37,* 1139–1144.

Miksztal, M. W. (1956). Chlorpromazine (Thorazine) and reserpine in residential treatment of neuropsychiatric disorders in children. *Journal of Nervous and Mental Disease, 123,* 477–479.

Millichap, J. G., Aymat, F., Sturgis, L. H., Larsen, K. W., & Egan, R. A. (1968). Hyperkinetic behavior and learning disorders III. Battery of neuropsychological tests in controlled trial of methlphenidate. *American Journal of the Diseases of Children, 166,* 235–244.

Millichap, J. G. (1973). Drugs in management of minimal brain dysfunction. *Annals of the New York Academy of Science, 205,* 321–334.

Mills, I. H. (1976). Amitriptyline therapy in anorexia nervosa (letter). *Lancet, 2,* 687.

Molitch, M., & Eccles, A. K. (1937). The effect of benzedrine sulfate on the intelligence scores of children. *American Journal of Psychiatry, 94,* 587–590.

Molitch, M., & Poliakoff. S. (1937). The effect of benzedrine sulfate on enuresis. *Archives of Pediatrics, 54,* 499–501.

Molitch, M., & Sullivan, J. P. (1937). The effect of benzedrine sulfate on children taking the new Stanford Achievement Test. *American Journal of Orthopsychiatry, 7,* 519–522.

Morselli, P. L., Bianchetti, G., Durand, G., Le Huzey, M. F., Zarifian, E., & Dugas, M. (1979). Haloperidol plasma level monitoring in pediatric patients. *Therapeutic Drug Monitoring, 1,* 35–46.

Munster, A. J., Stanley, A. M., & Saunders, J. C. (1961). Imipramine (Tofranil) in the treatment of enuresis. *American Journal of Psychiatry, 118,* 76–77.

Needleman, H. L., & Waber, D., (1977). The use of amitriptyline in anorexia nervosa. In R. Vigersky (Ed.), *Anorexia nervosa* (pp. 341–348). New York: Raven Press.

Ney, P. G. (1967). Psychosis in a child associated with amphetamine administration. *Canadian Medical Association Journal, 97,* 1026–1029.

Oettinger, L. Jr. (1962). Chlorprothixene in the management of problem children. *Diseases of the Nervous System* (Oct.), 568–571.

Oettinger, L., & Simonds, R. (1962). The use of thioridazine in the office management of children's behavior disorders. *Med. Times. 90,* 596–604.

Page, J. G., Janicki, R. S., Bernstein, J. E., Curran, C. F., & Michelli, F. A. (1974). Pemoline in the treatment of childhood hyperkinesis. *Journal of Learning Disorders, 7,* 498–503.

Pasamanick, B. (1951). Anticonvulsant drug therapy of behavior problem with abnormal electroencephalograms. *Archives of Neurology and Psychiatry, 65,* 752–766.

Petti, T. A., & Campbell, M. (1975). Imipramine and seizures. *American Journal of Psychiatry, 132,* 538–540.

Petti, T. A., & Law, W., III (1982). Imipramine treatment of depressed children: A double-blind pilot study. *Journal of Clinical Psychopharmacology, 2*(2), 107–110.

Polizos, P., Engelhardt, D. M., Hoffman, S. P., & Waizer, J. (1973). Neurological consequences of psychotropic drug withdrawal in schizophrenic children. *Journal of Autism and Childhood Schizophrenia, 3,* 247.

Porrino, L. J., Rapoport, J. L., Behan, D., Scevy, W. Ismond, D. R., & Bunney, W. E. (1983). A naturalistic assessment of the motor activity of hyperactive boys. *Archives of General Psychiatry, 40,* 681–687.

Poussaint, A. F., & Ditman, K. S. (1965). A controlled study of imipramine (Tofranil) in the treatment of childhood enuresis. *Journal of Pediatrics, 67,* 283–290.

Poznanski E. O., Carroll B. J., Banegas M. C., et al. (1982). The dexamethasone suppression test in prepubertal depressed children. *American Journal of Psychiatry, 139,* 321–324.

Psychopharmacology Bulletin (1973). Special Issue, Pharmacotherapy of children. NIMH, DHEW publication No. (HSM) 73-9002.

Puig-Antich, J. (1980). Affective disorders in childhood. *Psychiatric Clinics of North America, 3,* 403–424.

Puig-Antich J., Blau S., Marx N., Greenhill, L. L., & Chambers, W. J. (1978). Prepubertal major depressive disorder. A pilot study. *Journal of the American Academy of Child Psychiatry, 17,* 695–707.

Puig-Antich, J., Perel, J. M., Lupatkin, W., Chambers, W. J., Shea, C., Tabrizi, M. A., & Stiller, R. (1979). Plasma levels of imipramine (IMI) and desmethylimipramine (DMI) and clinical response in prepubertal major depressive disorder. A preliminary report. *Journal of the American Academy of Child Psychiatry, 18,* 616–627.

Puig-Antich J., Tabrizi M. A., Davies, M., Goetz, R., Chambers, W. J., Halapern, F., & Sachar, E. J. (1981). Prepubertal endogenous major depressive hyposecrete growth hormone in response to insulin-induced hypoglycemia. *Biological Psychiatry, 16,* 801–807.

Quinn, P., & Rapoport, J. L. (1975). One year followup of hyperactive boys treated with imipramine or methylphenidate. *American Journal of Psychiatry, 132,* 241–245.

Rapoport, J. (1965). Childhood behavior and learning problems treated with imipramine. *International Journal of Neuropsychiatry, 1,* 635–642.

Rapoport, J. L., Buchsbaum, M. S., Zahn, T. P., Weingartner, H., Ludlow C. & Mirkkelser, E. L. (1978). Dextroamphetamine: Cognitive and behavioral effects in normal prepubertal boys. *Science, 199,* 560–562.

Rapoport, J., Mikkelson, E. J., Zavadil, A., Nee, L., Gruenau, C., Mendelson, W. & Gillin, J. C., (1980). Childhood enuresis II. *Archives of General Psychiatry, 37,* 1146–1152.

Rapoport, J. L., Quinn, P. O., Bradbard, G., Riddle, D., & Brooks, E. (1974). Imipramine and methylphenidate treatments of hyperactive boys. *Archives of General Psychiatry, 30,* 789–793.

Remschmidt, H., (1976). The psychotropic effect of carbamazepine in non-epileptic patients with particular reference to problems posed by clinical studies in children with behavior disorders. In W. Birkmayer (Ed.), *Epileptic seizures-Behavior-Pain* (pp. 253–258). Baltimore: University Park Press.

Rettig, J. H. (1955). Chlorpromazine for the control of psychomotor excitement in the mentally deficient. *Journal of Nervous and Mental Disease, 122,* 190.

Rogers, W. J. B. (1965). Use of haloperidol in children's psychiatric disorders. *Clinical Trials Journal, 2,* 162–164.

Rosenblum, S., Buoniconto, P., & Graham, B. D. (1960). "Campazine" vs. placebo: A controlled study with educable, emotionally disturbed children. *American Journal of Mental Deficiency, 64,* 713.

Safer, D., Allen, R., & Barr, E. (1972). Depression of growth in hyperactive children on stimulant drugs. *New England Journal of Medicine, 287,* 217–220.

Saletu, B., Simeon, J., Saletu, M., Itil, T. M., & DaSilva, J. (1974). Behavioral and visual evoked potential investigations during trihexyphenidyl and thiothixene treatment in psychotic boys. *Biological Psychiatry, 8,* 177–189.

Salgado, M. A., & Kierdel-Vegas, O. (1963). Treatment of enuresis with imipramine. *American Journal of Psychiatry, 119,* 990.

Saraf, K., Klein, D., Gittelman-Klein, R., & Groff, S. (1974). Imipramine side effects in children. *Psychopharmacologia, 37,* 265–274.

Sargant, W., & Blackburn, J. M. (1936). The effect of Benzedrine on intelligence scores. *Lancet,* Dec. 12, 1385–1387.

Satterfield, J. B., Satterfield, B. T., & Cantwell, D. P. (1981). Three years multimodality treatment study of 100 hyperactive boys. *Journal of Pediatrics, 98,* 650–655.

Seignot, J. J. N. (1961). A case of the syndrome of tics of Gilles de la Tourette controlled by R1625. *Annales Medico-Psychologiques,* 1961. 119:578–579.

Schain, R. J., & Reynard, C. L. (1975). Observations on effects of a central stimulant drug (methylphenidate) in children with hyperactive behavior. *Pediatrics, 55,* 709–716.

Shaffer, D., Costello, A. J., & Hill, I. D. (1968). Control of enuresis with imipramine. *Archives of Diseases in Children, 43,* 665–671.

Shapiro, A. K., & Shapiro, E., (1982). Clinical efficacy of haloperidol, pimozide, fenfluridol, and clonidine in the treatment of Tourette Syndrome. New York: Raven Press.

Shapiro, A. K. & Shapiro, E. (1981). Do stimulants provoke, cause or exacerbate tics or Tourette's Syndrome. *Comprehensive Psychiatry, 22,* 265–273.

Shapiro, A. K., Shapiro, E., & Wayne, H. (1973). Treatment of Tourette's syndrome. *Archives of General Psychiatry, 28,* 92–97.

Shaw, C. R., Lockett, H. J., Lucas, A. R., Lamontagne, C. H., & Crimm, F. (1963). Tranquilizer drugs in the treatment of emotionally disturbed children: I. Inpatients in a residential treatment center. *Journal of the American Academy of Child Psychiatry, 2,* 725–742.

Sheard, M. H., Marini, J. L., & Bindger, C. I. (1976). The effect of lithium on impulsive aggressive behavior in man. *American Journal of Psychiatry, 133,* 1409–1413.

Sherwin, A. C., Flach, F. F., & Stokes, P. E. (1958). Treatment of psychoses in early childhood with triiodothyronine. *American Journal of Psychiatry, 115,* 166–167.

Silver, A. A. (1955). Management of children with schizophrenia. *American Journal of Psychotherapy, 9,* 196.

Silver, L. B. (1981). The relationship between learning disabilities, hyperactivity, distractibility and behavior problems, a clinical analysis. *Journal of the American Academy of Child Psychiatry, 20,* 385–397.

Simmons, J. Q., III, Leiken, S. J., Lovaas, O. I., Schaeffer, B., & Perloff, B. (1966). Modification of autistic behavior with LSD-25. *American Journal of Psychiatry, 122,* 1201–1211.

Sprague, R. L., & Sleator, E. K. (1977). Methylphenidate in hyperkinetic children: Differences in dose effects on learning and social behavior. *Science, 198,* 1274-1276.

Stores, G. (1978). School children with epilepsy at risk for learning and behavior problems. *Developmental Medicine and Child Neurology* 20:302–308.

Sykes D. H., Doyles, V. I., Weiss, G., & Minde, K. K. (1971). Attention in hyperactive children and the effect of methylphenidate. *Journal of Child Psychology and Psychiatry, 12,* 129–139.

Swanson, J., Kinsbourne, M., Roberts, W., & Zucker, K. (1978). Dose response analysis of the effect of stimulant medication on the learning ability of children referred for hyperactivity. *Pediatrics, 61,* 21–29.

Tarjan, G., Lowery, V. E., & Wright, S. W. (1957). Use of chlorpromazine in two hundred seventy-eight mentally deficient patients. *American Journal of Diseases of Children, 94,* 294–300.

Ucer, E., & Kreger, K. C., (1969). A double-blind study comparing haloperidol and thioridazine in emotionally disturbed, mentally retarded children. *Current Therapeutic Research, 11,* 278–283.

Waizer, J., Polizos, P., Hoffman, S. P., Engelhardt, D. M., & Margolis, R. A. (1972). A singleblind evaluation of thiothixene with outpatient schizophrenic children. *Journal of Autism and Childhood Schizophrenia, 2,* 378–386.

Waizer, J., Hoffman, S. P., Polizos, P., & Engelhardt, D. M. (1974). Outpatient treatment of hyperactive school children with imipramine. *American Journal of Psychiatry, 131,* 587–591.

Walker, C. F., & Kirkpatrick, B. B. (1947). Dilantin treatment for behavior problem children with abnormal electroencephalograms. *American Journal of Psychiatry, 103,* 484–492.

Weinberg W. A., Rutman J., & Sullivan, L. (1973). Depression in children referred to an educational diagnostic center: Diagnosis and treatment. *Journal of Pediatrics, 83,* 1065–1072.

Weingartner, H., Langer, D., Gria, J., & Rapoport, J. L. (1982). Acquisition and retreival of information in amphetamine-treated hyperactive children. *Psychiatry Research, 6,* 21–26.

Weiss, G., Werry, J., Minde, K., Douglas, V., & Sykes, D. (1968). Studies on the hyperactive child V: The effects of dextroamphetamine and chlorpromazine on behavior and intellectual functioning. *Journal of Child Psychology and Psychiatry, 9,* 145–156.

Weller, E B., Preskorn, S. H., Weller, R. A., & Croskell, M. (1983). Childhood depression: Imipramine levels and response. *Psychopharmacology Bulletin, 19*(1), 59–62.

Wender, Paul (1971). *Minimal brain dysfunction in children.* New York: Wiley.

Werry, J. S., Weiss, G., Douglas, V., & Martin, J. (1966). Studies on the hyperactive child III: The effect of chlorpromazine upon behavior and learning ability. *Journal of the American Academy of Child Psychiatry, 5,* 292–312.

White, J. H., & Schnaulty, N. L., (1977), Successful treatment of anorexia nervosa with imipramine. *Diseases of the Nervous System, 38,* 567–568.

Winsberg, B. G., Beater, I., Kupietz, S., & Tobias, J. (1972). Effects of imipramine and dextroamphetamine on behavior of neuropsychiatrically impaired children. *American Journal of Psychiatry, 128,* 1425–1431.

Winsberg, B. G., Goldstein, S., Yepes, L. E., & Perel, J. M. (1975). Imipramine and electrocardiographic abnormalities in hyperactive children. *American Journal of Psychiatry, 132*, 542–545.

Wolpert, A., Hagamen, M. B., & Merlis, S. (1966). A pilot study of thiothixene in childhood schizophrenia. *Current Therapeutic Research, 8*, 617–620.

Wolpert, A., Hagamen, M. B., & Merlis, S. (1967). A comparative study of thiothixene and trifluoperazine in childhood schizophrenia. *Current Therapeutic Research, 9*, 482–485.

Wolpert, A., Quintos, A., White, L., & Merlis, S. (1968). Thiothixene and chlorprothixene in behavior disorder. *Current Therapeutic Research, 10*, 566–569.

Yepes, L., Balka, B., Winsberg, B., & Bialer, I. (1977). Amitriptyline and methylphenidate treatment of behaviorally disordered children. *Journal of Child Psychology and Psychiatry, 18*, 39–52.

Youngerman, J., & Canino, I. A. (1978). Lithium carbonate use in children and adolescents. *Archives of General Psychiatry, 35*, 216–224.

Zier, A. (1959). Meprobamate (Miltown) as an aid to psychotherapy in an outpatient child guidance clinic. *American Journal of Orthopsychiatry, 29*, 377–382.

Zimmerman, F. T., & Burgemeister, B. B. (1958). Action of methylphenidate (Ritalin) and reserpine in behavior disorders in children and adults. *American Journal of Psychiatry, 115*, 323–328.

Developmental Considerations in Psychopharmacology: The Interaction of Drugs and Development

THEODORE SHAPIRO, M.D.

DEFINITION OF A PROBLEM

Child psychiatrists use pharmacological agents in order to affect behavior. Insofar as that behavior occurs in a growing and changing organism, the medication can be said to influence developmental patterning. Most child psychiatrists consider themselves practitioners of developmental psychiatry suited by their training to deal with the interplay of drugs with changing behavior. Physiological concepts such as "inhibiting" and "disinhibiting" sound too mechanistically gruff in a human context. The notion of "modulating" behavior in order to encourage a new adaptive state or phase might be more salutary.

These preliminary comments are made to highlight the child psychiatrist's problem in defining an appropriate framework for the use of medication for children. Stated in this form the problem requires the integration of language from disciplines learned during medical training with the language of developmental propositions that has become the major scaffolding of child psychiatry. It is clear that in using pharmacological agents, we are attempting to change some substrate and have therefore tacitly accepted a mechanistic contribution to the emergence of behavior. On the other hand, day to day work with children requires an observational stance that accounts for psychosocial and dynamic factors in change.

During the past 10 years of active psychopharmacological research on children there has been a tendency toward polarization within the child psychiatry community, similar to that which has occurred among certain general psychiatrists. There are those who claim to be childhood psychopharmacologists, while others resist prescribing a medication because they feel they do not know enough about pharmacologic action. There are also sectarians in both groups who feel alternatively that not to use a medication is tantamount to malpractice, while others feel that the use of pharmacological agents mechanizes the practice of child psychiatry so as to compromise their role as humanistically oriented physicians.

How can we extricate ourselves from the paradox that a group of clinicians devoted to the well-being of children, humanistically oriented, and geared toward developmental principles will avoid or minimize the use of medication, because doing so implies a firm brain-behavior correlation as though it were exclusive of other approaches?

Perhaps the antagonism is a pseudoconflict! Bastardized phrases such as clinical psychopharmacology are attempts to solve the implied antagonisms. A breakdown of that term may help us define our task: Pharmacology pertains to the rational use of medicines in biological systems and the study of their rates of absorption, excretion, sites of action, toxicity, etc. Psycho refers to the mind, clinical to ministrations at the bedside. Joined together they give a compound term that attests to the Anglo-Saxon origins of our English language. But the reconciliation that really demands the most from us as physicians using medication is not linguistic; it is that we not only have to bring together the mind, the body, and the behavior, but also have to bring together these sectors in relation to a growing organism, in a changing social milieu with different requirements at different stages of the life cycle. The latter is what renders the developmental point of view unique from others and warrants a separate disciplinary definition of child psychiatry.

Development implies and includes concepts such as growth, differentiation, maturation and, finally, integrated development itself. The first two terms are borrowed from biology, the third is a fiction of heuristic value to help us to make rational some of what we do. Growth pertains to the accretion of cells and changing size or mass; differentiation refers to specialization of more general cellular elements or differentiation of behavior from more global, syncretic beginnings to more highly specialized and articulated functions. Maturation refers to the natural unfolding of genetic potentials in "average expectable environments" (Hartmann et al., 1947). Development refers not only to maturation, but also to the milieu in which maturation emerges. As such, development pertains to the species-specific potentials of an organism, and also to the variations in the environment at different stages. The hierarchic structuralization of mind is the synthesis of all these forces impinging on the organism and serves as the background for creative and new behaviors in aging systems. In addition, child psychiatry includes affective components in its view of development, unlike some cognitive psychologies that exclude such factors to decrease the number of parameters to be considered in their experimental work.

While these general principles clarify some of the training biases of developmental psychiatrists, they do not cover the methodological biases that are inherent in the techniques used to study development. We can look at development from the standpoint of cross-sectional norms, which indicate that this child ought to be this or that weight and height or have this and that variety of behavior at such and such an age. These normative approaches are characteristic of testing devices used to arrive at intelligence or developmental quotients. Normalizing developmentalists of this ilk utilize bell-shaped distribution curves showing the relative presence or absence of behaviors in relation to chronological age. They are not usually interested in the structural underpinnings of changing capacity. There are also longitudinal techniques designed to alert us to the sequences and precursors of behavior in their increasing complexity as development ensues toward its ends as highly integrated and differentiated behaviors. In addition to these approaches, child psychiatrists also utilize the concepts of "developmental lines" or "aims of development" outlined in terms of more general concepts of maturity not based on the usual, but on the desirable and adaptive. It is hard to separate such schemes from developmental Utopianism, but they are useful in pinpointing the fulfillment of human capacity and determining prolongation of arrest or regression. Anna Freud's scheme of developmental lines (1965) is one such program. Erikson (1963) offers another. He refers to the reconciliations that individuals are expected to make at each stage of development between their concomitant needs and capacities to adapt in an ecological balance with the rest of society and nature.

Our discussion to this point presents us not only with the problem of bringing together substrate with behavior and epiphenomena of mind in consideration of the use of pharmacological agents, but also with various views of development that may not converge at the same focus. How can we reconcile these into a holistic program so that the child psychiatrist can still maintain the distinctivenes of his or her essential training as a developmental clinician? Clearly, such an approach would involve describing a process that is not so one-sided as to divide us into sectarian organicists or functionalists with their concomitant nasty definitions as "brain changers" or "mind manipulators." Rather we should be able to describe a context in which we can function as physicians with a developmental bias that enables us to treat children as they are growing up with rational concern for their adaptation no matter which level of inquiry is favored. In practice we see children with actual worries and wishes in real or imagined trouble with a real environment of parents and society with similar or dissimilar desires and concerns. How can we succeed therapeutically using the enabling principles of our training?

DEVELOPMENTAL VIEW IN THEORY AND PRACTICE

A careful look at our particular training will enable us to outline further how we approach problems. We are all trained dualistically in medical schools as applied physiologists believing in the possibility of altering structure and function through mechanistic means, while at the same time, we depend heavily on the doctor–patient relationship and the capacity of individuals to respond to talking, relationship, and insight therapies that range from psycho to transactional analysis. It is exactly here that the developmental principles not only tolerate the presumed dualism, but offer theoretical reconciliations. Developmental observation does not permit a stand that is either all nature or all nurture. In order to make the variety of disorders we see in childhood understandable, we have been trained to be alert to factors that we may (for the sake of ease) call inner and outer influences. The weight we give to each sector is highly dependent on the existing knowledge and information available within our science.

Freud's early interest in distinguishing actual neuroses from psychoneuroses reflected a strongly organismic and organic bias. On the other hand, the insistence on trauma as real and external showed his willingness to shift his focus to the external world as a source of pathological influence. Both of these concepts only came together when he explicated the notion of psychic reality and could postulate the possibilities of exploring the individual, who behaved neurotically. Furthermore, when he made the etiological inferences about causes in the past, his guidelines for practice were posed as hypotheses yet to be tested by clinical observation.

Similarly, concepts within child psychiatry have undergone change. A diagnosis such as "minimal brain dysfunction" (MBD) is but one example of where we hedge our bets in reasoning by analogy to the presenting clinical picture of known orgaic mental syndromes with actual tissue damage. Yet, as child psychiatrists, we are aware that children bearing this formidable diagnosis can be helped clinically by a number of techniques that include substrate manipulation (medication) as well as learning techniques (tutoring) and, frequently, psychotherapy. Indeed, no one treatment is generally enough. When confronted by reality we are practical empiricists. DSM-III (1980) is an apt testimony to this idea insofar as it has helped take the onus off the brain by changing MBD to Attention Deficit Disorder (ADD). Now attention is the most important behavior to be considered, not hyperactivity, and the brain, though involved, is now out of the name.

The adaptive point of view espoused by Hartmann and others talks about average biological equipment in an average expectable environment with a notion that the individual can come into homeostasis within himself as well as with his environment. He is fitted to adaptation in the ecological interplay within the family and the smaller community as well as the larger community if he is at least averagely endowed. And currently developmental knowledge suggests a great deal more "prewiring" than we ever suspected. However, a thoroughgoing developmentalist must take the theoretical view that influencine one sector in a system may affect something within that system, but may also affect other systems. Thus, a child psychiatrist must be alert to all sectors of development. There is continuous interplay between soma, psyche, and society. Drug therapy applies knowledge and skills to one or more sectors but may not be sufficient by itself to affect all systems uniformly or beneficially. Multiple approaches are needed.

In order to explicate these developmental principles, let us look at a number of practical examples commonly seen in child psychiatry and how the use of medication may alter the vital balance within and between subsystems and also require other therapeutic considerations.

During the second year of life, many children show interrupted sleep. Should such children be given some mild bedtime medication such as diphenhydramine (Benadryl), if to do so might interfere with working out and arriving at a satisfactory resolution of a phase-specific conflict? In some children a need to establish control, perhaps in response to toilet training or as a feature of the new negativism that emerges at the end of the second year is clearly operative. While the drug may interfere with the mother–infant interface stimulated by a new training demand, the parents and the child are also in a balance developmentally. If the sleep disturbance interferes with the mother's sense of well-being and affects her attitudes and concerns about the child, how will she respond to the continuing nighttime intrusions and will they evolve into a sense of battle? A sadomasochistic model could ensue, as well as one where control is offered by a drug. A developmental psychopharmacologist asks if a mild sedative would change the scenario to the developmental advantage of the infant at that level of patterning.

At a still simpler level, we have been told that ADD, especially in children who have encephalographic changes, is influenced favorably by the use of stimulant drugs (Satterfield et al., 1972, 1973). In fact, some argue that it may be reprehensible to withhold such medication from a child who needs help in focussing attention and increasing learning potential. Not only do the matters that concern mother-child interface apply as in the first instance, but we are aware also that the medication itself may have an effect on the growth potential of the child (Safer & Allen, 1973), and that interfering with one biological system must be considered in light of the benefits that the medication might offer. Moreover, a recent study suggests that the drug is not specific to the disorder and may help anyone to achieve better attention (Rapoport et al., 1978). The more recent discovery that tardive dyskinesia occurs in children of neuroleptics has also led to increased concern about the weight of therapeutic effect versus side effects of drug use (Gualtieri & Hawk, 1981).

The more extreme circumstance of childhood psychosis provides the example of a child who behaves bizarrely and has tantrums at times. The child may be using the only adaptive means available to attract the caretaker's attention. We may be tempted to interfere with the radical behaviors, frequently at the behest of distraught parents. Should we do so if these are the child's *only* human interactions? Such an intervention (if it were possible to be handled with medication) would quiet the child, to be sure. However, we could not be certain that while the complaining environment might welcome the quieting, it might also deprive the child of the only interaction he is, at that juncture, able to elicit. So often, medication is wrongly used to quiet so as not to disturb, rather than as an adjunct to, or concomitant with, other methods designed to enhance developmental progress. These examples and others are presented to remind those who are interested in using medication for children that the medication alone is rarely sufficient. Parents and children's shorthand designations such as a "reading pill" are just as bad as the physician's "he'll grow out of it," because each conveys the implication that one factor or one therapeutic intervention will suffice. The fact is that neither is sufficient in itself but requires adjunctive help for other developmental systems in producing a well-functioning child in an adapted state with a minimum of useful anxiety.

The organismic view of development does not easily accede to dividing functions into varying sectors, but some more clarity may be gained by discussing each level of the human organization separately, largely on the justification that each level may be studied by a different method. This is done with the general caution that there is no mind without a brain, there is no behavior without stimuli, and childhood dependency is a feature of human development. These factors notwithstanding, we can look in a rational way at the individual child in relation to these varying sectors in order to explicate aspects of drug use according to known developmental principles.

We will first address biological development. We will then look at developmental lines as the significant feature of the ego's adaptive organization and consider the influence of medication on such functions, and finally take those functions which are more largely under the sway of the pleasure principle and look at the influence of drugs on fantasy formation, capacity for compromise, etc. Within each sector we will try to attend to the child's interactional homeostasis of the child at each stage of development with reference to his caretakers, ranging from mother through teacher and reaching to the extended community. Their developmental expectations and normative values will be looked at as feeding back to and influencing the maturing and developing child. The changing meaning of the developing child to his parents and community as well as the changing meaning of varying techniques available for modulating development will be examined with special reference to the use of medication.

INDEPENDENT AND INTEGRATED SECTORS OF DEVELOPMENT

Biological Features

The child is in a biological process of growth, maturation, and development. These may be measured by height and weight curves, physiological responses that clinically include blood pressure and pulse rate, temperature control, at the biochemical level by the techniques that are available for observing the changes that occur, for example, in liver and thyroid function with progressive chronological maturation. In addition, whatever organ system is potentially affected by a medication can itself be monitored along with behavior. In order to keep close track on developmental biological issues, one must have a working knowledge and empirical understanding of the supposed sites of action of each drug as well as their potential side effects, and utilize available measures as a means of monitoring both drug dosage and their potential side effects, as well as drug dosage and drug effectiveness. Because we are interested in behavioral alterations, it is all too easy to forget that the medication itself works on a biochemical substrate and that the substrate alteration may be sufficiently distressing to warrant changing either the drug used or its dosage.

A developmentally alert clinician also attends to biological sectors because slow psychological development may be secondary to slow physical maturation. When looking for target symptoms to influence by drug use, the clinician must consider the organism's developmental underpinnings. For example, it has been shown that early adolescent development of secondary sexual characteristics influences social competence (McCandless, 1960). However, direct measurement of hormonal changes may not be significantly related to socialization.

Another important developmental factor to be considered is that although we may be altering an undesirable developmental trait by medicating, there may be secondary or long term effects of the drug that are less desirable. For example, fluorides are useful to strengthen the enamel of teeth, but they also may lead to mottling, which is unsightly later in life. Chlorpromazine is certainly useful as an antipsychotic neuroleptic but also has a tendency to lower the seizure threshhold; it is often sedating at therapeutic dosage levels but may interfere with learning, and now we know that it may give rise to tardive dyskinesia in some children.

The third factor to be considered concerns the natural thrust of maturation itself, which is relatively independent of external environmental influences. We must always ask whether it is medication that is providing the change or do we have developmental and maturation on our side to do the job? Is it the specificity of the particular agent or the general attention-focusing effect it provides? For example, a child who first begins to speak while a drug is being administered cah provide us with the "therapeutic fallacy" that "the drug did it." Our conclusion must be tempered with developmental skepticism and the consistent use of careful measurement of results. Moreover, when a developmental landmark is achieved during pharmacologic treatment, it not only could be argued that the medication did it, or set it in motion, but that the child has attained a critical hierarchic integration and can now go ahead on his own steam without further need for a boost. These are the factors that lead us to question whether or not medications ought to be discontinued intermittently; whether or not their long term effects are or are not desirable; and whether interruption will negate the new ground gained. Our models must include "developmental boosters" designed to prod development along, "developmental sustainers" designed to modulate development on a continuous basis, and placebos that function as "environmental suggestives" to permit auxiliary support to children in human milieus.

Even a biological view of development depends on behavioral evidence of effectiveness. As physicians, we know it is not enough to treat the diabetic's urine but the patient with diabetes. We may look at children as having a number of characteristics from infancy on that require monitoring. Many investigators have chosen their own favorites (Fries & Woolf, 1953; Fish, 1967; Thomas et al., 1963). I would choose four as having particularly biological significance: Anergy-energy, modulated-unmodulated, attention-inattention, and predictive patterning versus randomness. From the developmental point of view, each of these features may be a factor in temperamental and characterological disposition. One expects that as development proceeds there will be an increasing balance among all these sectors: The child ought to be energetic enough, sufficiently modulated and attending in his behavior, and with predictable rhythmicity. We expect that there may be periods of crankiness and difficulty and show decreases in attention (at times), but the general trend should be toward more predictability in balance and toleration of frustration as well as capacity for pleasure. The description of Thomas et al. (1968) of the difficult child or slow to warm up child permits the view that the pathology that is more likely to be seen is added to by poor interaction with parents, rather than being wholly temperamental in origin.

When using medication one must have in mind some developmental norms, but also be prepared to allow for individual stylistic variation. For eample, the attention span of an infant of six months is clearly shorter than the attention span of a two-year-old who may be operating within the context of the omnipotence of the practicing period (Mahler et al., 1975). Yet such a child's attention disposition may be insufficiently unresponsive to society's demands as compared to the attention span available to a four-year-old who is expected to attend and even cooperate in a nursery program. Clinicians would have to take into account the richness of variation in children's behavior that may be based on maturational factors, but also on other influences, when they consider whether or not a medication should or ought to be used. One would not want incorrectly to convert exuberance to hyperactivity, because exuberance is desirable whereas hyperactivity is definitionally fraught with undesirable connotations.

Behavioral Measures

Now we must again confront the difficulty alluded to before of assaying which method or model of development we should use as a yardstick to measure drug effect on behavior. There are many global severity rating scales available; there are also symptom checklists and there is the developmental lines vantage point. One also can break development into hypothetical stages such as libidinal organization or ego integrations. Any or all of these methods have and may be used to verify change, but we ought to recognize that changes that take place at one stage of development might not be considered desirable or may even be undesirable at another, and also that any checklist or global scale omits features present in others. For example, many checklists have an item for "separating easily from the parent." This is desirable at four if nursery school is the order of the day, but one would like to see protest and separation anxiety in a 12-month-old as an index of attachment behavior, which we consider a significant precursor of future object relations. An example of this problem is the tendency to over extend paradigms designed for one stage to use at another, as the Ainsworth et al. (1978) "strange situation" has been extended despite warnings to the contrary.

Similarly, although in our current state of culture we send our children to school at three or four, enlightened teachers do not expect our children to be able to play reciprocally at age three. Moreover, the measure of a developmental landmark must be seen in the context of the demands of the teacher coordinated with the requirements of the home. "Sesame Street" and similar environmentally enriched cognitive nutriments may invite, even excite the child to read at three but, as Piaget and others point out, it is not necessary that reading begin at three so long as age-appropriate developmental landmarks for cognitive development are achieved when "their time comes." Moreover, early reading does not guarantee enjoyment from reading. Indeed, Piaget has quipped that the American question is "can we do it earlier," whereas he was more interested in the invariance of and processes underlying the sequences of development that enable reading and other skills. While we are able to pick up reading disabilities earlier and earlier, there are as yet no decent studies suggesting accuracy in predicting which child will or will not have a frank reading disability even in those with minimal perceptual lags. From a developmental standpoint, the issue is one of distinguishing a lag in maturation from a fixed or developmental "lesion." Recent work has clearly shown that appropriate tutoring in appropriately diagnosed learning disabled children is not enhanced by medication (Gittelman et al., 1983).

Nonnormative Developmental Lines Approach

Generally, child psychiatrists utilize a broader definition of developmental disorders than the simple normative index of the presence of symptoms or cognitive deficits. Some functions are clearly in the biological maturational scheme of things, but these also interact with other psychic and social structures. A developmental position within psychiatry views symptom formation as way stations in solving conflicts not only with the external world, but also within. Transient identifications or transient compromises may result in new ego adaptations. Enuresis provides an interesting example of a common symptom that may have a number of roots and may be examined developmentally. Some families insist that the child be placed on the potty as soon as he can sit and use "gastrocolic reflexology" as their ally in toilet training, figuring that bladder training follows bowel training. Other families, on the advice of enlightened physicians, insist that the "myelinization route" be followed, and that one should not put pressure on a child until 18 months of age when the sphincter is supposedly innervated. Other families who feel children should never be coerced do not really toilet train their children and trust that somehow the socialization process will include toilet training by shame or social constraint. With this variability of possible environmental impositions or lack of impositions, the central notion of the move from body tyranny to body control as a developmental line has gained in attractiveness to developmentally alert clinicians. "When is the child able to participate in the control of his bowels and bladder for his own purposes?" becomes the central query for such a frame of reference. On the other hand the force of numbers should not hold sway. It is estimated that seven-eighths of the world's children are reflexly toilet trained, yet that does not recommend it to all cultures.

In still another vein, at what stage and in what kind of community should we expect the child to have less separation anxiety rather than more, and in what communities would it be wiser if the child stuck close to an adult's side because of actual environmental dangers. To what degree should a child be expected to yield his egocentric wishes and move toward more cooperative approaches? However, maturation also may make a child more capable of moving away from his own primary demands toward social demands. If we accept Piaget's frame of reference, it is a distinct step in development when the child can decentrate and cognitively take the other individual's vantage point. Does this achievement itself influence the capacity to move out of the egocentric position or is it a prerequisite to achieving the social step of cooperation?

This brief excursion into the developmentalists' conceptual framework now permits a better basis for understanding drug use in children.

If parents and/or schools ask for drugs as an adjunct in helping the overassertive, egocentric, unsocialized child, they may in fact be asking for a drug to increase the speed of development of a cognitive process that may be slower in this specific child on a maturational basis. It may be that the use of the drug for nonpharmacological effects in quieting the complaining community or school may influence the child indirectly by a trickle-down effect resulting in a less threatened and anxious child. Clearly, the facts are that ego developmental lines or ego functions themselves will be only secondarily influenced by medication, insofar as medications somehow affect the substrate, the background music, the noise factor, and/or the resultant anxiety that underlies the symptoms that may accrue. On the other hand, a relieved community puts less pressure on a child.

The developmental line of movement from body to toy to work enables us to observe a gradual reorganization of a child's thinking as well as the encroachment of reality factors on pleasure factors. These can be directly inferred clinically from the vantage point of "capacity to attend to play," which might be considered an ego function, and also from inferences concerning how much and what kind of libidinal or aggressive organizations are expressed in the fantasies themselves. This could lead us to a method of understanding the drive factors from the standpoint of how a drug modulates wishes and what the balance is in a regression–progression continuum. Moreover, such observation can be used to infer how the child distortedly or realistically interprets the medication itself and how it fits into his fantasies.

First, we may inquire on a cognitive level whether the child is using predominantly mediational or associational thinking, and whether the level is appropriate for the stage of development. Second, we may assay the "relative abundance" of aggressive themes. Third, is there too much fusion or defusion of drives. Moreover, we can observe how much expression of the drive is tolerated as opposed to dampened and inhibited, and how this expression emerges relative to expectations at each developmental stage. As clinicians, we have certain normative standards of how well a child ought to be able to control or express his fantasies. All in all, we are looking for the happy balance at each stage and age that represents an appropriate equilibrium between drive factos and their organization in goal-oriented wishes in an adaptive relationship with the requirements of the child's community.

For some children the pressures of wishes may be insistent, persistent, and oppressive to their own sense of well-being. For other children the inhibitions may be strong, because of excessive social demands. Either of these states (too much or too little) may lead the clinician to prescribe medication. Usually, in neurotic compromises there is a tendency to dampen excessively and create substitutive symptoms that in themselves reveal a pressure similar to the drives, as in obsessional questioning or tics. However, when drives in the form of bizarre fantasies encroach on reality, a child may act in an uninhibited manner that tends to disrupt his relationships to peers and adults alike. Clinicians should be neither activity "makers" nor "dampeners," but seek to establish better homeostatic mechanisms from within that ultimately can be trusted. The developmental notion that modulation from without has to be replaced by controls from within is another form of this developmental proposition. We assume that as ego apparatuses develop, gratification of the drives become possible in and along socially acceptable channels and that each stage of development is seen to have its appropriate pleasures and controls.

Descriptive Diagnoses and Development

Yet another area of developmental concern has recently arisen involves the issue of childhood manifestations of adult disorders. There is much controversy regarding whether we see the same picture in childhood as we do in adults. One view suggests that each developmental stage will provide a different manifestation of a disorder, and one has to consider the stage–phase related capacities for social response as more central to phenomenology than the issue of whether a descriptive syndrome can be identified as such. Two examples present themselves from the most recent literature. The offspring of manic depressive families have been studied by a number of investigators (Kron et al., 1982; Kestenbaum, 1982)—this is so largely because there is a pharmacologic treatment for mania and also many first admission manics were called schizophrenics during recent years (Carlson et al., 1978). Studies of the progeny of bipolar parents suggest abnormality and unusual behavior, but nothing that corresponds to what mania looks like in adulthood.

Similar questions have been raised with respect to the early manifestations of frank depressive disorders. Many (Carlson & Cantwell, 1979, 1980, 1982; Cytryn & Bunney, 1980; Puig-Antich, 1982) have suggested and shown that we do have both pubertal and prepubertal depression. Assessment instruments (Poznanski et al., 1979; Puig-Antich, 1982) can certainly pick them up. The criteria of each assessment instrument differ some, but even using careful assessment instruments does not uncover a high prevalence of frank depressive disorders in the prepubertal years. Indeed, even those conduct disorders that respond to antidepressants (Puig-Antich, 1982) must satisfy research criteria for depression (RDC) to be considered for drug trials. Thus, the landscape is somewhat muddied by the developmental process because each stage of development will provide its own repertoire of behaviors that can be affected by whatever disorder intervenes.

The general trends described make it difficult to study forms of adult disorder in cildhood if we continue to require the simple-minded notion that children have to have the same characteristics as the adults. Instead developmental propositions provide us with a new research line that suggests that we need some method or metric of detecting diathesis, the biological, or genetic factors as they interact with social and behavioral observations during the early life cycle.

The Meaning of Taking Drugs

We are not only what we eat or how we act. Instead we also are as our fantasies dictate.

If a child's fantasies are laden with aggression and fears of penetration and/or oral impregnation, a medication taken by mouth may be fraught with unhappy meaning. According to his capacity for reality testing, he may fancy that he is being poisoned, that one is putting foreign substances into him, that he is being given a magical strengthening potion, and so on. If the mother is in charge of the drug administration, she may be looked upon as the object from whom the evil or balm is dispensed. Giving medication also may be perceived according to prior patterns of interaction in families; for example, as a continuation of an earlier pattern of oral assault—being forced to eat, or being duped into a dishonest relationship. The background of basic trust would have to be assessed before one decides that it is she rather than the child himself who is to administer it. If the level of conflict is centered about toilet training, giving drugs can deteriorate into a sadomasochistic struggle, or taking medicine can be construed as pleasing mother by being submissive. Conversely administration of drugs may become a nonparticipating pseudoalliance enveloped in denial of passivity.

Giving medication by injection or in suppository form offers even more possibility for misinterpretation. Anal sadistic assault is easily read into such routes. Phallic level interpretations may be dominant no matter what the route of administration. The notion of being intruded on, seduced, or having one's manhood taken away or feminity mocked are all possible modes of interpretation for a vulnerable child who has been made to feel less than adequate by whatever symptom he or she has that requires pharmacological treatment.

The hope that fantasy life and reality organization will become modulated by the administration of medication also depends on what life problems have to be solved by the child at what stage of his development.

SUMMARY

A drug used to treat a symptom without some understanding of the nature of the disorder in developmental terms is not only poor clinical practice, but also antithetical to the developmental propositions that guide the work of child psychiatrists. These developmental principles mesh with the old pharmacological rule of thumb that suggests one use the appropriate drug in the appropriate dose for the right child who has a given symptom that is the target for a desired effect. Developmentally, we must add the caution that the drug be used for as long a time as necessary and titrated to the current needs of our patients based on what is known to be different about them because they are children.

Not only must a child be considered at each stage of her development for her maturity in accepting the medication, but also for the maturity of her detoxification methods—her routes of absorption and excretion and end-organ responses. The therapeutic effects expected must be potentially better than the toxic or side effects and the therapeutic/toxic ratio must be satisfactory for the stage of development of the young patient. One cannot simply compare the responses of adults to the responses of children. We must take into account the "paradoxical" differences that accrue at different stages of development and that may be very discreetly demarcated by chronological (maturational) age (Fish, 1967). Extrapolation of dose by body weight simply does not apply in children, just as indices of severity are more important than diagnosis per se in some instances. Level of I. Q. will also be determining because as psychic organization becomes more complex, drug effect is less clearly dependent on biological effect. For example, diphenhydramine is well tolerated in very high doses with good effect on modulating behavior until age 10, following which it may have the same soporific effect as in adults and, more important, not effect the target behavior. Moreover, it tends to be effective in the disorders of minor severity. Developmentaly, we are required to look at toxicity not only as toxicity to the physiological biological system, but toxicity in the sense of behavioral deterioration that interferes with the desired "good functioning" of the child (Fish & Shapiro, 1964). Again, this diversion into biology amidst a discussion of psychological factors points up the need to look for developmental balance, not simple effects on one sector of behavior. Parents must be guided not only by their wish that the child lose a symptom, but by the fact that the symptom may signify developmental turmoil or temperamental variety as well as pathology.

One must also be guided by the fact that the use of medication is something that is neither desirable or undesirable in itself according to preconceived notions, but something that may help a child to be able to accept available educational and social opportunities. If a clinician can bring a parent into this kind of cooperative participation, drug therapy will be much more successful and less prone to failure due to conflict between the child and parents or parents and physician. While a physician may have authority on his side and want to provide placebo effect by lending the weight of that authority, he must always take into consideration that overselling a medication leads to disappointments for the parents as well as the children and encourages a lack of confidence for future therapeutic enterprises.

The developmentally alert clinician should maximize his therapeutic relationship before any medication is used. This requires careful and prolonged consultation as well as accurate dose regulation in a particular child. Now, because there are an increasing number of pharmacological agents being touted as effective for troubled behavior, children will be subjected to an increasing likelihood of having drugs offered to take care of their problems by psychiatrically unsophisticated practitioners. If the public mind associates giving drugs to children with the illegal and illicit "drug scene," a detrimental effect is projected onto the possibility of influencing the therapy of children who need medication and who may otherwise be subjected to prolonged suffering. Moreover, if a contaminated view of drug administration prevails within the family, the developmental effect on the growing child will be to establish attitudes against a "pill pushing" culture. On the other hand, drug administration in the context of the developmental principles outlined should make giving medicines to children more reasonable and provide a framework of limits, aims, and constraints as well as a well-tempered appropriate optimism.

REFERENCES

Ainsworth, M. D. S., Blehar, M. D., & Waters, E. (1978). *Patterns of attachment: A psychological study of the strange situation.* Hillsdale, NJ: Erlbaum.

The American Psychiatric Association. (1980). *Diagnostic and statistical manual of mental disorders.* (3rd ed.). Copyright Division of Public Affairs, APA, 1700 18th Street, N.W., Washington, D.C. 20009.

Carlson, G. A., & Cantwell, D. P. (1979). A survey of depressive symptoms in a child and adolescent psychiatric population. *Journal of the American Academy of Child Psychiatry, 18,* 587–599.

Carlson, G. A., & Cantwell, D. P. (1980). Unmasking masked depression in children and adolescents. *American Journal of Psychiatry, 137,* 445–449.

Carlson, G. A., & Cantwell, D. P. (1982). Diagnosis of childhood depression: A comparison of the Weinberg and DSM III criteria. *Journal of the American Academy of Child Psychiatry, 21*(3), 247–250.

Carlson, G. A., & Strober, M. (1978). Manic depressive illness in early adolescence. *Journal of the American Academy of Child Psychiatry, 17,* 138–153.

Cytryn, L., & Bunney, W. (1980). Diagnosis of depression in children: Reassessment. *American Journal of Psychiatry, 137,* 22–25.

Erikson, E. H. (1963). *Childhood and society* (2nd ed.) (pp. 247–274). New York: Norton.

Fish, B. (1967). Methodology in child psychopharmacology. In D.H. Efron et al. (Eds.), *Psychopharmacology, review of progress.* Public Health Publication No. 1836.

Fish, B., and Shapiro, T. (1964). A descriptive typology of children's psychiatric disorders, II. A behavioral classification in child psychiatry. *American Psychiatric Association Research, 18,* 75–86.

Freud, A. (1965). The concept of developmental lines. *Normality and pathology in childhood: Assessments of development* (pp. 56–92). New York: International University Press.

Fries, M., & Woolf, P. (1935). Some hypotheses on the role of congenital activity type in personality development. *Psychoanalytic study of the child.* New York: International University Press, *8,* 48–62.

Gittelman, R., Klein, D. F., & Feingold, I. (1983). Children with reading disorders, II. Effects of methylphenidate in combination with reading remediation. *Journal of Child Psychology and Psychiatry, 24*(2), 193–212.

Gualtieri, C. T., & Hawk, B. (1981). Tardive dyskinesia and other drug-induced movement disorders among handicapped children and youth. *Annual Progress in Child Psychiatry and Child Development* (pp. 617–632). New York: Brunner/Mazel.

Hartmann, H., Kris, E., & Lowenstein, R. M. (1947). Comments on the formation of psychic structure. *Psychoanalytic study of the child* (pp. 11–38). New York: International University Press.

Kestenbaum, C. J. (1982). Children and adolescents at risk for manic-depressive illnesses: Introduction and overview. *Adolescent Psychiatry: Development and Clinical Studies.* Vol X (pp. 245–255). Chicago: The University of Chicago Press.

Kron, L., Decina, P., Kestenbaum, C. J., et al. (1982). The offspring of bipolar manic depressives: Clinical features. *Adolescent Psychiatry: Developmental and Clinical Studies.* Vol X (pp. 273–291). Chicago: The University of Chicago Press.

McCandless, B. (1960). Rate of development: Body build and personality. *Child Development and Child Psychiatry. American Psychiatric Association Research, No. 13,* p. 42.

Mahler, M. (1952). On child psychosis and schizophrenia: Autistic and symbiotic infantile psychoses. *Psychoanalytic Study of the Child* (pp. 286–305).

Mahler, M. S., Pine, F., & Bergman, A. (Eds.) (1975). *The psychological birth of the human infant.* New York: Basic Books.

Poznanski, E. O., Cook, S. C., & Carroll, B. J. (1979). A depression rating scale for children. *Pediatrics, 64,* 442–450.

Puig-Antich, J. (1982). Major depression and conduct disorder in prepuberty. *Journal of American Academy of Child Psychiatry, 21,* 118–128

Puig-Antich, J., & Chambers, W. J. (1982). Schedule for affective disorders and schizophrenia for school age children (6–16), (K-SADS-P) (present episode version).

Rapoport, J., Buchsbaum, M., & Weingartner, H., et al. (1978). Dextroamphetamine: Behavioral and cognitive effects in normal prepubertal boys. *Science, 199,* 560–563.

Safer, D. J., & Allen, R. P. (1973). Factors influencing the suppresant effects of two stimulant drugs on the growth of hyperactive children. *Pediatrics, 51,* 660–667.

Satterfield, M. D., Cantwell, D. P., & Lesser, L. I. (1972). Physiological studies of the hyperkinetic child. *Journal of the American Journal of Psychiatry, 128,* 1418–1424.

Satterfield, H. H., Lesser, L. I., & Saul, R. E. (1973). EEG aspects in the diagnosis and treatment of minimal brain dysfunction. *Annuals of New York Academy of Science, 205,* 274–282.

Thomas, A., Chess, S., & Birch, H. G. (1968). *Temperament and behavior disorders in children.* New York: New York University Press.

Thomas, A., Chess, S., Birch, H. G., Hertzig, M. E., & Korn, S., (1963). *Behavioral individuality in early childhood.* New York: International University Press.

Methodological and Assessment Issues in Pediatric Psychopharmacology

C. KEITH CONNERS, Ph.D.

"We are not free from the techniques, the methods, from the means by which we know, we see."

—MAHASI SAYADAW

DESIGN ISSUES

Chapters on methodology tend to be like sermons that exhort one to be virtuous and to lead the good life; they provide general principles but fail to tell one how to behave in particular problematic circumstances. Are there methodological issues unique to psychopharmacology? If so, are there particular problems associated with the pediatric age group? Probably not. Little can be said of methodological issues in drug studies that is not true of problems in research in clinical psychopathology in general. But it is the translation from the general rules to the specific applications that pose difficulty. [A recent chapter by Goldberg & Hamer (1983) provides an excellent overview of these issues written by a psychopharmacologist–statistician team.]

Establishing control over experimental variables is the fundamental problem of all research investigations. One response to the typical dilemmas of the pediatric psychopharmacologist/clinical researcher, charmingly described by Loney and Halmi (1980), is to collect a lot of information about everything, stop worrying, and start regressing (in the statistical sense). Thus, one is exhorted to provide more detailed descriptions of background variables, exclusion criteria, treatments, and subject expectancies. This naturally will lead to large data sets that can be managed only by a combination of judicious use of statistical technique and "balanced consideration of alternative interpretations" (Loney & Halmi, 1980, p. 151).

At the other end of the spectrum are those authors who decry bigness and statistical designs as inimical to individuality, novelty, and originality. The particularity of the phenomenon of drug response in an individual patient is said to be disguised by the average effects obtained in large numbers. Along with Lord Rutherford they declare that if you need statistics for your experiment, you need to do a better experiment.

Some argue that drug research, having become governmentalized and institutionalized, operates on several false assumptions: that drugs are specific for and should be tested against individual nosologic entities; that a given dose or dose range is suitable for all patients; that age, duration of illness, living circumstances, object relations and the attitude of the physician are unimportant (Ostow, 1965). The proposed remedy is the careful observation of the individual case over time.

It should be clear, however, that the methods of the case study and the group design are appropriate to different questions, not alternative methods for answering the same questions. Group studies attempt to generalize beyond the individual symptom to the general processes that give rise to the symptom. The clinician, however, is seldom interested in

70

a *class* of symptoms that respond to a drug, but rather particular exemplars of that case. The clinician will want to know what dosage of a drug is optimal for *this* child, while a group study will necessarily only specify a dosage range for a *sample* that represents some theoretical population. The problem comes in believing that methods suitable for the one question are also applicable to the other.

Therefore, it is important at the outset to eschew the temptation to opt for the *one* right design, dosage, response measure, or subject selection procedure. The kind of methodologic imperialism which decrees that a particular strategy of investigation of drug effects is superior usually arises from a disease that Donald Klein has referred to as "premature hardening of the categories." Good methodology, like life, ought to be a dance that skillfully adjusts to the changing nature of the problem.

Some problems require large numbers and elaborate statistical designs; others do not. But the rules of scientific inference remain the same in both circumstances. These rules arise from the need to avoid kidding oneself about assertions that are in fact mistaken or that are true for reasons other than what one supposed. The fact that these rules of causal inference are fundamentally *statistical* is one of the important philosophical conclusions underlying modern science (Russell, 1948). But this conclusion has often naively been taken to imply that *inferential statistics* are always required in a scientific study.

One of the most useful analyses of the factors that influence causal inferences in clinical research is provided by Campbell and Stanley (1966). They make the distinction between experimental and quasi-experimental designs and call attention to the fact that in behavioral science there is a wide continuum of designs available, depending upon which sources of error one is willing to tolerate in a particular investigation. Some of these sources of error are described in Tables 3.1 and 3.2.

Almost all of the sources of possible error are unprotected in the case study, which is more appropriate for *hypothesis finding* than *hypothesis testing*. On the other hand, there are many sources of error that can be controlled in the single subject by the application of single-case experimental designs. A review of these studies as applied to psychopharmacology shows that some important discoveries as well as answers to clinical problems have been made using these designs (Conners & Wells, 1982). Tables 3.3 and 3.4 review applications of single-case designs for drug studies of depression and hyperactivity in children. They are highlighted here because of their relative neglect in the literature.

Typical problems encountered with the application of single-subject designs in psychopharmacology are carryover effects of treatments that

Table 3.1. Sources of Internal Validity as Related to Therapy Outcome Research

Source	Definition	Examples	
		General	Specific Instance
History	Events other than therapy that occur during the time period when therapy is provided; simultaneous occurrence of extratherapy events.	Informal counseling by peers; important life-style change.	A long phone call from a former roommate relieves a client's depression and gives a new meaning to his life. The phone call comes about the time that the therapist begins an important part of treatment. The depression is relieved.
Maturation	Psychological or biological changes that appear to occur naturally with the passage of time.	Children's development of the capacity for abstract thought; menopausal effects.	The normal cognitive development of a child may result in an increased ability to take another person's perspective, and therefore behave in a more sensitive and empathic manner. The child displays less aggression.
Testing	The impact of repeated exposure to the assessment measures.	Increased skill due simply to the practice provided by repeated testing; reduced anxiety due to repeated exposure to the feared stimulus; increased self-disclosure due to multiple instances of asking personal questions.	A client becomes more interpersonally skilled in social situations as a result of the researcher's role-play tests. Performing the role-play test over and over has beneficial effects. The client more comfortably interacts with members of the opposite sex.

Table 3.1. (Continued)

		Examples	
Source	Definition	General	Specific Instance
Instrumentation	Decay in the sensitivity–accuracy of the assessment instruments.	Fatigue on the part of observers; decreased sensitivity of psychophysiological equipment due to usage.	Children's attentiveness in the classroom appears to show less off-task behavior due to the observers paying less attention after having observed for several weeks. The observers are not seeing or recording the off-task behavior. The child appears to be paying more attention, but only because the off-task behavior is not being noticed.
Statistical regression	The tendency for persons whose initial scores on assessment measures are extreme (high or low) to have later scores that drifted toward the mean.	Extreme depression (bottom of the scale) is more likely to rise, since it cannot drop further; hyperactive children are more likely to show less activity.	A client who scores particularly high on a measure of anxiety before therapy is statistically more likely to score nearer the mean on a second testing than to score even higher.
Mortality	Attrition of participants–clients.	Clients who drop out from therapy and for whom posttherapy assessments are not available.	Clients in a study of the treatment of depression terminate prematurely. Their data is lost, even though they may have terminated because of a sense of already achieved relief. The client has not returned to complete the assessments.

Table 3.1. (*Continued*)

		Examples	
Source	Definition	General	Specific Instance
Selection	Utilization of partici-pants—clients who might appear to change simply be-cause of personal factors that pre-dispose them to do so rather than due to the intervention.	Clients who volun-teer for a therapy program advertised in a local newspaper may be on the verge of changing due to a high level of personal motivation.	Using adolescents in studies of peer pres-sure or persuasion. The characteristics of adolescent subjects tend to make them especially susceptible to peer pressure and persuasive maneuvers.

Source. P. C. Kendall and L. N. Butcher, (Eds.). (1982). *Handbook of research methods in clinical psychology* (pp. 438–439). New York: Wiley. Copyright © 1982 by John Wiley & Sons, Inc. Reprinted by permission.

Table 3.2. *Threats to External Validity as Related to Therapy Outcome Research*

		Examples	
Threat	Definition	General	Specific Instance
Interactions of the environ-ment and testing	Preintervention as-sessments may sensitize clients to the intervention, thus po-tentiating the intervention's influence.	When clients who are to receive a therapy for fear are asked to role play the feared situation, this action may increase their motivations to change.	An otherwise ineffec-tive treatment may appear to alleviate fear, but the fear re-duction is due to increased motivation from some aspect of the study. This in-creased motivation would not be present when the treatment is provided outside of the context of a study and would then be ineffective.

Table 3.2. *(Continued)*

Threat	Definition	Examples	
		General	Specific Instance
Interaction of selection and intervention	If all clients selected are a special subgroup who are particularly amenable to participation, these clients cannot be considered comparable to the rest of the population.	If only two of the four clinics that are asked to be involved in a therapy outcome study agree to do so, the results cannot be generalized to all clinics. The two that refused might be significantly different from the two that agreed.	A project designed to compare psychological therapy, medications, and a control condition for the treatment of hyperactivity requires parents to give their informed consent. Many parents refuse to participate, not wanting their child assigned to the control condition. This selection problem reduces the researcher's ability to generalize the results to all hyperactive children.
Reactive arrangements	Clients may change due to a reaction to the fact of participating in a novel experience, rather than due to the therapy interaction.	Clients may change due to an expectancy on their parts or on the part of their therapist. Therapy must, or should, cause change, and clients change simply because they expect they ought to.	A father's physical abuse of family members is reduced by therapy: not as a result of the therapist's actions, but a function of the father's belief that going to therapy will make him stop being abusive.

Table 3.2.   *(Continued)*

Threat	Definition	Examples	
		General	Specific Instance
Multiple intervention interference	When several kinds of intervention are combined in one experience, the total effect may be very different from the outcome of any one of them in isolation.	Clients involved in multicomponent therapies may fail to change because the plethora of intervention obscures the positive impacts of each separate component.	A child's acting-out aggressive behavior pattern elicits aggression from his father rewarding attention from his mother and his peers, and attempts at rational discussion by school authorities. A single consistent approach designed to reduce the aggression would be more effective when not interfered with by other effort

Source. P. C. Kendall and L. N. Butcher, (Eds.). (1982). *Handbook of research methods in clinical psychology* (pp. 440). New York: Wiley. Copyright © 1982 by John Wiley & Sons, Inc. Reprinted permission.

occur in reversal designs, and indeterminate interaction effects among successive treatment conditions. Problems of external validity (generalizability) are, of course, intrinsic to these designs. Multiple baseline designs—in which subjects are given a staggered start with the treatment—have seldom been used in psychopharmacology but might be particularly useful in clinical settings where placebos cannot be used or where the nature of the condition mitigates against reversal of the experimental treatment. Much research is not done because of the ethical problems of using placebos, and the single-case designs offer some advantage under these conditions.

ORGANISMIC VARIABLES

Subject Selection

DSM-III and Diagnosis.   Interview methods for clinical diagnosis continue to form the foundation of research in child psychiatry. A com-

Table 3.3.   Single-Case Design for Drug Studies of Hyperactive Children

Study	Ss	Design	Dependent Dependent Measures	Distinctive Findings	Drugs
Martin, 1971	1	A-B₁-B-C (B = drug C = token program)	*Behavioral:* 1. Appropriate and inappropriate social behavior 2. *Task performance:* 2. Pegboard, stimulus matching, block design, picture naming	Decrease in appropriate behavior on placebo. Increase in rate and variability of appropriate social behavior on drug. Increased variability in task performance on drug.	Dexedrine: 5 mg b.i.d.
Ayllon et al. 1975	3	Combined design: Multiple baseline across behaviors on ABA design (B = drug)	*Behavioral:* 1. "Hyperactivity," for example, gross motor behavior, noise. *Academic:* 2. Percentage of correct math and reading responses	Hyperactivity increased when drug withdrawn and decreased when academic responses reinforced.	S_1: Ritalin: 5 mg q.i.d. S_2: Ritalin: 5 mg b.i.d. S_3: Ritalin: 5 mg t.i.d.

Table 3.3. *(Continued)*

Study	Ss	Design	Dependent Measures	Distinctive Findings	Drugs
Stableford et al. 1976	2	S_1:B_3-B_2-B_1-A_1-A-C (B_3-B_1 = decreasing doses of drug C = behavioral program) S_2:B_5-B_4-B_3-B_2-B_1-A_1-A (B_5-B_1 = decreasing dose of drug)	*Behavioral:* 1. Out of seat 2. On task 3. Appropriate 4. Inappropriate	Behavior did not deteriorate till placebo removed in A phase. 1 primary observer not blind. No dramatic increase in negative behavior when drug decreased. Decrease when pills withdrawn.	Ritalin: 15, 10, 5 mg Dexedrine: 25, 20, 15, 10, 5 mg
Wells et al., 1981	1	A-B-A-C-CD-A_1D-CD (B = Dexedrine C = Ritalin D = self-control program)	*Behavioral:* 1. Off task 2. Gross motor 3. Deviant behavior *Physiological:* 1. Finger temperature 2. EMG	Combination better than either alone on behavioral measures. Only study to collect physiological measures. Helped in decision as to effectiveness of Ritalin over Dexedrine.	Ritalin: 15 mg, b.i.d. Dexedrine: 5 mg. b.i.d.

Study		Design	Measures	Results	Drug/Dose
Horn et al. 1982	1	A-A_1-B_1-A_1-C-B_1C-B_2C-A_1C-B_1C-B_2C (B = Dexedrine program)	*Behavioral:* 1. Off task $\longrightarrow$ 2. Gross motor $\longrightarrow$ 3. Noise and vocalization $\longrightarrow$	Dexedrine and self-control best. Equivocal effects. Equivocal effects.	Dexedrine: B_1 = titrating drug, B_2 = 10 mg
			Teacher Report: 1. Conners teacher questionnaire $\longrightarrow$	Drug and self-control best.	
			Academic Measures: 1. Match performance $\longrightarrow$ 2. Spelling performance $\longrightarrow$	Direct reinforcement only produced effects.	
			Laboratory Measures: 1. Continuous performance test $\longrightarrow$	Dexedrine alone best.	
Rose, 1978	2	A-A_1-B-A_1-B-A_1 (B = food additives, tartrazine #5)	*Behavioral:* 1. Out of seat 2. On task 3. Aggression	Increased. Decreased. Unclear.	Tartrazine #5; 0.5 mg/kg

Table 3.3. (*Continued*)

Study	Ss	Design	Dependent Measures	Distinctive Findings	Drugs
Wulbert & Dries, 1977	1	B-A_1-B-A_1 (B=drug)	*Behavioral:* 1. Rituals 2. Aggressive behavior	No drug effects on behavior in clinic. Increased aggression and increased ritualistic behavior in home.	Ritalin: 10 mg q.i.d.
Shafto & Sulzbacher, 1977	1	A-B_2-B_2^2-C-A-B_1-B_3-C-A Alternating tx design phase in an additive design (B=drug C=behavioral intervention)	*Behavioral:* 1. Activity changes⟶ 2. Nondirected or ⟶ indistinct verbals 3. Isolate play⟶ 4. Wandering⟶ 5. Attending⟶ 6. Compliance⟶	Both together better than either alone. Increased during drug. Decreased during behavioral intervention Equivocal. Decreased with behavioral intervention. Increased with drug. Increased with low dose drug.	Ritalin: B_1 = 5 mg, B_2 = 10 mg, B_3 = 15 mg

| Pelham, 1977 | 1 | BC-C (B=drug C=behavioral program) | *Teacher report:* 1. IMH Global rating scale | Continued improvement with behavior program after drug withdrawn. | Ritalin: 10 mg |
| Williamson et al. 1981 | 1 | A-B-A-B-BC-BCD-BCDEF B=drug C=instructions D=practice E=feedback F=reinforce-ment) | *Behavioral:* 1.• On task ⟶ 2. Gross motor ⟶ 3. Appropriate ⟶ *Monitor:* 1. Arm activity ⟶ 2. Foot activity ⟶ | Increased best with drug. Decreased best with Dexe-drine, feedback and reinforce. Equivocal. Decreased best with Dexe-drine, feedback, and reinforcement. Decreased best as above. | Dexedrine: increased to 20 mg |

Note. The author is indebted to Karen C. Wells, Ph.D. for the compilation of this table.

Table 3.4. Single-Case Design for Drug Studies of Depressed Children

Study	Ss	Design	Measures	Distinctive Findings	Drugs
Petti, et al. 1980	1	AB (B = drug)	*Ward observations:* 1. CBI total deviant	Decrease	Imipramine: 100 mg
			Behavioral analog measures 1. Eye contact	Increase	
			2. Smiles	Increase	
			3. Speech duration	Increase	
			4. Requests for new behavior	Increase	
Petti & Unis, 1981	1	$A\text{-}A_1\text{-}B_1\text{-}B_2\text{-}B_1\text{-}A_1\text{-}B_2$ (B = drug)	*Behavioral:* 1. Adaptive peer	Increase	Imipramine: $B_2 = 125$ mg/day, full dose; $B_1 =$ titrating up and down
			2. Bizarre vocalizations	Decrease	
			3. Unusual movements	Decrease	
			4. Activities of daily living	Increase	
			5. Adaptive mealtime behavior	Increase	
			6. Compliance	Increase	
			7. Number of seclusion orders	Decrease	
Michelson, et al., in press	1	A-B-A	*Behavioral:* 1. On task in class	Increase; no reversal	Imipramine: 150 mg
			2. Disruptive in class	Decrease: no reversal	
			3. Activities of daily living	Increase: no reversal	
			4. Enuretic episodes	Decrease: no reversal	

Note. The author is indebted to Karen C. Wells, Ph.D. for the compilation of this table.

plete discussion of the methodological issues associated with interviewing is beyond the scope of this chapter, but two excellent general sources are recent papers by Matarazzo (1978) and Garfield (1978). Following a similar trend in adult psychopharmacology, it is likely that the new diagnostic rules for childhood diagnoses will have an important effect upon psychopharmacological research.

The first important issue with the DSM-III system is how its reliability will vary as a function of a number of variables, including the training of the raters, the age of the subjects, the setting, and the range and the severity of psychopathology. Rutter and Shaffer (1980) argue that reliability is limited to major categories. Despite enthusiasm by proponents of DSM-III, reliabilities of 50 percent on major categories for modestly trained raters generally are reported (Cantwell et al., 1979a and b).

Still the standard method in the field is the traditional clinical method of assembling a wide array of historical, observation, psychometric, and unstructured interview data, and then using a case-conference approach to achieve diagnoses. Werry et al. (1983) studied 195 admissions to a child psychiatric inpatient unit. Children were diagnosed by two to four clinicians well-versed in the rules of DSM-III. Some of the categories of most interest to pediatric psychopharmacologists, such as Attention Deficit Disorder, Conduct Disorder, and Anxiety disorders have satisfactory interdiagnostician reliability (Kappa values = .76, .53, .67, respectively).

However, important subcategories are highly unreliable. For example, it is known that aggressive behavior is a highly important predictor of drug outcome in children (Loney et al., 1978), yet the category of socialized aggressive conduct disorder has a Kappa reliability of −0.04! Similarly, the much-heralded distinction of Attention Deficit Disorder Without Hyperactivity has a reliability of .05. Clearly, better methods are needed for selecting these subjects for pharmacological investigation.

Another approach to the problem limits the variance attributable to the clinical interviewing method by using a structured interview. A number of structured clinical instruments more or less tied to DSM-III have recently appeared. These instruments attempt to satisfy the requirements of epidemiological research, to more satisfactorily operationalize dimensions of affective disorder, and to provide a research basis for psychopharmacology studies within the prepubertal range. The characteristics of several such instruments now available are shown in Table 3.5.

As an instrument becomes more structured, with probes and skip patterns completely determined, differences in diagnostic reliability among interviewers become trivial. At the same time, the meaningfulness and *validity* of the results come into question. In a recent study of 20 cases seen in our child psychiatry outpatient study (Conners & Makari, un-

Table 3.5. Characteristics of Assessment Instruments: Psychiatric Interviews

	DICA Herjanic & Welner	PI Herjanic & Welner	MHAF Kesten-baum & Bird	ISC Kovacs et al. (unpub-lished)	SI Langner et al. (1976)	K-SADS Puig-Antich & Chambers	BSQ Richman & Graham (1971)	IWS Rutter & Graham (1968)
Purpose:								
Diagnostic	X	X		X		X		
Screening			X		X		X	X
Method:								
Self-report								
In-person interview								
Structured	X	X		X	X	X		
Semi-structured		X	X			X	X	
Informant:								
Child	X		X	X	X	X		X
Parent (or surrogate)		X			X	X	X	
Teacher (or school)								
Other (records, clinicians)								
Scale Properties:								
Number of items	About 200	About 100	About 180	About 37	83	About 100	12	About 100
Items: Defined (D) Global (G)	D	D G	D	D	D	D	D	D G
Time period assessed	Lifetime	Unclear	Unclear	Past 2 weeks	Current	Past month	Past 4 weeks	Unclear

Age assessed	9–17 yrs.	6–16 yrs.	7–12 yrs.	8–13 yrs.	6–18 yrs.	6–16 yrs.	Pre-schoolers	7–12 yrs.
Completion time	1½ hrs.	1 hr.	45 min.	35 min.	20 min.	1½ hrs.	10 min.	30 min.
Forms: Precoded (P) Uncoded (U)	P	U	P	P	P	P	P	P
Scoring system	X	No	X	X	X	X	X	Unknown
Content:								
Interpersonal functioning	X	X	X	X	X	X	X	X
School functioning	X	X	X	X	X	X	X	X
Mood disturbances	X	X	X	X	X	X	X	X
Psychosis	X	X	X	X		X		X
Anxiety	X	X	X		X	X	X	X
Phobias/fears	X	X	X	X		X	X	X
Obsessive/compulsive	X	X	X	X		X		X
Conduct disorder	X	X	X	X	X	X		X
Hyperactivity/attention		X	X		X		X	X
Drug/alcohol abuse	X	X		X		X		X
Delusions/hallucinations	X	X	X	X		X		X
Enuresis/encopresis	X	X		X			X	
Somatic concerns	X	X		X	X	X		X
Psychometric properties:								
Reliability	X	X	X	X	X	X	X	X
Validity	No	No	No	X	X	No	X	X

Source. H. Orvaschel, D. Sholomskas, & M.M. Weissman (1980). *The Assessment of Psychopathology and Behavioral Problems in Children: A Review of Scales Suitable for Epidemiological and Clinical Research (1967–1979).* Monograph for NIMH Series AN No. 1, DDHS Publication No. (ADM) 80-1037, Superintendent of Documents, U.S. Government Printing Office, Washington, DC pp. 76–77.

published), 17 children were diagnosed as conduct disorders, and 11 as paranoid. The interviewing schedule, administered by a medical student, precisely followed the DSM-III diagnostic rules and was scored by a computer algorithm. An example of the problems created by this method is that all a child has to do to fit criteria for paranoia is feel that he or she has ever been followed or spied on or attacked, hardly an unlikely occurrence in today's urban environment. Unless the clinician filters the response with appropriate understanding of what a true paranoid condition is, the results are misleading.

Clinicians will note that the interview methods have significant qualitative differences and, hence, are appropriate for different types of investigation. Some instruments, like Puig-Antich's Kiddie-Sads (Puig-Antich et al., in press), modeled after the adult version of the SADS, retain the flexibility of multiple probes in order to elicit information that the psychiatrist then rates on a judgmental scale. The method assumes that the rater is capable of sophisticated judgments, both with regard to the nature of psychopathology and how to conduct the interview in a skillful fashion. This is an appropriate method *in the hands of a well-trained rater.*

Slightly more structured, but with some of the same clinical flexibility, the Interview Schedule for Children (ISC) by Kovacs (Kovacs et al., unpublished) provides reasonable reliability for most categories. There is still considerable flexibility regarding probes for further information, and the emphasis is still upon an informed rating of symptomatology.

On the other hand, with untrained interviewers, the NIMH Diagnostic Interview Schedule for Children (DISC) (Costello et al., unpublished) and Herjanic's Diagnostic Interview for Children and Adolescents (DICA) (Herjanic et al., 1975) totally remove the variance due to rater training, and indeed have shown good reliability in the hands of nonprofessional or paraprofessional interviewers. However, recent results from the Pittsburgh validation study of the DISC (Costello et al., unpublished) demonstrate very low levels of test-retest and parent-child agreement on many of the major diagnostic categories. Thus, there is a tradeoff between item reliability and validity.

Despite their limitations, these interview methods begin to bring some comparability and order into methods of subject selection for psychopharmacology with children. Because these instruments are undergoing rapid changes, no final recommendations based upon reliability and validity can be made at this time. However, based upon its overall characteristics, this author recommends the NIMH DISC (Conners, Herjanic, & Puig-Antich, unpublished) or its predecessor, the DICA, for clinicians.

In the hands of a skilled interviewer using the instrument flexibly, the fixed format has distinct utility. It provides comprehensive coverage of symptomatology and standard rules of classification. Whether increased diagnostic specificity will reveal more specific drug/diagnosis interactions remains to be demonstrated. A computer program has been written for the Apple II that simplifies the task of obtaining multiple diagnoses from the DISC (Conners & Blouin, unpublished).

Dimensional Methods. Following the publication of the NIMH Psychopharmacology Bulletin Special Issue on Children (1973), the use of rating scales for subject selection, sample description, and drug response has become commonplace. Characteristics of the more frequently used scales are presented in Table 3.6.

The American Psychological Association recently commissioned Achenbach, Conners, and Quay to develop a clinical instrument that combines the knowledge gained from many studies into a single scale. Eleven clinical syndromes identified from previous factor analyses are incorporated into the instrument, which is currently being validated. These instruments have a role as subject selection measures, as well as in the measurement of important dependent variables. Because of their wider use in clinical drug studies, currently use of the Conners Teacher and Parent symptom questionnaires is recommended where dimensional methods are needed for screening and drug effect measurement (NIMH, 1973).

One of the most important subject selection problems in drug studies is whether there are in fact separate syndromes of hyperactivity and conduct disorder. Most previous studies that identify subjects by rating scales confound important dimensions of activity, aggression and achievement (Routh, 1983). One reason for this is the high degree of correlation among the factor dimensions of Conduct Disorder and Hyperactivity. This overlap leads some (Quay, 1979; Lahey et al., 1980; O'Leary & Johnson, 1979; Shaffer and Greenhill, 1979) to question the existence of separate syndromes. In many factor analytic studies of childhood behavior ratings, symptoms of hyperactivity and conduct disorder load heavily on the same factor, with conduct disorder symptoms usually obtaining the highest loadings.

Both the high correlation between factors derived by orthogonal extraction techniques and the multiple loadings of items have recently been shown to be artifacts of the factor scoring methods (Blouin & Conners, 1983). Separate syndromes in fact do emerge when large enough samples are explored for their existence (Trites & Laprade, 1983).

Table 3.6. Characteristics of Assessment Instruments: General Psychopathology Scales

	CBCL Aohenbach	CBC-P Arnold & Smeltzer	CBCS* Borgatta & Fanshel	CBDI* Burdock & Hardesty	CPS Cohen et al.	PQ Conners	TQ Conners	TBRS Cowen
Purpose:								
Diagnostic								
Screening	X	X	X	X	X	X	X	X
Method:								
Self-report	X	X	X	X	X	X	X	X
In-person interview								
Structured								
Semi-structured								
Informant:								
Child								
Parent (or surrogate)	X	X	X		X	X		
Teacher (or school)			X	X			X	X
Other (records, clinicians)			X	X				
Scale properties:								
Number of items	130	74	115	137	48	94	41	25
Items: Defined (D) Global (G)	D	D	D	D	D	D	D	D
Time period assessed	Past 12 months	Not stated	Past 3 months	Not stated	Past 2 months	Past month	Past week	Not stated
Age assessed	4–16 yrs.	2–18 yrs.	Birth–17 yrs.	1–12 yrs.	Preschool	3–17 yrs.	6–15 yrs.	6–12 yrs.

Completion time	17 min.	Not stated	Not stated	Not stated	Not stated	15 min.	10 min.	10 min.
Forms: Precoded (P) Uncoded (U)	\P	U	Unknown	Unknown	P	P	P	U
Scoring system	X	X	X	X	X	X	X	X
Content:								
Interpersonal functioning	X		X	X	X	X	X	X
School functioning	X	X	X				X	X
Mood disturbances	X	X		X			X	X
Psychosis	X							
Anxiety	X		X			X		X
Phobias/fears	X	X			X	X		X
Obsessive/compulsive	X	X				X		
Conduct disorder	X	X	X		X	X	X	
Hyperactivity/attention	X	X		X		X	X	X
Drug/alcohol abuse	X							
Delusions/hallucinations	X							
Enuresis/encopresis	X	X				X		
Somatic concerns	X	X				X		
Psychometric properties:								
Reliability	X	No	X	X	X	X	X	X
Validity	X	No	No	X	No	X	X	X

*Detailed information on content is lacking, since scale was not obtained in time for report.

89

Table 3.6. (Continued)

	CAP Cytrynbaum & Snow	ALAC Gleser et al.	MCDI* Ireton & Thwing	SCL* Kohn & Rosman	LBCL Miller	SBCL Miller	BPC Quay & Peterson	QBC Reinherz & Kelfer
Purpose:								
Diagnostic								
Screening	X	X	X	X	X	X	X	X
Method:								
Self-report	X	X	X	X	X	X	X	X
In-person interview								
Structured								
Semi-structured	X							
Informant:								
Child	X	X						
Parent (or surrogate)	X	X	X		X		X	X
Teacher (or school)	X			X		X	X	X
Other (records, clinicians)	X						X	
Scale Properties:								
Number of items	About 287	40	320	58	164	96	55	38
Items: Defined (D) Global (G)	D G	D	D	D	D	D	D	D
Time period assessed	Unclear and variable	Recent weeks	Not stated	Not stated	Not stated	Past 2 months	Not stated	Past 2 months
Age assessed	Not stated	11–19 yrs.	6 months –6½	3–6 yrs.	3–18 yrs.	3–13 yrs.	5–17 yrs.	4–5 yrs.

Completion time	not stated	Not stated	45 min.	Not stated	30 min.	20 min.	Not stated	25 min.
Forms: Precoded (P) Uncoded (U)	U	P	P	Unknown	P	P	P	P
Scoring system	Unknown	X	X	X	X	X	X	X
Content:								
Interpersonal functioning	X	X	X	X	X	X	X	X
School functioning	X	X			X	X		
Mood disturbances	X	X			X	X	X	X
Psychosis								
Anxiety	X	X			X	X	X	X
Phobias/fears	X	X			X			X
Obsessive/compulsive	X							X
Conduct disorder	X	X			X		X	
Hyperactivity/attention					X	X	X	X
Drug/alcohol abuse		X			X			
Delusions/hallucinations					X			
Enuresis/encopresis		X			X		X	X
Somatic concerns		X			X	X	X	X
Psychometric properties:								
Reliability	No	X	X	X	X	X	X	X
Validity	No	X	No	X	X	No	X	No

*Detailed information on content is lacking, since scale was not obtained in time for report.

92

Table 3.6. (Continued)

	BCL Richman & Graham	CBQ-T Rutter	DESB Spivak & Swift	DCB Spivak & Swift	DAB Spivak & Swift
Purpose:					
Diagnostic					
Screening	X	X	X	X	X
Method:					
Self-report					
In-person interview	X	X	X	X	X
Structured					
Semistructured					
Informant:					
Child					
Parent (or surrogate)	X			X	
Teacher (or school)		X	X	X	
Other (records, clinicians)				X	X
Scale Properties:					
Number of Items	19	26	47	97	84
Items: Defined (D) Global (G)	D	D	D	D	D
Time period assessed	Past 4 weeks	Past year	Past month	Past 2 weeks	Past 2 weeks
Age assessed	Preschool	6–13 yrs.	5–12 yrs.	5–12 yrs.	13–18 yrs.

	Not stated P	Not stated P	Not stated P	15 min. P	15 min. P
Completion time Forms: Precoded (P) Uncoded (U)					
Scoring system	X	X	X	X	X
Content:					
Interpersonal functioning	X			X	X
School functioning			X		
Mood disturbances	X	X		X	X
Psychosis					X
Anxiety	X				
Phobias/fears	X	X			
Obsessive/compulsive				X	X
Conduct disorder	X	X	X	X	X
Hyperactivity/attention	X	X		X	X
Drug/alcohol abuse					
Delusions/hallucinations				X	X
Enuresis/encopresis	X				
Somatic concerns		X			
Psychometric properties:					
Reliability	X	X	X	X	X
Validity	X	X	No	X	X

Source. H. Orvaschel, D. Sholomskas, & M. M. Weissman (1980). *The assessment of psychopathology and behavioral problems in children: A review of scales suitable for epidemiological and clinical research (1967–1979).* Monograph for NIMH Series AN No. 1, DDHS Publication No. (ADM) 80-1037, Superintendent of Documents, U.S. Government Printing Office, Washington, DC, pp. 78–79.

*Detailed information on content is lacking, since scale was not obtained in time for report.

Nevertheless, the fact that in clinical samples aggressive and hyperactive symptoms co-occur more often than not argues for the importance of careful sampling and/or the statistical separation of these two sources of variance in drug outcome studies.

An important issue in the diagnosis of ADD/Hyperactivity is whether the problem is pervasive (cross-situational) or limited to a specific setting, such as home or school. One scholarly opinion argues that confirmation of the disorder across more than one setting is required (Barkley, 1981). On the other hand, the fact that similar pharmacological responses are found in both normal and hyperactive children suggests that the distinction may not matter as far as stimulant drug effect is concerned (Rapoport et al., 1978). Recent work indeed demonstrates that "borderline hyperactive" and cross-situationally defined hyperactive children do not differ in attentional performance or cortical evoked potential response to stimulant treatment (Klorman et al., 1983). Thus, an organismic variable that ought to make a difference appears not to as far as drug treatment is concerned. (Such differences might, however, be highly relevant in studies that evaluate *combinations of treatment,* such as behavioral and pharmacological treatments.)

The Independent Variable

Compliance.   In most psychopharmacological studies the independent variable of interest is the level of the drug. Ultimately brain levels rather than blood levels or dosage are of interest, but one usually settles for the latter two in human studies. Prescribing the drug is usually assumed as a sufficient condition to ensure that the appropriate variable is being manipulated. Recent studies of drug noncompliance make it increasingly clear that this is not the case.

It is estimated that approximately one-half of all patients in chronic drug treatment do not adhere to their prescribed regimens (Epstein & Cluss, 1982). In an earlier well-known survey, Solomons (1973) reports that only about 43 percent of children receiving stimulants were being properly monitored.

In an important recent study, 12 male hyperactive children, 6–12 years of age, were randomly assigned to placebo, dextroamphetamine, or methylphenidate (MPH) for six weeks in a triple-blind crossover design (Kauffman et al., 1981). Weekly urine samples were obtained and assayed for MPH and dextroamphetamine. Individual compliance varied from 0 to 100 percent, with a mean of 67 percent, with the percent of patients compliant for a given week varying from 55 to 80 percent (mean of 67 percent). More interestingly, significant *positive noncompliance* was found in that MPH was found in the urine of 5 of the 12 subjects during what was supposedly their placebo period.

As the authors correctly note:

> *failure of the patient to take medication as dictated by the investigational protocol has gone totally unrecognized as a potential contributor to the confusion and contradiction among studies. . . . The relatively high rate of noncompliance observed in this study raises serious questions regarding the reliability of behavioral and learning data obtained from even relatively well-controlled studies. (p. 236)*

Firestone (1982) investigated several variables that might relate to patient noncompliance with medication requirements. He followed 76 families over a 10-month period. Children were randomly assigned to either MPH treatment or a behavior modification program. By the end of the 10 months 44 percent of the children were no longer taking medication. "Nonadherents" tended to be slightly younger and less intelligent, but no significant pretreatment factors were found that were characteristic of these children. It did appear that families of female rather than male children were more likely to discontinue medication. No differences in family psychopathology were found, but nonadherent parents were significantly younger and showed a trend to being less intelligent on a standardized measure. These predictors are similar to those previously found in studies of adherence to behavioral programs.

Another important finding was that 26 percent of the parents originally assigned medication refused this treatment. This could be an extremely important biasing factor for subject selection in drug studies. Noncompliance in many studies may represent resistance to subtle coercion to be in a drug study in the first place. There seems to be little doubt that compliance with a drug regimen may be one of the most significant variables in the outcome of pediatric drug trials, particularly among outpatients.

Drug Plasma Levels

STIMULANTS. Kinetic studies of psychostimulants in childhood indicate that, as in adults, MPH is rapidly metabolized to ritalinic acid and that the half-life is relatively short. Volumes of distribution appear to be relatively large, suggesting extensive distribution of the drug to body tissues (Coffey et al., 1983).

Recent studies provide important though contradictory information regarding the role of drug plasma levels of MPH and clinical response in hyperactive children. If drug plasma levels could be shown to be important in clinical response, it would have important implications for both research and clinical issues with this drug. Gualtieri et al. (1982) carried out two investigations using a modification of the single-ion monitoring gas chromotography–mass spectrometric procedure. Twelve children were treated with .3 mg/kg and 16 children with .3 mg/kg and .6 mg/kg in double-blind placebo crossover studies. Two important findings emerge. First, there is considerable inter *and* intraindividual variability in serum levels at one-hour postingestion. Second, there are no differences between responders and nonresponders in peak serum levels.

Published almost simultaneously, work from the Yale group (Shaywitz et al., 1982) finds similar pharmacokinetic half-life results, but different peak concentration and clinical results. They report peak plasma concentration occurring at about 2.5 hours in contrast to Gualtieri et al.'s peak at about 1 hour. In addition, they find a significant relationship between peak plasma MPH levels (at 2 hours) and the same measure of clinical response that failed to correlate in the Gualtieri et al. study (Fig. 3.1).

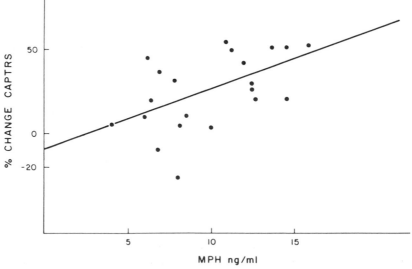

Fig. 3.1. Percentage change in Conners abbreviated (ten-item) parent–teacher rating (CAPTRS) in relationship to peak single samples of plasma methylphenidate (MPH) obtained at two hours after administration. Relationship is statistically significant ($r = .771$, $p < .001$). (*Source:* S. E. Shaywitz, R. D. Hunt, et al. Psychopharmacology of attention deficit disorder: Pharmokinetic, neuroendocrine, and behavioral measures following acute and chronic treatment with methylphenidate. *Pediatrics, 69*, 693, 1982.)

The authors also note that all three of the drug nonresponders have the lowest plasma concentration levels.

In another study with five children, Kupietz et al. (1982), report that one child had peak levels at one hour, one at two hours, and three at three hours. Using a sensitive paired-associate verbal learning method, they find a significant correlation between plasma peak concentration values and learning.

Whether the puzzling contradictory results of these new studies relate to different assay methods or other factors is unclear. One thing is certain, however; the short time-action curve and the high intrasubject variability of plasma concentration peaks obviously have implications for research methodology in the further study of the behavioral effects of MPH. At the moment, it appears that dosage level is as good a predictor of effect as plasma levels.

The variability in diagnosis and individual plasma response to stimulants leads to the interesting proposal to use single dose probes with provocative agents such as MPH and clonidine as a method of exploring the responsivity of dopaminergic and noradrenergic mechanisms in ADD (Hunt et al., 1982). These authors suggest that subsequent sequential measures of plasma levels of neurotransmitters, their metabolites, and hormones may help define the responsivity of neurochemical systems.

ANTIDEPRESSANTS. Imipramine and other antidepressants probably act through several different mechanisms in their effects upon a wide variety of childhood disorders (Gualtieri, 1977). Recent work suggests that plasma levels of tricyclic antidepressants (TCA) may be important predictors of clinical response in treatment of childhood depression. Preskorn et al. (1982) find an almost identical therapeutic window for hospitalized depressed children treated with imipramine as has been reported for adults. These results support an earlier preliminary report by Puig-Antich et al. (1979). However, to date no convincing studies of a drug-placebo difference for TCAs in childhood depressive disorder have appeared. Part of the problem is the high spontaneous improvement rate in hospitalized children. There are convincing well-controlled *single-case* design studies, which strongly support, but do not confirm, the value of this treatment modality (Petti & Unis, 1981; Petti et al., 1980). The effect of TCA on cognition in depressed children may be highly significant (Staton et al., 1981).

Plasma concentration of TCAs and their metabolites are important in the therapeutic response in the treatment of enuresis (Jorgensen et al., 1980; Rapoport et al., 1980; Dugas et al., 1980). Considerably lower concentrations are required for therapeutic effect than in the treatment of depression. But not all nonresponse is due to inadequate plasma levels (Rapoport et al., 1980).

NEUROLEPTICS.   Children require larger doses of chlorpromazine (CPZ) than adults to achieve comparable plasma concentrations. On the other hand, the apparent therapeutic plasma concentration in children, estimated at about 40–80 ng/ml, is lower than that reported for adults (50–300 ng/ml). Plasma concentrations appear to decline in many children despite maintaining the same dosage level, perhaps because of autoinduction of CPZ metabolism. Doses of less than 6 mg/kg/day frequently fail to produce the desired plasma CPZ levels in children (Rivera-Calimlim et al., 1979). It is well-established that toxic reactions to neuroleptics in children are closely related to plasma concentrations (Tsujimoto et al., 1982).

Important developments in the assessment of neuroleptic-related dyskinesias have come from the NIMH Psychopharmacology Branch, including the Modular Algorithm for Tardive Dyskinesia Diagnosis (MALTD) developed by Schooler and Kane (1982), and the Abnormal Involuntary Movement Scale of AIMS (Fann et al., 1980).

Dosage.   Since Sprague and Sleator's (1977) claim that the optimal dose of MPH for cognitive function is .3 mg/kg while the optimal level for social behavior and activity is 1 mg/kg, it has become something of a *de facto* standard of dosing in treatment studies. However, this important work was never replicated by the authors, using the same measures, and considerable contrary evidence now exists. Charles et al. (1981) studied 42 hyperactive children with doses ranging from .2 mg/kg of MPH to .8 mg/kg over an 18-week period. Measures of sustained attention and behavioral ratings both showed a linear improvement with increased dosage.

On the other hand, Klorman et al. (1983) report that .3 mg/kg is the optimal dosage for affecting both the P300 component of the visual evoked response and the continuous performance measures obtained concurrently with the brain measures.

An interesting theoretical analysis of this problem is provided by Ackerman et al. (1983), who find that response to dosage level interacts with whether the subject is a "strong" or "weak" type, based upon the Pavlovian classification of nervous system strength.

In a recent critical review, Pelham (1983) carefully re-examines the relationship between dosage and a number of other methodological factors as they relate to academic achievement in stimulant drug studies with hyperactive children. One may recall that Barkley and Cunningham (1978) had more or less appeared to conclusively demonstrate that stimulants had little or no effect on measures of academic achievement. This also is an oft-repeated shibboleth of clinical practice. The article, however, leaves many puzzled clinicians wondering whether the dramatic school improvements of children being treated by them are flukes or unusually profound placebo effects.

Pelham's review (1983) concludes with a tongue-in-cheek set of recommendations on how *not* to find a drug treatment effect on academic measures:

> (a) Select a group of HA (hyperactive) children, some of whom are also LD and/or have academic deficits and need an academic intervention and some of whom do not; (b) administer a psychostimulant drug to all of these children at a dose that is 2 to 5 times higher than the level known to maximize improvement in cognition in most children. If doses are individually titrated, make certain that they are titrated on measures of global improvement rather than measures of cognition, thereby insuring that the majority of children in the study will be overmedicated with respect to cognitive performance; (c) entrust drug administration to the children's parents, thus guaranteeing that more than half of the children will not follow the prescribed regimen; (d) administer the medication in such a way that there is very little overlap between the medication's time of peak effectiveness and the child's performance of daily academic tasks; (e) do not systematically arrange for concurrent interventions and instructional conditions that will maximize potential drug effects; (f) utilize dependent measures that are not sensitive to treatment effects; (g) finally, ignore individual differences in drug and dose response, academic deficits, and all other relevent dimensions, and average results across all of these variables, thus obscuring any positive results that would otherwise have been evident. (p. 32–33)

Much of the work with stimulants in childhood needs to be reevaluated with these considerations in mind.

SETTING VARIABLES

Virtually no attention has been paid to the interaction of the drug effects and the social or stimulus environment of the child treated with drugs. Indeed, awareness of these variables arrived late upon the adult scene as well until an important stimulus was given by the findings with adult schizophrenics that significant drug treatment variance is accounted for by aspects of the social environment in aftercare (Hogarty et al., 1974).

In an extended multiple-treatment single-case design, Wells et al. (1981) showed an interaction between drug treatment, behavioral treatment (self-control), and stimulus setting. The drug treatment (MPH) and the behavioral treatment have different effects upon behavior, depending whether classroom or ward settings are examined.

An important point regarding comparative efficacy studies of antidepressants and stimulants is made by Garfinkel et al. (1983). They find that although MPH is generally superior in the treatment of ADD, TCAs have more effect on mood and provide more improvement across settings because of the longer half-life of these drugs compared with MPH. Comparative studies clearly need to consider the impact of different dose-time-action profiles of drugs as they relate to when and where a particular target symptom will be observed.

DEPENDENT VARIABLES

Barkley (1981) provides a characteristically thorough account of the existing rating, observational, and psychometric measures that are useful in drug research with hyperactive children. Abikoff et al. (1980) report a highly reliable and valid direct observational measure of hyperactivity that has proven to be drug sensitive. Campbell et al. (1981) have thoroughly reviewed the methodological issues in the pharmacotherapy of autistic and severely disturbed children. They provide important automated operant discrimination learning and direct observational techniques that begin to clearly identify the nature of neuroleptic drug response in these children (Cohen et al., 1978; Cohen et al., 1980). The series of recent studies from this group, including work on haloperidol, lithium, and behavioral treatments, provides a number of important new methods for the study of this most difficult population. Among these are the TBRS (Time Behavioral Rating Sheet; Cohen et al., 1980). This instrument is a useful measure of both adaptive and maladaptive behaviors of severely impaired young children. Their methods are an excellent model for investigators seeking to do drug studies with severely impaired or psychotic children.

The increasing availability of the microcomputer insures that many methods formerly dependent upon highly specialized laboratory facilities will become more common in children's drug studies. For example,

Klee and Garfinkel (unpublished) report the successful use of a computerized continuous performance test in drug studies. We have also computerized much of the ECDEU (NIMH Early Clinical Drug Evaluation Unit) battery, including rating scales, a structured interview, and a battery of cognitive tests. These instruments are adapted for the Apple II computer and currently are being field tested in two multicenter collaborative studies.

STATISTICAL ISSUES

Placebo Contingency

An interesting phenomenon in stimulant drug research is the finding that the best predictor of drug response across many different measures is the pretreatment level of the particular measure being studied (Conners, 1972). Commonly used rating scales, such as our Hyperkinesis Index, frequently produce substantial regression effects between pre and posttreatment testing (Milich et al., 1980). However, pretreatment symptom levels provide prediction over and above what would be expected from regression to the mean, since they appear even when placebo response is controlled.

Hicks et al. (1983) report that an individual child's response to MPH can be predicted by his level of performance in the drug-free condition. The so-called *placebo contingent* effects are found across a wide range of measures in short-term studies (Gualtieri et al., 1982) and appear to hold in chronic treatment conditions as well (Gualtieri et al., in press). Figure 3.2 shows the powerful nature of this phenomenon for several of the most frequently employed measures. By analyzing a number of published studies, these authors are able to conclude that the placebo contingency effects accounts for 25–99 percent of the MPH variance on various measures.

Data Analysis

Two recent statistical contributions to psychopharmacologic problems deserve mention. One of the most common issues in the analysis of drug-placebo effects is how to handle the change scores that characterize the pre to postdrug and pre to postplacebo change effects. Simple algebraic difference scores have been criticized since they produce scores that are correlated with both pre and postscores, and in which the re-

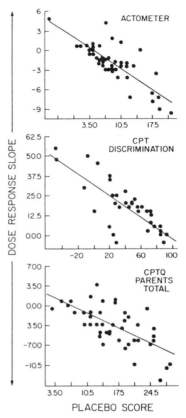

Fig. 3.2. Dose response slope versus placebo score. (*Source:* **R. E. Hicks, C. T. Gualtieri, et al. Methylphenidate and homeostasis: Drug effects are inversely related to placebo levels of response. In press.**)

gression weight of these correlations is assumed, often incorrectly, to be unity. Analysis of covariance, on the other hand, while appropriately adjusting for the regression of pre and postscores, makes many assumptions that are frequently violated in typical drug studies (e.g., differential dropout in drug and placebo groups due to side effects can lead to inequality of regression slopes in the two treatment conditions, a fundamental violation of required assumptions).

Klein et al. (1975) provide a demonstration of the utility of the Kappa coefficient as an alternative method of analysis. One advantage of this method is that it provides an estimate of the proportion of drug-treated patients who actually benefit from drug treatment—a statistic somewhat more meaningful in many cases than the size of mean difference between drug and placebo.

Another method has particular applicability to the complex problem of detecting patterns of effect of a drug in clinical laboratory measures. Typically, drug studies will examine the impact of a drug upon renal, hepatic, hematological, endocrine, or other variables one at a time, counting the number of patients showing an abnormality, or the number of abnormalities in drug vs. placebo conditions. This method is obviously meaningless with respect to the issue of the *pattern* of effect that a drug might have. The problem is more akin to detecting the difference between individuals by their fingerprint than by a list of independent characteristics. Moreover, much of the information is lost since each laboratory value is counted only in terms of its normal to abnormal classification rather than its actual level.

Ryback et al. (1982) recently demonstrated that a relatively new technique, quadratic discriminant analysis, is a useful method for discriminating among medical conditions that are symptomatically very similar. The technique "is a nonlinear form of discriminant analysis which does not assume that the variability present in the discriminating variables (e.g., clinical laboratory tests) is the same for each medical condition but rather takes into account the finding that heterogeneity is very common in medical data" (p. 2342). This technique has been successfully used to demonstrate subtle clinical laboratory differences between alcoholics and nonalcoholics. However, it appears to be ideally suited as a method of examining the impact of a drug compared with a placebo on the overall pattern of side effects in a drug study.

Quitkin et al. (in press, a, b), have shown how traditional pre–post change measures may obscure the effect of pharmacological agents that are slow-acting and effect only a subgroup of responders. They provide simple methods of pattern analysis that clarify the effects in samples containing true responders to an antidepressant. Such methods have typically been ignored in childhood studies where slow-acting drugs are predominant.

ETHICAL ISSUES

The United States Department of Health and Human Services (DHHS) recently proposed new guidelines regarding the protection of children involved as subjects in research. In these new guidelines children must give *assent*, while parents must give *permission*. The age and capability of the child to give assent is determined by the institutional review board (IRB) on an individual basis. If there is direct benefit to the child only through the research or if the child is not capable of assent, the IRB may decide that assent is not required.

One advantage of these regulations is that they require investigators to assure that children are more psychologically involved and agreeable to participation when they are in drug studies, possibly one of the important variables relating to whether the child adheres to the treatment protocol. Obvious problems occur when the cognitive limitations of the child render assent meaningless, but IRBs must now make a more discriminating evaluation of how pediatric drug protocols relate to the wellbeing and trust of the children serving as study subjects.

REFERENCES

Abikoff, H., Gittelman, R., & Klein, D. F. (1980). Classroom observation code for hyperactive children: A replication of validity. *Journal of Consulting and Clinical Psychology, 48*, 555–565.

Achenbach, T. The child behavior profile: An empirically based system for assessing children's behavioral problems and competencies. *International Journal of Mental Health* (in press).

Ackerman, P. T., Dykman, R. A., Holcomb, P. J., & McCray, D. S. (1983). Effects of high and low dosages of methylphenidate in children with strong and sensitive nervous systems. *Pavlov Journal of Biological Science, 18*, 36–38.

Arnold, L. E., & Smeltzer, D. I. (1974). Behavior checklist factor analysis for children and adolescents. *Archives of General Psychiatry, 30*, 799–804.

Ayllon, T., Layman D., & Kandel, H. J. (1975). A behavioral-educational alternative to drug control of hyperactive children. *Journal of Applied Behavior Analysis, 8*, 137–146.

Barkley, R. A. (1981). *Hyperactive children : A handbook for diagnosis and treatment.* New York: Guilford Press.

Barkley, R. A., & Cunningham, C. E. (1978). Do stimulant drugs improve the academic performance of hyperactive children? *Clinical Pediatrics, 17*, 85–92.

Blouin, A., Conners, C. K., & Seidel, W. T. (in press). The independence of hyperactivity from conduct disorder: Methodological considerations. *Journal of Abnormal Child Psychology.*

Borgatta, E. F., & Fanshel, D. (1970). The child behavior characteristics (CBC) form: Revised age specific forms. *Multivariate Behavioral Research, 5*, 49–82.

Burdock, E., & Hardesty, A. (1964). A children's behavior diagnostic inventory. *Annals of the New York Academy of Sciences, 105*, 890–896.

Campbell, D. T., & Stanley, J. C. (1966). *Experimental and Quasi-Experimental Design for Research.* Chicago: Rand McNally.

Campbell, M., Cohen, I. L., & Anderson, L. T. (1981). Pharmacotherapy for autistic children: A summary of research. *Canadian Journal of Psychiatry, 26*, 265–273.

Cantwell, D. P., Russell, A. T., Mattison, R., & Will, L. (1979a). A comparison of DSM II and DSM III in the diagnosis of childhood psychiatric disorders. I. Agreement with expected diagnosis. *Archives of General Psychiatry, 36,* 1208–1213.

Cantwell, D. P., Russell, A. T., Mattison, R., & Will, L. (1979b). A comparison of DSM II and DSM III in the diagnosis of childhood psychiatric disorders. IV. Difficulties in use, global comparisons and conclusions. *Archives of General Psychiatry, 36,* 1227–1228.

Charles, L., Schain, R., & Zelniker, T. (1981). Optimal dosages of methylphenidate for improving the learning and behavior of hyperactive children. *Journal of Developmental and Behavioral Pediatrics, 2,* 27–81.

Children's Assessment Package: A Psychosocial Evaluation Procedure for Child and Family Mental Health Services (CAP). New Haven, Connecticut: Yale University School of Medicine and Hill Health Center. Copyright January, 1977.

Coffey, B., Shader, R. I., & Greenblatt, D. J. (1983). Pharmacokinetics of benzodiazepines and psychostimulants in children. *Journal of Clinical Psychopharmacology, 4,* 217–225.

Cohen, D. J., & Dibble, E. (1977). Father's and mother's perceptions of children's personality. *Archives of General Psychiatry, 34,* 480–487.

Cohen, I. L., Anderson, L. T., & Campbell, M. (1978). Measurement of drug effects in autistic children. *Psychopharmacology Bulletin, 14,* 68–70.

Cohen, I. L., Campbell, M., Posner, D., Small, A. M., Triebel, D., & Anderson, L.T. (1980). Behavioral effects of haloperidol in young autistic children. *Journal of the American Academy of Child Psychiatry, 19,* 665–677.

Conners, C. K. (1970). Symptom patterns in hyperkinetic, neurotic, and normal children. *Child Development, 41,* 667–682.

Conners, C. K. (1972). Stimulant drugs and cortical evoked responses in learning and behavior disorders in children. In W. L. Smith (Ed.), *Drugs, development and cerebral function.* Springfield, Illinois: Charles C. Thomas.

Conners, C. K., & Makari, G. (1983). Problems in clinical diagnosis with the DISC. Unpublished manuscript. Children's Hospital National Medical Center, 111 Michigan Avenue, NW, Washington, DC 20010.

Conners, C. K., & Wells, K. C. (1982). Single-case designs in psychopharmacology. In A. E. Kazdin and A. H. Tuma (Eds.), *New directions for methodology of social and behavioral sciences: Single-case research designs, Number 13.* San Francisco: Jossey-Bass.

Cowen, E., Darwin, D., & Orgel, A. (1971). Interrelations among screening measures for early detection of school dysfunction. *Psychology in the Schools, 8,* 135–139.

Dugas, M., Zariflan, E., Leheuzey, M. F., Rovei, V., Durand, G., & Moselli, P. L. (1980). Preliminary observations of the significance of monitoring tricyclic antidepressant plasma levels in the pediatric patient. *Therapeutic Drug Monitoring, 2,* 307–314.

Epstein, L. H., & Cluss, P. A. (1982). A behavioral medicine perspective on adherence to long-term medical regimens. *Journal of Consulting and Clinical Psychology, 50,* 950–971.

Fann, W. E., Smith, R. C., Davis, J. M., & Domino, E. F. (Eds.) (1980). *Tardive dyskinesia: Research and treatment.* New York: Spectrum Publications.

Firestone, P. (1982). Factors associated with children's adherence to stimulant medication. *American Journal of Orthopsychiatry, 52,* 447–457.

Garfield, S. L. (1978). Research problems in clinical diagnosis. *Journal of Consulting and Clinical Psychology, 46,* 596–607.

Garfinkel, B. D., Wender, P. H., Sloman, L., & O'Neill, I. (1983). Tricyclic antidepressants and methylphenidate treatment of attention deficit disorder in children. *Journal of the American Academy of Child Psychiatry, 22,* 343–348.

Gleser, G., Seligman, R., Winget, C., & Rauh, J. L. (1977). Adolescents view their mental health. *Journal of Youth and Adolescence, 6,* 249–263.

Goldberg, S. C., & Hamer, R. M. (1983). Problems in statistics and experimental design in clinical psychopathology. In C. E. Walker (Ed.), *The handbook of clinical psychology: Theory research and practice.* Homewood, Illinois: Dow Jones-Irwin.

Gualtieri, C. T. (1977). Imipramine and children: A review and some speculation about the mechanism of drug action. *Diseases of the Nervous System, 38,* 368–375.

Gualtieri, C. T., Hicks R. E., Mayo, J. P., & Schroeder, S. R. (1982). The clinical effects of methylphenidate are placebo-contingent. Annual Meeting, American Academy of Child Psychiatry, Washington, DC, October, 1982.

Gualtieri, C. T., Hicks, R. E., Mayo, J. P., Schroeder, S. R., & Lipton, M. A. (in press). The persistence of stimulant effects in chronically treated children: Further evidence of an inverse relationship between drug effects and placebo levels of response, *Psychopharmacology.*

Gualtieri, C. T., Wargin, W., Kanoy, R., Patrick, K., Shen, C. D., Youngblood, W., Mueller, R.A., & Reese, G. (1982). Clinical studies of methylphenidate serum levels in children and adults. *Journal of The American Academy of Child Psychiatry, 21,* 19–26.

Herjanic, B., Herjanic, M., Brown, F., & Wheatt, T. (1975). Are children reliable reporters? *Journal of Abnormal Child Psychology, 3,* 41–48.

Hicks, R. E., Gualtieri, C. T., Mayo, J. P., Schroeder, S. R., & Lipton, M. A. (1983). Methylphenidate and homeostasis: Drug effects are inversely related to placebo levels of response. Unpublished manuscript, University of North Carolina School of Medicine, Chapel Hill, NC 27574.

Hogarty, G. E., Goldberg, S. C., Schooler, N. R., & Ulich, R. F. (1974). Drug and sociotherapy in the aftercare of schizophrenic patients. II. Two year relapse rates. *Archives of General Psychiatry, 31,* 603–608.

Horn, W. F., Chatoor, I., & Conners, C. K. (1983). Additive effects of dexedrine and self-control training: A multiple assessment. *Behavior Modification, 7*(3), 383–402.

Hunt, R. D., Cohen, D. J., Shaywitz, S. E., & Shaywitz, B. A. (1982). Strategies for study of the neurochemistry of attention deficit disorder in children. *Schizophrenia Bulletin, 8,* 236–252.

Ireton, H., & Thwing, E. (1972). The Minnesota child development inventory in the psychiatric development evaluation of the preschool age child. *Child Psychiatry and Human Development, 3,* 102–114.

Jorgensen, O. S., Lober, M., Christiansen, J., & Gram, L. F. (1980). Plasma concentration and clinical effect in imipramine treatment of childhood enuresis. *Clinical Pharmacokenitics, 5,* 386–393.

Kauffman, R. E., Smith-Wright, D., Reese, C. A., Simpson, R., & Jones, F. (1981). Medication compliance in hyperactive children. *Pediatric Pharmacology, 1,* 231–237.

Kendall, P. C., & Norton-Ford, J. D. (1982). Therapy outcome research methods. In P. C. Kendall and J. N. Butcher (Eds.), *Handbook of research methods in clinical psychology.* New York: Wiley.

Kestenbaum, C. J., & Bird, H. R. (1978). A reliability study of the mental assessment form for school age children. *Journal of the American Academy of Child Psychiatry, 17,* 338–347.

Klee, S. H., & Garfinkely, B. D. The computerized continuous performance task: A new measure of inattention. Unpublished manuscript. E. P. Bradley Hospital, 1011 Veterans Memorial Parkway, East Providence, RI 02915.

Klein, D. F., Ross, D. C., & Feldman, S. (1975). Analysis and display of psychopharmacological data. *Journal of Psychiatric Research, 12*, 125–147.

Klorman, R., Salzman, L. F., Bauer, L. O., Coons, H. W., Borgstedt, A.S., & Halpern, W. I. (1983). Effects of two doses of methylphenidate on cross-situational and borderline hyperactive children's evoked potentials. *Electroencephalography and Clinical Neurophysiology, 56*, 169–185.

Kohn, M., & Rosman, B. (1973). A two factor model for emotional disturbance in the young child: Validity and screening efficacy. *Journal of Child Psychology and Psychiatry, 14*, 31–56.

Kovacs, M., Betof, N. G., Celebre, J. E., Mansheim, P. A., Petty, L. K., & Raynak, J. T. Childhood depression: Myth or clinical syndrome? Unpublished manuscript.

Kupietz, S., Winsberg, B. G., & Sverd, J. (1982). Learning ability and methylphenidate (Ritalin) plasma concentration in hyperkinetic children: A preliminary investigation. *Journal of the American Academy of Child Psychiatry, 21*, 27–30.

Lahey, B., Green, K. D., & Forehand, R. (1980). On the independence of hyperactivity, conduct problems and deficits in children: A multiple regression analysis. *Journal of Consulting and Clinical Psychology, 48*, 566–574.

Langner, T. S., Gersten, J. C., McCarthy, E. D., Eisenberg, J. G., Greene, E. L., Herson, J. H., & Jameson, J. D. (1976). A screening inventory for assessing psychiatric impairment in children 6 to 18. *Journal of Consulting Clinical Psychology, 44*, 286–296.

Loney, J., & Halmi, K. A. (1980). Clinical treatment research: Its design, execution, analysis and interpretation or how I stopped worrying and learned to love regressing. *Biological Psychiatry, 15*, 147–156.

Loney, J., Prinz, R. J., Mishalow, J., & Joad, J. (1978). Hyperkinetic/aggressive boys in treatment: Predictors of clinical response to methylphenidate. *American Journal of Psychiatry, 135*, 1487–1491.

Martin, M. (1971). Single-subject designs for assessment of psychotropic drug effects in children. *Child Psychiatry and Human Development, 2*, 102–115.

Matarazzo, J. D. (1978). The interview: Its reliability and validity in psychiatric diagnosis. In B. B. Wolman (Ed.), *Clinical diagnosis of mental disorders.* New York: Plenum Press.

Michelson, L., DeLorenzo, T., & Petti, T. (in press). Behavioral assessment of imipramine effects in a depressed child. *Journal of Behavioral Assessment.*

Milich, R., Roberts, M. A., & Loney, J. (1980). Differentiating practice effects and statistical regression on the Conners Hyperkinesis Index. *Journal of Abnormal Child Psychology, 8*, 549–552.

Miller, L. (1972). Social behavior checklist: An inventory of deviant behavior for elementary school children. *Journal of Consulting Clinical Psychology, 22*, 134–144.

O'Leary, K. D., & Johnson, S. B. (1979). Psychological assessment. In H.C. Quay and J. S. Werry (Eds.), *Psychopathological disorders of children* (2nd ed.). New York: Wiley.

Orvaschel, H., Sholomskas, D., & Weissman, M.M. (1980). The assessment of psychopathology and behavioral problems in children: A review of scales suitable for epidemiological and clinical research (1967–1979). Monograph for NIMH Series No. 1, DDHS Publication No. (ADM) 80-1037, Superintendent of Documents, U.S. Government Printing Office, Washington, DC.

Ostow, M. (1965). Method and madness: A critique of current methodology in psychiatric drug research. *Journal of New Drugs, 5,* 3–8.

Pelham, W. E. (1977). Withdrawal of a stimulant drug and concurrent behavioral intervention in the treatment of a hyperactive child *Behavior Therapy, 8,* 473–479.

Pelham, W. (1983). The effects of psychostimulants on academic achievement in hyperactive and learning-disabled children. *Thalmus, 3,* 1–48.

Petti, T., Bornstein, M., Delamater, A., & Conners, C.K. (1980). Evaluation and multimodality treatment of a depressed prepubertal girl. *Journal of the American Academy of Child Psychiatry, 19,* 690–702.

Petti, T. A., & Unis, A. (1981). Imipramine treatment of borderline children: Case reports with a controlled study. *American Journal of Psychiatry, 138,* 515–518.

Preskorn, S. H., Weller, E. B., & Weller R. A. (1982). Depression in children: relationship between plasma imipramine levels and response. *Journal of Clinical Psychiatry, 43,* 450–453.

Psychopharmacology Bulletin, Special Issue on Children (1973). National Institute of Mental Health.

Puig-Antich, J., Perel, J. M., & Lupatkin, W. (1979). Plasma levels of imipramine (IMI) and desmethylimipramine (DMI) and clinical response in prepubertal major depressive disorder. *Journal of the American Academy of Child Psychiatry, 18,* 616–627.

Quay, H. C. (1977). Measuring dimensions of deviant behavior: The behavior problem checklist. *Journal of Abnormal Child Psychology, 5,* 277–287.

Quay, H. C. (1979). Classification. In H. C. Quay and J. S. Werry (Eds.), *Psychopathological disorders of children* (2nd ed.). New York: Wiley.

Quitkin, F. M., Rabkin, J. G., Ross, D., & McGrath, P. J. (in press). Duration of antidepressant drug treatment: What is an adequate trial?

Quitkin, F. M., Rabkin, J. G., Ross, D., & Stewart, J. W. (in press). Identification of true drug response to antidepressants: use of pattern analysis.

Rapoport, J. L., Buchsbaum, M. S., Zahn, T. P., Weingartner, H., Ludlow, C., and Mikkelson, E. J. (1978). Dextroamphetamine: Cognitive and behavioral effects in normal prepubertal boys. *Science, 100,* 560–563.

Rapoport, J. L., Mikkelsen, E. J., Zavadil, A., Nee, L., Gruenau, C., Mendelson, W., & Gillin, J. C. (1980). Childhood enuresis. II. Psychopathology, tricyclic concentration in plasma, and antienuretic effect. *Archives of General Psychiatry, 37,* 1146–1152.

Reinherz, H., & Kelfer, D. Identifying preschool children at risk. National Institute of Mental Health Progress Report, September 23, 1976 to June 30, 1977, NIMH Grant #R01 MH27458-02.

Richman, M., & Graham, P. (1971). A behavioral screening questionnaire for use with three year old children. Preliminary findings. *Journal of Child Psychology and Psychiatry, 12,* 5–33.

Rivera-Calimlim, L., Griesbach, P. H., & Perlmutter, R. (1979). Plasma chlorpromazine concentrations in children with behavioral disorders and mental illness. *Clinical Pharmacology and Therapeutics, 26,* 114–121.

Rose, T. L. (1978). The functional relationship between artificial food colors and hyperactivity. *Journal of Applied Behavior Analysis, 11*(4), 439–446.

Routh, D. K. (1983). Attention deficit disorder: Its relationships with activity, aggression and achievement. In *Advances in developmental and behavioral pediatrics* (Volume 4, pp. 125–163). New York: JAI Press, Inc.

Russell, B. (1948). *Human knowledge: Its scope and limits.* London: George Allen and Unwin, Ltd.

Rutter, M. (1965). Classification and categorization in child psychiatry. *Journal of Child Psychology and Psychiatry, 6,* 71–83.

Rutter, M., & Graham, P. (1968). The reliability and validity of the psychiatric assessment of the child. I. Interview with the child. *British Journal of Psychiatry, 114,* 563–579.

Rutter, M., & Shaffer, D. (1980). DSM III: A step forward or back in terms of the classification of child psychiatric disorders. *Journal of the American Academy of Child Psychiatry, 3,* 371–394.

Ryback, R. S., Eckardt, M. J., Rawlings, R. R., & Rosenthal, L. S. (1982). Quadratic discriminant analysis as an aid to intepretive reporting of clinical laboratory tests. *Journal of American Medical Association, 248,* 2342–2345.

Schooler, N. R., & Kane, J. M. (1982). Research diagnoses of tardive dyskinesia (Letter to the editor). *Archives of General Psychiatry, 39,* 486–487.

Shaffer, D., & Greenhill, L. A. (1979). A critical note on the predictive validity of the hyperkinetic syndrome. *Journal of Child Psychology and Psychiatry, 20,* 61–72.

Shafto, F., & Sulzbacher, S. (1977). Comparing treatment tactics with a hyperactive preschool child: Stimulant medication and programmed teacher intervention. *Journal of Applied Behavior Analysis, 10,* 13–20.

Shaywitz, S. E., Hunt, R. D., Jatlow, P., Cohen, D. J., Young, J. G., Pierce, R.N., Anderson, G. M., & Shaywitz, B. A.(1982). Psychopharmacology of attention deficit disorder: Pharmacokinetic, neuroendocrine, and behavioral measures following acute and chronic treatment with methylphenidate. *Pediatrics, 69,* 688–694.

Solomons, G. (1973). Drug therapy: Initiation and follow-up. *Annals of the New York Academy of Sciences, 205,* 335–344.

Spivack, G., Haimes, P. E., & Spotts, J. (1967). Devereux adolescent behavior scale manual. Devereux Foundation, Devon, Pennsylvania

Spivack, G., & Spotts, J. (1966). Devereux child behavior rating scale manual. Devereux Foundation, Devon, Pennsylvania

Spivack, G., & Swift, M. S. (1967). Devereux elementary school behavior rating scale maual. Devereux Foundation, Devon, Pennsylvania.

Sprague, R. L., & Sleator, E. K. (1977). Methylphenidate in hyperkinetic children: Differences in dose effects on learning and social behavior. *Science, 198,* 1274–1276.

Stableford, W., Butz, R., Hasazi, J., Leitenberg, H., & Peyser, J. (1976). Sequential withdrawal of stimulant drugs and use of behavior therapy with two hyperactive boys. *American Journal of Orthopsychiatry, 46,* 302–312.

Staton, R. D., Wilson, H., & Brumback, R. A. (1981). Cognitive improvement associated with tricyclic antidepressant treatment of childhood major depressive illness. *Perceptual and Motor Skills, 53,* 219–234.

Trites, R. L., & Laprade, K. (1983). Evidence for an independent syndrome of hyperactivity. *Journal of Child Psychiatry and Psychology and Related Disciplines, 24,* 573–586.

Tsujimoto, A., Tsujimoto, G., Ishizaki, T., Nakasawa, S., & Ichihashi, Y. (1982). Toxic haloperidol reactions with observation of serum haloperidol concentration in two children. *Developmental Pharmacological Therapy, 4,* 12–17.

Wells, K. C., Conners, C.K., Imber, L., & Delamater, A. (1981). Use of single-subject methodology in clinical decision making with a hyperactive child on the psychiatric inpatient unit. *Behavioral Assessment, 3*, 359–369.

Werry, J. S., Methven, R. J., Fitzpatrick, J., & Dixon, H. (1983). The interrater reliability of DSM III in children. *Journal of Abnormal Child Psychology, 11*, 341–354.

Williamson, D. A., Calpin, J. P., DiLorenzo, T. M., Garris, R. P., & Petti, T.A. (1981). Treating hyperactivity with dexedrine and activity feedback. *Behavior Modification, 5*, 399–416.

Wulbert, M., & Dries, R. (1977). The relative efficacy of methylphenidate (Ritalin) and behavior modification technique in the treatment of a hyperactive child. *Journal of Applied Behavior Analysis, 10*(1), 21–31.

The Clinical Disorders

Schizophrenic Disorders and Pervasive Developmental Disorders/Infantile Autism

MAGDA CAMPBELL, M.D.

DEFINITION AND INDICATIONS

Schizophrenic disorders and pervasive developmental disorders are the most severe clinical conditions in child psychiatry. The prognosis of these disorders is at best guarded. Various treatment interventions for these conditions have been developed over the years; several are currently in use. Experience has shown that pharmacotherapy can be a valuable addition or an essential modality in the total treatment of these children. Pharmacotherapy is the only treatment modality that has been assessed for efficacy in a critical and systematic way, but this is so only for infantile autism. There is little research-based knowledge about the effectiveness of psychoactive drugs for schizophrenia in childhood. The advent of neuroleptics changed the practice of adult psychiatry; their efficacy and superiority over psychosocial treatments alone in schizophrenics has been confirmed (GAP, 1975; Klein et al., 1980). In addition to symptom reduction, these drugs also affect the course of the adult illness (WHO, 1967). This does not seem to be true for schizophrenic disorder of childhood onset; there is also a paucity of data concerning schizophrenia with onset in adolescence.

The goals of treatment in child psychiatry are to decrease maladaptive behaviors and promote development. In addition, in infantile autism (often associated with mental retardation), nonexistent or rudimentary language, self-care, adaptive and social skills have to be developed. Clearly, no single treatment can accomplish these goals. Comprehensive treatment programs are necessary for these children. Combined pharmacotherapy and behavior therapy might prove more effective than either treatment alone (Sprague, 1972). Behavior therapy and pharmacotherapy are quantifiable and readily subjected to statistical analyses; therefore, their efficacy can be measured. Behavioral symptoms may be reduced in a relatively short period of time with the administration of an effective psychoactive drug. When this is achieved, the child may become more amenable to other interventions, such as behavior therapy or special education. Behavior therapy, a rather costly treatment intervention, can reduce maladaptive behavior and teach complex behaviors such as language (Lovaas & Newsom, 1976).

Neuroleptics are most effective in diminishing psychomotor excitement. This is a direct and usually predictable effect on a target behavior. More indirect effects develop slowly, probably as a result of the modified interaction of the individual with the environment (Irwin, 1968). The enduring effects of drug therapy on behavior are due to concurrent environmental and psychosocial treatments. The hyperactive child with short attention span, when calmed down by a drug, may be able to focus

114

attention on a task and thus acquire some reading and writing skills. The agitated, assaultive, or self-mutilating patient, whose symptoms are eliminated or reduced with an effective psychoactive medication, may develop more adaptive social interactions that, in turn, will improve learning. Drugs themselves do not create learning or intelligence, nor do they necessarily alter parental attitudes, but they can make the patient more amenable to environmental treatments or manipulations. It is important to institute drug treatment early rather than after other and frequently inappropriate therapies have failed. Children with symptoms of hyperactivity, aggressiveness, and/or agitation may respond well to neuroleptics, while those who are anergic and hypoactive often get worse and/or excessively sedated at doses that yield little or no improvement. The aliphatic phenothiazines (chlorpromazine) are usually not beneficial for these children (Campbell et al., 1972b and c; Fish, 1960, 1970). The more "stimulating" piperazine phenothiazine (trifluoperazine) proves to be somewhat better in this respect (Fish et al., 1966), with haloperidol as particularly effective (Anderson et al., 1984; Campbell et al., 1978, 1982; Cohen et al., 1980). Fish et al., (1966) observed that less impaired (not profoundly retarded) psychotic children may show clinical improvement on placebo and/or milieu therapy, while the more severely disturbed and impaired (lower IQ) children respond to the high-potency neuroleptics such as trifluoperazine (Fish et al., 1966) and haloperidol (Anderson et al., 1984; Campbell et al., 1978, 1982; Cohen et al., 1980).

In the formative years of the individual, drugs alone never suffice. The choice of other treatments (environmental manipulations, behavior therapy, special education, individual psychotherapy, group therapy, parental counseling, as well as hospitalization) depends on contributing factors, associated handicaps of the individual patient, and the family. Many patients, after cessation of symptoms such as hyperkinesis, stereotypies, aggressiveness, agitation, hallucinations, no longer need drug therapy, but require continuation of other treatment(s) and extended follow-up.

Pharmacotherapy is one, often very important, modality in the comprehensive treatment program in these severely disturbed children. Short term and long term efficacy and safety of psychoactive drugs in schizophrenic and autistic children will be discussed, with emphasis on more recent findings.

DIAGNOSTIC CONSIDERATIONS AND VARIATIONS

The most recent *Diagnostic and Statistical Manual* (DSM-III) of the American Psychiatric Association (1980) represents a marked improvement over its predecessors concerning these groups of psychopathologies in children. In regard to chizophrenic disorder, a child has to meet the criteria listed for adults: loosening of associations or incoherence, hallucinations, delusions, continuous signs of the disease for at least six months and deterioration in functioning as shown in Table 4.1. Labels such as childhood schizophrenia (Bender, 1942), schizophrenic reaction, childhood type (APA, 1952) and schizophrenia, childhood type (APA, 1968) have been deleted from DSM-III. It has been shown that prepubertal children can meet the adult criteria for schizophrenic disorder (Green et al., 1984, in press; Kydd & Werry, 1982), including deterioration from a previous level of functioning (Green et al., 1984). According to DSM-III, schizophrenic disorder with onset in childhood is a discrete entity and can be different from the pervasive developmental disorders, based on comparative studies of carefully diagnosed children (Kolvin, 1971; Green et al., 1984), though not all agree with this classification (Fish, 1975). On the other hand, children previously diagnosed as schizophrenic syndrome of childhood using the Nine Points (Creak, 1964) would now be labeled infantile autism by DSM-III, rather than schizophrenia.

Table 4.1. Diagnostic Criteria for Schizophrenic Disorders

A. *At least one of the following:*
   1. Bizarre delusions.
   2. Somatic, grandiose, or other delusions without persecutory or jealous content.
   3. Delusions with persecutory or jealous content is accompanied by hallucinations.
   4. Auditory hallucinations in which either one voice keeps talking about the patient's thoughts or behavior, or more voices converse.
   5. Auditory hallucinations heard several times consisting of more than one or two words, with no apparent relation to depressed or elated mood.
   6. Incoherent speech, pronounced loosening of associations, and illogical thinking, or poverty of content of speech if associated with at least one of the following:
      (a) Blunted, flat, or inappropriate affect.
      (b) Hallucinations or delusions.
      (c) Catatonic or other grossly disorganized behavior.
B. *Deterioration of functioning such as work, self-care, and social relations.*
C. *Duration:* Continuous manifestation of illness for at least six months at some time, with some manifestations currently.

Source. Adapted from American Psychiatric Association, 1980, *Diagnostic and Statistical Manual of Mental Disorders,* (3rd ed.) by Campbell and Green (1985).

Under pervasive developmental disorders, DSM-III lists the following conditions: infantile autism, childhood onset pervasive developmental disorder, and atypical pervasive developmental disorder. Each of these may be present as a full syndrome or in the residual state. Autism was first described and delineated by Kanner (1943). Its chief symptoms are failure to develop relatedness (autism), absence of or severe delays and distortions in language development, insistence on sameness, peculiar interests in or attachments to objects, and stereotypies (Table 4.2). While schizophrenia rarely if ever starts before the age of five years and is very infrequent before puberty, onset of autism takes place during the first 30 months of life. Other discriminators between the two conditions include: increased incidence of schizophrenia in families of schizophrenic children, an increase in pre- and perinatal complications, seizure disorder, and mental retardation with erratic functioning in infantile autism and outcome (Kolvin, 1971; Green et al., 1984). The labels of childhood onset and atypical pervasive developmental disorders have yet to be validated. For the use of DSM-III, a book by Rapoport and Ismond (1983) is recommended.

It is difficult to evaluate some of the literature, because the diagnostic criteria were not spelled out, and the distinction between infantile autism and prepubertal schizophrenic disorder was not always made. DSM (1952) and DSM-II (1968) did not include the diagnosis of infantile autism. Thus, in many research reports, autistic children were diagnosed "schizophrenic," and the qualifier "with autistic features" was usually added. This was so until the advent of DSM-III, which included infantile autism and differentiated the two conditions.

Table 4.2. *Pervasive Developmental Disorders of Childhood*

299.00   *Infantile Autism, Full Syndrome Present*
Currently meets the criteria for Infantile Autism.
Diagnostic criteria for Infantile Autism
  A.   Onset before 30 months of age.
  B.   Pervasive lack of responsiveness to other people (autism).
  C.   Gross deficits in language development.
  D.   If speech is present, peculiar speech patterns such as immediate and delayed echolalia, metaphorical language, pronominal reversal.
  E.   Bizarre responses to various aspects of the environment, e.g., resistance to change, peculiar interest in or attachments to animate or inanimate objects.
  F.   Absence of delusions, hallucinations, loosening of associations, and incoherence as in Schizophrenia.

Source.   Diagnostic and Statistical Manual of Mental Disorders, pp. 89–90.

REVIEW OF THE LITERATURE

Schizophrenic Disorder

Table 4.3 gives some of the study characteristics of the representative literature in schizophrenic children and adolescents. As shown, there are only a few studies addressing these age groups; some of the samples are diagnostically heterogeneous along with other methodological deficiencies. The study by Pool et al. (1976) is an exception. The patient sample of hospitalized acute schizophrenics or chronic schizophrenics with acute exacerbation is adequate and the methodology is sound. There was a minimum 5-day washout period prior to the study. The patients were receiving loxapine (mean dose 87.5 mg/day), haloperidol (mean dose 9.8 mg/day) or placebo over a period of four weeks. There were only a few statistically significant differences between the two drugs, but both were superior to placebo. Hallucinations, delusions, thought disorder, and social withdrawal were among the symptoms which decreased in response to these drugs. The patients were carefully monitored; except for excessive sedation and parkinsonian side effects both drugs were shown to be safe during this short-term drug administration.

Realmuto et al. (1984) compared the therapeutic effects of a high-potency neuroleptic, thiothixene, to a low-potency neuroleptic, thioridazine, in 21 chronic schizophrenic adolescents. The subjects, whose ages ranged from 11 years 9 months to 18 years 9 months, were randomly assigned to one or the other treatment; one of the two raters was blind to the treatment. As in the above study, ratings were done on the Brief Psychiatric Rating Scale (BRPS) and on the Clinical Global Impressions scale (CGI). Optimal daily doses of thiothixene ranged from 4.8 to 42.6 mg (mean, 16.2) and those of thioridazine from 91 to 228 mg (mean, 178); on both drugs there were statistically significant decreases in rating scores. Though there were no statistically significant differences in the efficacy between the two drugs, more of these chronic patients were sedated by thioridazine than by thiothixene. Only about half of the sample showed improvement.

Le Vann (1969) also found haloperidol to be beneficial in 40 schizophrenics, ages 9–21, who represented part of a sample of 100 hospitalized and diagnostically heterogeneous patients. They received haloperidol from 2–82 days (mean, 42 days) in doses of .75–12.0 mg/day (mean, 3.0). Symptoms of hyperactivity, assaultiveness, self-injury, excitability, insomnia and poor appetite decreased significantly within the first two weeks of treatment. Mental alertness, as measured by the Tulane Behavioral Test, did not change, or showed improvement at

Author(s) and Year	Sample	Age in Years	Design	Drug and Dosage (mg/day)	Measures
Le Vann, 1969	Heterogeneous N = 100 (46 schizo-phrenics?)	6–22	Open	Haloperidol (.72–12)	Target symptoms; global changes; Tulane Behavioral Test
Pangalila-Ratulangi, 1973	Heterogeneous N = 10 (8 schizo-phrenics?)	9–14	Open and single-blind (placebo)	Pimozide (1–2) or .05 mg/kg	Global clinical impressions; target symptoms; developed questionnaire; projective tests
Simeon et al., 1973	Heterogeneous N = 10 (4 schizo-phrenics)	5–15	Open	Thiothixene (6–30, miaximum 60)	Clinical Global Impressions (CGI); developed scale; Treatment Emergent Symptoms Scale (TESS)
Pool et al., 1976	Homogeneous N = 75	13–18	Double-blind, placebo controlled, random, 3 groups	Haloperidol (M = 9.8, maximum 16) vs. loxa-pine (M = 87.5, maximum 200)	Brief Psychiatric Rating Scale (BPRS); Clinical Global Impressions (CGI); Nurse's Observation Scale for Inpatient Evaluation (NOSIE)
Realmuto et al., 1984	Homogeneous N = 21	11–18	Double-blind, random, 2 groups	Thioridazine (M = 178, maximum 228) vs. thiothixene (M = 16.2, maximum 42.6)	BPRS, CGI

the end of the third week of treatment. Laboratory tests (complete blood count, SGOT, SGPT, alkaline phosphatase, and urinalysis) remained unchanged over a period of one and one-half years. (Adverse effects are listed in Table 4.6.)

The study by Faretra et al. (1970) involved 60 hospitalized children under 12 years of age, treated with fluphenazine or haloperidol. The sample was diagnostically heterogeneous; it seems that some of the children were schizophrenic, though definite statements cannot be made.

Pimozide, a diphenylbutylpiperidine, was investigated in a sample of 10 children, ages 9–14 years. Eight of the children were said to have "schizophrenia or schizophrenia-like symptomatology" (Pangalila-Ratulangi, 1973). In all patients indication for pimozide treatment was blunted affect; in two children, paranoid thoughts, in one child "hallucinatory disorientation," and in four, learning disturbances. The study design was problematic: an open study followed by single-blind. Five of these patients had a "striking improvement in target symptoms"; in two, this was accompanied by normalization of the EEG.

Simeon et al. (1973) reported on the effects of thiothixene in 10 children, four of whom were diagnosed as schizophrenic. The children first received placebo for 3–9 weeks (mean, 5.2 weeks) followed by 2 mg of trihexyphenidyl daily for 1–3 weeks. This latter drug was given in order to prevent the emergence of extrapyramidal symptoms. Thiothixene was administered for 6–46 weeks (mean, 16.5) in doses of 6–60 mg/day (mean, 27); the optimal daily dose ranged from 6–30 mg (mean, 14). The children were carefully monitored both clinically and by a variety of laboratory measures. As a group, the children showed improvements in motor activity, verbal production, thinking, and social relationships with adults, with decreases in anger, mood lability, emotional unresponsiveness, attentional problems and feeding difficulties.

Infantile Autism

Tables 4.4 and 4.5 detail some of the study characteristics of the representative literature involving autistic children. There is considerably more research on infantile autism than schizophrenic disorder in children and adolescents, including phenomenology, diagnosis, classification, biochemical research and investigations into underlying pathology and treatment (Campbell & Green, 1985; Green et al., 1984). As recent reviews of the literature indicate, a great variety of drugs was administered to autistic children over the past 30 years (Campbell et al., 1977, 1981). However, with one exception, the older reports suffer from methodological deficiencies (Fish et al., 1966). Only in the past few years

Table 4.4. Therapeutic and Untoward Effects of Amphetamine, L-Dopa and Fenfluramine in Patients with Infantile Autism

Author(s) and Year	Sample	Age in Years	Design	Measures	Drug and Dosage (mg/day)	Clinical Effects	
						Therapeutic	Untoward
Campbell et al., 1972c	Hetero-geneous	2–5	Crossover, acute, double-blind, placebo con-trolled	Developed scale	Dextroamphetamine (1.2–10, M=4.6)	None	Irritability, motor excitement, excessive sedation
Campbell et al., 1972a	Hetero-geneous (N=16)	3–6	Crossover, double-blind	Developed scale; CGI	Dextroamphetamine (1.25–10)	Slight; increases of attention span and verbal production, decrease of hyperactivity	Marked irritability, hyperactivity, worsening of withdrawal, stereotypies, loss of appetite (all patients had untoward effects)
Ritvo et al., 1971	Homo-geneous (N=4)	3–13	Pilot, two-week placebo baseline, open	Clinical Observation	L-Dopa (2000–4000)	None	Vomiting

Table 4.4. (*Continued*)

Author(s) and Year	Sample	Age in Years	Design	Measures	Drug and Dosage (mg/day)	Clinical Effects	
						Therapeutic	Untoward
Campbell et al., 1976	Hetero-geneous (N = 12) (11 autistics)	3–6/9	Crossover, double-blind	Developed scale; CGI	Levoamphetamine (3.5–42)	Slight; decrease of hyperactivity	Worsening of stereotypies or stereotypies de novo, loss of weight and appetite, worsening of irritability, of aggressiveness, and of psychosis, excessive sedation
					vs.		
					L-Dopa (900–2250)	Slight in five children: decrease in negativism, increases in play, energy, verbal production, and affective responsiveness	Increase of stereotypies or stereotypies de novo, decrease of appetite, vomiting, worsening of irritability, motor retardation

| Ritvo et al., 1983 | Homogeneous | 2–18 | Double-blind and placebo controlled crossover, without randomization (ABA) | Serial IQ testing, Alpern-Boll Developmental Profile; developed scales: Behavior Observation Scale, and Ritvo-Freeman Real Life Rating Scale; parent interviews; family daily diaries | Fenfluramine (1.5 mg/kg/day) | Decreased motility disturbances, increased attention span, language and relating to objects | Weight loss, lethargy, irritability, restlessness, awakening at night |

Table 4.5. *Therapeutic and Untoward Effects of Neuroleptics in Patients with Infantile Autism*

Author(s)	Sample	Age in Years	Design	Measures	Drug and Dosage (mg/day)	Clinical Effects	
						Therapeutic	Untoward
Fish et al., 1966	Homogeneous N = 22	2–6	Controlled double-blind, matching	Developed scale (Fish, 1968)	Trifluoperazine (2–20)	In the more retarded children: increased alertness, social responsiveness, and energy	In the higher functioning children: slower motor activity, lethargy, less interest in environment, and decreased verbal production
Wolpert et al., 1967	Homogeneous N = 16	8–15	Double-blind, random	Developed scale, global impressions, draw a person, Bender Motor Gestalt	Trifluoperazine (13–20) vs. thiothixene (6–30)	Decreases in withdrawal and stereotypies, improved appetite	

Faretra et al., 1970	Heterogeneous N=60	5–12	Double-blind, random	Target symptoms; global improvement	Haloperidol (.75–3.75)	Reduction of anxiety, autism, and provocativeness, improvement in social and motor behavior; 24% of children showed moderate to marked improvment.	Parkinsonian extrapyramidal effects, akathisia, dystonia rash
					vs.		
					Fluphenazine (.75–3.75)	Reduction of anxiety, improvement in social and motor behavior; 34% of children showed moderate to marked improvement	Akathisia, rash

Table 4.5. (*Continued*)

Author(s)	Sample	Age in Years	Design	Measures	Drug and Dosage (mg/day)	Clinical Effects	
						Therapeutic	Untoward
Campbell et al., 1970	Heterogeneous N = 10 (9 autistic)	3–7	Pilot, double-blind	Developed scale (Fish, 1968)	Thiothixene (1–6, M = 2)	Decreases in withdrawal, stereotypies, excitability and psychotic speech; increases in affective responsiveness, attention span, speech, social and play behavior	Excessive sedation, motor retardation, irritability, Parkinsonian extrapyramidal effects, insomnia, anorexia, worsening of psychosis
Campbell et al., 1971	Heterogeneous N = 10 (8 autistic)	3–5	Pilot, double-blind	Developed scale (Fish, 1968)	Molindone (1–2.5, M = 1.5)	Decreases in withdrawal, negativism, and stereotypies; increases in affective responsiveness and communicative speech	Parkinsonian extrapyramidal effects, acute dystonic reactions, increases in impulsivity, crying, euphoria, excessive sedation

Study	Sample	Age	Design	Scale	Drug (dose)	Effects	Side effects
Campbell et al., 1972b	Heterogeneous N = 10 (7 autistic)	3–6	Controlled, double-blind, crossover	Developed scale (Fish, 1968), CGI	Chlorpromazine (9–45 mg; maximum dose 60)	Slight decreases in psychotic speech, withdrawal, stereotypies; increases in affective responsiveness, vocabulary, attention span and initiation of speech	Excessive sedation, motor excitation, irritability, insomnia, worsening of psychosis, catatoniclike states, rash (1).
Waizer et al., 1972	Homogeneous N = 18	5–13	Pilot, single-blind	Developed scale (CPRS-1), CGI	Thiothixene (2–24, M = 16.9)	Decreases in stereotypies, improvement in motor activity, coordination, sleeping, affect and exploratory behavior, concentration and eating habits	Parkinsonian extrapyramidal side effects, excessive sedation, head rocking
Engelhardt et al., 1973	Homogeneous N = 30	6–12	Double-blind, random	Developed scale (CPRS-1) CGI	Haloperidol (2–16, M = 10.4) vs.	Improvement in coordination, self-care, affect, and exploratory behavior	Parkinsonian extrapyramidal effects, akathisia, drowsiness, dizziness

Table 4.5. (Continued)

Author(s)	Sample	Age in Years	Design	Measures	Drug and Dosage (mg/day)	Clinical Effects	
						Therapeutic	Untoward
					Fluphenazine (2–16, M = 10.4)	Improvement in self-awareness, constructive play; decreases in compulsive acts, and self-mutilation	Parkinsonian extrapyramidal effects, acute dystonic reaction, tremor, drowsiness, dizziness, anorexia, polyuria
Campbell et al., 1978	Homogeneous N = 40	2.6–7.2	Placebo controlled, double-blind, random	CPRS, CGI, CBI, NGI, DOTES, TESS-Write-In; Cognitive Battery; assessment of effects of behavior therapy	Haloperidol (.5–4.0, M = 1.65)	Significant decreases of stereotypies and withdrawal; facilitation of acquisition of speech with conjoint language therapy	Excessive sedation, excitement–agitation, insomnia, acute dystonic reaction (2), increased motor activity, increased irritability, depressive affect
Cohen et al., 1980	Homogeneous N = 10	2.1–7.0	Placebo controlled, double-blind, random, ABAB	Developed scales (TBRS and Look at Me)	Haloperidol (.5–4.0, M = 1.78)	Significant decrease of stereotypies and withdrawal	Excessive sedation, increased irritability, hyperactivity, drooling, acute

Study	Sample	Age	Design	Measures	Drug (Dose)	Results	Side Effects
Naruse et al., 1982	Heterogeneous N = 87 (34 autistic)	3–16	Placebo controlled, double-blind, random, crossover	Developed scales	Haloperidol (.75–6.75) vs. Pimozide (1–9)	Significant decreases of hyperactivity, emotional lability, withdrawal, aggressiveness	Excessive sedation
Anderson et al., 1984	Homogeneous N = 40	2.33–6.92	Placebo controlled, double-blind, random, ABA	CPRS, CGI, PTQ, discrimination learning, and measurement of motor activity and duration of stereotypies in automated laboratory; DOTES; TESS-Write-In, AIMS, Simpson abridged (1979)	Haloperidol (.5–3.0, M = 1.11)	Significant decreases of withdrawal, stereotypies, hyperactivity, abnormal object relationships, fidgetiness, negativism, angry affect and lability of affect; significant decreases of severity of illness and greater behavior improvement	Excessive sedation, irritability, acute dystonic reaction (11), tremor, decreased motor activity

have studies included an adequate and diagnostically homogeneous patient sample and sound or even sophisticated methodology (Table 4.5). This work is mainly a systematic study of haloperidol: a critical assessment of its efficacy, effect on learning, and safety.

Perhaps three goals characterize pharmacotherapy research in autism. First, a search for "less sedative" neuroleptics: drugs that decrease symptoms without excessive sedation at the same doses, since sedation may interfere with cognition and learning (Fish, 1960, 1970). This resulted from the clinical observation that chlorpromazine was sedative for the autistic child at doses that yielded only a slight decrease in symptoms (Campbell et al., 1972b and c). For this purpose the following neuroleptics were explored: trifluoperazine, trifluperidol, haloperidol, thiothixene, and molindone. This avenue of research met with some success, particularly in regard to haloperidol, the drug which is now undergoing systematic investigation.

The second avenue of research was to explore more "stimulating" psychoactive drugs for the autistic child with serious delays in most areas of development, and particularly in language behavior. Agents such as LSD, methysergide, amphetamines, imipramine, and triiodothyronine (T_3) were administered to autistic children. These studies have methodological flaws. The exception is a recently completed double-blind placebo controlled crossover study of triiodothyronine (Campbell et al., 1978), with results much more modest than those of previous poorly controlled studies. L-amphetamine and D-amphetamine, both dopamine agonists, decrease hyperactivity and impulsivity and increase attention span in children diagnosed as having attention deficit disorder (Klein et al., 1980) with symptoms shared by many autistic children. In addition, their administration results in improved performance on a variety of cognitive tasks—an effect that all autistic children could benefit from. In our studies of D- and L-amphetamine in young autistic children, even though hyperactivity decreased, the positive effects were usually outweighted by untoward effects, including worsening of existing stereotypies, stereotypies *de novo* and irritability (Campbell et al., 1972a and c, 1976). In general, these drugs are not recommended for the treatment of autistic children: improvements were rated only in a small number of patients and worsening of behavior was reported (for a review, see Campbell et al., 1977, 1981).

The third approach related behavioral abnormality (symptoms) to underlying biochemical abnormalities, mainly those of serotonin, and attempted to decrease both simultaneously with an antagonist drug. The two drugs explored were L-dopa and fenfluramine. Studies of L-dopa consist of small patient samples and have methodological problems: one, based on four subjects, failed to show behavioral effects (Ritvo et al., 1971) while the other, consisting of 12 young children, suggested that further research was warranted (Campbell et al., 1976). In the latter study, therapeutic effects were accompanied by worsening of preexisting stereotypies, or stereotypies *de novo* (Campbell et al, 1976). L-dopa is a dopamine agonist, and so are D- and L-amphetamine: both yielded similar untoward effects in these children. More recently, fenfluramine, another serotonin antagonist, was administered to 15 autistic children; the data on 14 indicate that positive behavioral and cognitive effects are obtained in the presence of some untoward effects (Ritvo et al., 1983). Loss of weight was reported in three patients; weight loss was large in one. Interestingly, the behavioral changes with both L-dopa and fenfluramine are not necessarily related to baseline serotonin elevation. Further careful and systematic research is needed in this area.

Only the studies of the butyrophenone haloperidol, a potent dopamine antagonist, will be detailed here, since no other neuroleptic drug has been investigated as systematically in childhood psychopharmacology, specifically in infantile autism, both in terms of short and long term efficacy and safety.

Faretra et al. (1970) and Engelhardt et al. (1973) found marked decreases in a variety of symptoms in children ages 5–12 years related to administration of haloperidol. However, Faretra's large sample of patients ($N = 60$), was diagnostically heterogeneous; neither study employed placebo as control and diagnostic criteria were not specified. The dosages employed were quite different: .75–3.75 mg/day in the first study, and 2/16 mg/day in the second.

These two studies, and the encouraging results of an earlier pilot study with trifluperidol* (Campbell et al., 1972c), another butyrophenone, stimulated interest in haloperidol. Since the prognosis of infantile autism on the basis of follow-up studies is at best guarded and no known treatment produces dramatic results, we felt it important to critically assess haloperidol efficacy, to compare it to a psychosocial intervention focusing on language acquisition, and to determine whether the combination of both treatments is more effective than each treatment alone. Behavior therapy was employed since this treatment modality is quantifiable, as is pharmocotherapy. The study was double blind and placebo controlled. Children were randomly assigned to one of the four treatment conditions; some received contingent, while others received non-

---

*Trifluperidol is no longer in investigational use in the United States.

contingent reinforcement. The children were carefully diagnosed and studied; their chronological ages were within a narrow range. Forty children completed the study (Campbell et al., 1978). Haloperidol alone, in doses of .5 −4.0 mg/day was effective in decreasing stereotypies and withdrawal, while the combination of haloperidol and contingent reinforcement facilitated language acquisition in the laboratory. The children were inpatients; compliance was 100 percent. A variety of rating scales was used by independent raters. The drug had no effect on cognition as measured by a cognitive battery administered during the two-week placebo baseline and at termination. More important, at these therapeutic doses, children were free of untoward effects. Above therapeutic doses, excessive sedation was the most common adverse effect. The study was carried out over a period of 12 weeks.

We now wished to determine how haloperidol facilitates learning; by decreasing behavioral symptoms or by directly affecting attentional mechanisms, independently of symptom changes. For this purpose, we designed a new study, which also was double blind and placebo controlled, employing an ABA design and combining an intensive study of a single subject (within subjects) and extensive (between-groups) design. This seemed to be a most economical approach in a condition as rare as infantile autism, and its utility in this population was demonstrated in a previous ABAB clinical trial (Cohen et al., 1980). Following a two-week placebo and baseline assessment period, the patients were randomly assigned to one of the two treatment sequences: haloperidol-placebo-haloperidol or placebo-haloperidol-placebo. Each treatment period was of four weeks duration. Discrimination learning* was assessed in a computer controlled laboratory with an operant conditioning apparatus, presenting stimuli, recording responses, administering reinforcers according to schedule, and recording duration of stereotypies and hyperactivity. Various rating scales were employed to rate behavioral symptoms in various situations, and adverse effects were carefully monitored. Haloperidol levels and the effects of haloperidol on electroencephalogram were assessed. Forty children, diagnosed by the same criteria as in the two previous clinical trials, completed this study; those who were exclusively hypoactive, were not accepted (Anderson et al., 1984; Campbell et al., 1982). Haloperidol in daily doses of .5–3.0 mg yielded significant decreases of stereotypies, withdrawal, hyperactivity, abnormal object relationships, fidgetiness, negativism, angry affect, and labile affect. Severity of illness decreased and global improvement was

---

*Autistic children suffer from defects in attentional mechanisms (Kolko et al., 1980).

significantly superior with haloperidol than with placebo. Thus, the behavioral effects of haloperidol were replicated in this study. So were its positive effects on learning in the laboratory. We have also shown that facilitation of discrimination learning was independent of decrease of symptoms, since in the laboratory haloperidol had no effect on stereotypies and on hyperactivity. At doses that resulted in behavioral improvement and facilitation of discrimination learning, haloperidol had no untoward effects. Above these doses, excessive sedation and acute dystonic reactions were most commonly observed. In all three studies, dosage was individually regulated in each patient (Anderson et al., 1984; Campbell et al., 1978, 1982; Cohen et al., 1980).

In one of these studies (Anderson et al., 1984) six patients were challenged with insulin on baseline and at the end of treatment with haloperidol; there was no significant change of their growth hormone response (Deutsch et al., 1985). In the subsequent study involving 40 subjects (Anderson et al., 1984) plasma levels of haloperidol were determined in 28; plasma levels were significantly related to decrease of withdrawal and stereotypies on the Children's Psychiatric Rating Scale, CPRS (Poland et al., 1982).

Haloperidol was not only statistically superior to placebo, but also clinically effective. Thirty-six of the 40 children continued the treatment on a long term basis. Preliminary results from this ongoing study indicate that haloperidol remained effective from six months up to 2½ years (Campbell et al., 1983b). IQs were retested on follow-up in 15 children whose ages ranged from 3.3–9 years. Their intellectual functioning at baseline ranged from borderline to profoundly retarded. After 9 months and for up to 3.8 years (mean, 3 years) of haloperidol maintenance (.5–3.0 mg, mean, 1.3), 8 children had marked increases in IQ or DQ scores; in five there was significant improvement in language. In two children the IQs remained stable, while five moved to a lower category (Die Trill et al., 1984).

We speculated as to the mechanism of efficacy of haloperidol in our young autistic children. There are pilot data suggesting that retarded autistic children, with severe stereotypies and hyperactivity show evidence of excess dopaminergic activity (for review, see Young et al., 1982). The dopaminergic system of the brain affects motor behaviors; its excess results in stereotypies and hyperactivity. While dopamine agonists, L-dopa, L-amphetamine, and D-amphetamine even at "optimal," but particularly above optimal doses yielded worsening of preexisting stereotypies and stereotypies *de novo*, in addition to other behavioral toxicity, haloperidol, a potent antidopaminergic agent, decreased these and other behavioral symptoms. Furthermore, at the same doses, it facilitated learning in the absence of untoward effects.

DRUGS OF CHOICE AND CLINICAL USAGE

Schizophrenic Disorder

While in adults and adolescents with acute schizophrenia the diminution of reactivity achieved by administration of a neuroleptic is desirable (Himwich, 1960), this is considered to be an untoward effect in the child who is apathetic and anergic as are many young schizophrenic children. In prepubertal children, the type of schizophrenia with slow, insidious onset is more common than the acute type (Green et al., 1984; Kolvin, 1971). Fish (1970) found that the youngest age group of schizophrenic patients responds to drugs in a similar fashion as the adult chronic schizophrenics who are anergic, apathetic, and withdrawn.

As noted above, in prepubertal children, there is not a single well-designed drug study involving a carefully diagnosed and homogeneous sample of children who would meet the DSM-III criteria for schizophrenic disorder. However, in daily practice, drugs are routinely prescribed to these youngsters irrespective of measurable therapeutic results. Recommendations are based solely on clinical experience. Prepubertal schizophrenia is rare (over a period of five years, 24 such children were admitted to a busy acute inpatient psychiatric service, Green et al., 1984). Unless one conducts systematic research in this population, clinical experience remains limited even over a period of two decades as is the case with this author. It seems that these children respond to neuroleptics to a much lesser degree than their adult counterparts (Green et al., 1984) and are often sedated even at low doses. However, haloperidol has less sedative properties at therapeutic doses then chlorpromazine or thioridazine.

The study by Pool et al. (1976), which involves a relatively large sample of adolescents, ages 13–18 years, all of whom were diagnosed as acute schizophrenic or chronic with acute exacerbation demonstrated that both haloperidol and loxapine are superior to placebo in the treatment of these patients. Hallucinations, thinking disorder, and other symptoms decreased significantly on both drugs, and there were only a few significant differences in therapeutic profile between the two drugs. However, there were some differences in untoward effects between these drugs. While both drugs had a high rate of extrapyramidal side effects (19 of the 26 patients receiving loxapine and 18 of the 25 patients who received haloperidol) consisting mainly of cogwheel phenomena, sedation was noted in 21 of the 26 loxapine patients and only in 13 of the 25 in the haloperidol group.

A low initial dose (e.g., .5 mg of haloperidol) with slow and small increments (twice a week) is recommended in order to reduce the incidence of acute dystonic reactions. Dosage should be regulated individually for each child. For maximum dosage, the *Physicians Desk Reference* (PDR) should be consulted. The duration of drug administration will depend on whether the patient is diagnosed as having acute or chronic schizophrenia. It should be discontinued after a period of at least two and up to six months, in order to determine whether the patient requires further drug therapy and for the assessment of possible neuroleptic-induced abnormal involuntary movements. In case of parkinsonian side effects, dosage reduction rather than concurrent administration of antiparkinsonian drugs is recommended. Prior to drug administration, a baseline laboratory work-up (complete blood count, differential, liver profile, and urinalysis) should be done and repeated as indicated.

A recent single-case report suggested that a combination of chlorpromazine and methylphenidate was therapeutic in a schizophrenic boy who had associated "attention deficit symptoms" (Rogeness & Macedo, 1983). Though adding the stimulant to chlorpromazine reduced the psychotic symptoms in this child, this combination cannot be recommended as a routine pharmacotherapy for schizophrenic children. In adult schizophrenics, stimulants are known to produce worsening of symptoms.

Infantile Autism

At the present time, most knowledge of short and long term efficacy and safety of psychoactive drugs in infantile autism is based on studies of haloperidol and, to a lesser degree, of trifluoperazine. Both the early study of trifluoperazine (Fish et al., 1966) and the systematic and long term studies of haloperidol (Campbell et al., 1978, 1982; Cohen et al., 1980; Anderson et al., 1984) are based on carefully diagnosed preschool-age children.

Those autistic children who have low IQs and who are normoactive or hyperactive, disruptive, and/or have temper tantrums respond well to haloperidol, while those who are exclusively anergic and hypoactive do not. However, a young, extremely hypoactive and anergic girl was the best responder when given 20 mg/day of trifluoperazine, although for the remaining children in this sample, the dosage of 2–6 mg/day, was adequate (Fish et al., 1966). As for haloperidol, in preschool-age children, the starting dose should be .5 mg/day, or, even .25 mg/day, and it should be gradually increased, as discussed above, in schizophrenia. The same is true for dosage regulation, handling of untoward effects, duration of treatment, and laboratory work-up.

Though a clinical report suggests that D-amphetamine was effective in reducing the "attention deficit component" in two children with childhood onset developmental disorder (Geller et al., 1981), in larger patient samples untoward effects of amphetamines outweighed the positive effects in carefully diagnosed autistic children (Campbell et al., 1972a, c, 1976), as noted above.

ADVERSE EFFECTS

All psychoactive drugs can have untoward effects (Thompson & Schuster, 1968). These will vary, depending on the type or class of drug, dosage level, duration of drug administration, conditions under which the drug is administered, patient's age, diagnosis, and the presence or absence of brain damage or brain disease. The physician should be familiar not only with the possible therapeutic effects of a drug but also with its untoward effects. The parents and, if appropriate, the patient also should be informed. In addition to past history and history of drug sensitivity, baseline assessments should include urinalysis, complete blood count, differential, liver profile and other systems that may be adversely affected. Avoid polypharmacy and unnecessary dosage escalation. With careful clinical and appropriate (or required) laboratory monitoring most serious untoward effects usually can be avoided. The available assessment methods and instruments for the measurement of untoward effects were recently reviewed elsewhere (Campbell et al., 1985).

Only the untoward effects associated with neuroleptic treatment will be reviewed here. The psychomotor stimulants are in general not therapeutic for these children and their use is not recommended. L-dopa is not prescribed in daily practice. However, the untoward effects of both L-dopa and of amphetamines in infantile autism are listed in Table 4.4; for details, Campbell et al., 1972a, c, and 1976 are recommended. The use of fenfluramine in infantile autism is very recent; the untoward effects in 14 subjects (Ritvo et al., 1983) are listed in Table 4.4.

UNTOWARD EFFECTS OF NEUROLEPTICS

Behavioral Toxicity

DiMascio and Shader (1970) define behavioral toxicity as actions of a drug producing changes in perceptual and cognitive functions, psychomotor performance, mood, motivation, interpersonal relationships, or intrapsychic processes that interfere with functioning or may be a physical hazard, occurring within the dose range found to have clinical value.

Effects on Cognition. Most research on the effects of neuroleptics on cognition was done in nonpsychotic or mentally retarded children (for review, see Platt et al., in press). Findings in one diagnostic category cannot be extrapolated to another since the adverse or beneficial effects of a neuroleptic may not be only a function of dose (Werry & Aman, 1975) but also a function of diagnosis (Anderson et al., 1984; Campbell et al., 1982; Platt et al., 1984). To the best of our knowledge, there are no published studies of neuroleptic adverse effects conducted in schizophrenic children or adolescents. As noted above, in our work with young autistic children there were no ill effects on cognition or learning at doses that were effective in reducing behavioral symptoms (Campbell et al., 1978, 1982; Anderson et al., 1984). Above these optimal doses, excessive sedation was the most common untoward effect; though the children were not tested at these higher doses, one can assume that deterioration of cognitive functioning occurred. As indicated above, the doses were regulated individually for each child in these studies. Since the range of optimal doses was wide (.5–4.0 mg/day of haloperidol) and the mean dose relatively low (slightly above 1 mg/day) one can conclude that if a fixed dosage were used, deterioration of learning and cognition would have been obtained in a number of patients.

Behavior. Worsening of preexisting symptoms or the emergence of new symptoms are frequently seen in young children before any other untoward effects are observed. These are mainly of affecto-motor nature and include irritability, apathy, temper tantrums, hyper or hypoactivity. Decrease of verbal production is also reported.

Central Nervous System Untoward Effects

Extrapyramidal Effects. These include acute dystonic reactions, dyskinesias, parkinsonian reactions, akathisia and the "rabbit syndrome."

ACUTE DYSTONIC REACTIONS.   These include tonic contractions of muscles manifested as oculogyric crisis, torticollis, opisthotonus, and spasms of the tongue and of the torso. Their duration may be from a few minutes to several hours. Acute dystonic reactions are relieved by oral or intramuscular administration of 25 mg of Benadryl. As a rule, dystonic symptoms occur after the first dose, or within the first few days of neuroleptic administration, though there are reports of occurrence after long term drug administration (Gardos, 1981). Dystonic reactions are more frequently associated with high-potency neuroleptics (e.g., fluphenazine or haloperidol) than with those of low potency (e.g., chlorpromazine or thioridazine).

ACUTE DYSKINESIAS.   Like acute dystonic reactions, these are the earliest extrapyramidal untoward effects. They consist of clonic muscle spasms: blinking, facial tics, lip smacking, tongue movements, shoulder shrugging, and pedaling of lower extremities.

PARKINSONIAN REACTIONS.   These include muscular rigidity (cogwheel phenomenon), finger and hand tremor, drooling, masklike face, and akinesia. Shuffling gait is rarely, if ever, observed in children. Their occurrence is usually within the first three weeks of treatment. Dosage reduction is recommended, rather than administration of antiparkinsonian agents. These agents may reduce the level of the neuroleptic in blood and worsen preexisting psychotic symptoms (Rivera-Calimlim et al., 1976), and could contribute to the development of tardive or withdrawal dyskinesia. Parkinsonian reactions are rare in preschool-age children at therapeutic or even above-therapeutic doses (Campbell et al., 1978, 1982; Anderson et al., 1984); they are more common in school-age children (Campbell et al., 1984) and adolescents.

AKATHISIA.   This is characterized by agitation, constant pacing and inability to sit still; it usually develops in the first five weeks of treatment. In children, it is difficult to differentiate akathisia from certain forms of hyperactivity.

RABBIT SYNDROME.   A late-onset extrapyramidal untoward effect, it is quite rare. The movements involve the perioral muscles and are similar to the extremely rapid, chewinglike movements of the rabbit (Villeneuve, 1972).

Other Central Nervous System Untoward Effects.   These include excessive sedation, dizziness, confusion, headache, insomnia, depersonalization, ataxia, and grand mal or partial seizures. Excessive sedation is by far the most common untoward effect in children associated with administration of neuroleptics. Especially undesirable in children, sedation requires careful dose titration and monitoring. The incidence of neuroleptic-associated seizures in infantile autism is difficult to assess, since this population is known to have a relatively high (4–32%) rate of seizure disorder (Campbell & Green, 1985), even without neuroleptic administration. However, it is reported that chlorpromazine will increase the frequency of seizures in individuals who suffer from such disorder, or lower the threshold for seizures (Tarjan et al., 1957).

Tardive and Withdrawal Dyskinesias (TD & WD). A recent review of the literature indicates that 8–51 percent of children and adolescents who receive neuroleptics will develop TD & WD with long term neuroleptic administration (Campbell et al., 1983a). These abnormal involuntary movements usually involve the muscles of the face, tongue, and mouth, and may extend to eyelids, upper and lower extremities, fingers, toes, torso, and neck. The typical oro-facial-lingual movements are slow and rhythmical. Choreiform, athetotic, dystonic, rolling, myoclonic, tic-like and ballistic movements also can involve the muscles in various parts of the body. Diaphragmatic and laryngeal muscle involvement is manifested as peculiar vocalizations, respiratory dyskinesia, grunts, and dysarthria. These movements may be rhythmic or irregular, repetitive, transient, or persistent. They may develop during drug administration, after dose reduction or drug withdrawal. The earliest onset of these involuntary abnormal movements is after three months of cumulative drug administration (Campbell et al., 1983). Earlier retrospective reports suggested that these movements in children differ from those seen in adult psychiatric patients because of both outcome and topography (Engelhardt & Polizos, 1978, 1980). More recent research, including a well-designed prospective study, has shown that these dyskinesias are the same in children and adolescents as in adults (Campbell et al., 1983a and b; Gualtieri et al., 1980, 1982). They often involve the bucco-lingual-masticatory muscles (Campbell et al., 1983a, b, submitted for publication) and include the persistent, irreversible form (Paulson et al., 1975). The reason for the great discrepancy among different studies concerning the prevalence of this condition can be ascribed to a variety of factors, including methodology, type of instruments used, diagnostic criteria, study design, patient variables, and drug and dose related variables (for review, see Campbell et al., 1983a; Gardos & Cole, 1980; Gardos et al., 1977). Recent research conducted in the mentally retarded suggests that neuroleptic-related dyskinesias are more common in those individuals who fail to respond to drug treatment than in those who respond to a decrease in behavioral symptoms (Gualtieri et al., 1982). For review of neuroleptic-related dyskinesias in children and adolescents, Campbell et al., 1983a, and Gualtieri et al., 1980 are recommended.

Behavioral and Other Withdrawal Effects

These refer to the emergence of a variety of symptoms and signs that develop subsequent to discontinuation of psychoactive agents (for review, see Klein et al., 1980; van der Kolk et al., 1978). Manifestations include worsening of preexisting symptoms ("rebound phenomena"), insomnia, anxiety, restlessness, agitation, irritability, anorexia, weight loss, nausea, vomiting, stomach cramps, diarrhea, chills, and cold sweats. Gualtieri et al. (1982) conducted neuroleptic withdrawal studies in the mentally retarded; the sample included children and adolescents.

Supersensitivity Psychosis

There are reports in adults of insomnia, agitation, anxiety, and worsening of preexisting schizophrenic symptoms upon withdrawal of neuroleptic administration. These behavioral manifestations were described as supersensitivity psychosis (Chouinard & Jones, 1980). In our research involving autistic children we observed that behavior deteriorated in some after discontinuation of the neuroleptic, and even became worse than on baseline. Within a week the severity of symptoms usually returned to baseline or, in some, decreased to the drug treatment level. We considered these to be rebound phenomena. However, one child exhibited symptoms that were comparable to those seen in supersensitivity psychosis in adults: agitation, insomnia, aggressiveness directed against self and others, and worsening of preexisting symptoms (Campbell et al., 1983a).

Abnormal Laboratory Findings

These include hematologic, blood chemistry, liver, urinary endocrine and metabolic abnormalities. Review of the literature suggests that children are more resilient than adults in this respect. Liver damage and blood dyscrasias seem to be rare in this age group (DiMascio et al., 1970; Engelhardt & Polizos, 1978). However, most reports are based on short term studies and not all indicate whether or how frequently laboratory monitoring was carried out. In our studies of young autistic children, no serious deviations from baseline were found.

It was emphasized that part of assessment of the efficacy and safety of a new drug is to obtain baseline (prior to drug administration) clinical laboratory data and repeated determinations at fixed intervals or as indicated (Gershon, 1973). However, norms are needed in certain patient populations because their baseline laboratory values may show variation from textbook normative data (McGlashan & Cleary, 1975, 1976; Gershon, 1973). This is particularly true for such special populations as autistic and schizophrenic children. Nonmedicated disturbed children may show abnormal baseline values (LeVann, 1969) or greater fluctuation over time of certain laboratory values than expected in normals. For example, our data show that a subgroup of preschool autistic children has marked fluctuations of hematologic and liver profile values while receiving placebo (Campbell, unpublished data). For a review of abnormal laboratory findings associated with neuroleptic drug administration, see Ebert and Shader (1970a, b).

Engelhardt and Polizos (1978) reported gynecomastia in children and increases in prolactin levels have been recorded (Campbell et al., unpublished data). In a study involving 10 adolescent schizophrenic boys, administration of chlorpromazine for a period of at least six months resulted in low basal plasma testosterone levels, normal response to human chorionic gonadotropin (HCG) stimulation, mild elevation of prolactin, and blunted luteinizing hormone (LH) response to luteinizing-releasing hormone (LRH) stimulation (Apter et al., 1983).

Miscellaneous

Autonomic nervous system side effects include dry mouth, constipation, and diarrhea; these appear to be rare in children. Hypotension was reported in one child (Anderson et al., in press); in general this symptom does not seem to be a problem in children.

Effects on Height and Weight

There is no systematic research in regard to the effects on growth of long term neuroleptic maintenance. However, there is some suggestion that disturbed children may have different growth patterns than those without psychiatric illness (Eggins et al., 1975). Autistic children are significantly shorter than their siblings or the expected norm (Campbell et al., 1980; Simon & Gillies, 1964). Roche et al. (1979) have recently presented a critical analysis and review of the literature concerning the effects of stimulant medication on children's growth. They emphasize the need for accurate measurements, updated growth charts, and adequate study design.

Green et al. (1984) studied the long-term effects of haloperidol on height and weight of 42 autistic children, in a prospective design. The patients' ages ranged from 2.0 to 7.6 years: after 6 months maintenance (daily dose 0.5 to 3.0 mg) there was a 4.7 point decrement in mean height percentile, which was not significant. In mean weight percentile, there was an 8.2 point increase (p<0.05).

Simeon et al. (1977) related acceleration of growth secondary to neuroleptic administration in 13 psychotic children, aged 5–12 years (mean, 9.8 years). In the 6 boys who received drug treatment for a mean of 71 weeks, acceleration of linear growth was noted, while in the remaining 5, who received drug for only 39 weeks, no acceleration of growth was observed. The same was true for 2 children who received treatment for less than 11 weeks. Engelhardt and Polizos (1978) studied 20 autistic boys ages 4–11 years. After 1–6 (mean, 4) years of neuroleptic maintenance their mean weights and heights remained close to the fiftieth percentile, as they were on baseline. In a study involving thiothixene over a period of 11–46 weeks (mean, 20) at maximum daily doses of 10–60 mg (mean, 32) a weight gain of 6–20 lb (mean, 14) was reported. We are currently analyzing the data from a prospective, longitudinal study of preschool-age autistic children placed on a haloperidol maintenance.

The untoward effects of neuroleptics in schizophrenic children and adolescents are listed in Table 4.6, and in autistic children in Table 4.5 (for more details in autistic children, see Campbell et al., 1978, 1982 and Anderson et al., 1984). For additional reading on the use of neuroleptics in children, a chapter by Winsberg and Yepes (1978) is recommended.

PATIENT SAMPLE, DESIGN, AND ASSESSMENT

The outcome of a clinical trial will depend not only on the efficacy and safety of a psychoactive drug, but will be influenced or even determined by the methodology employed. A review of the literature (Tables 4.3 and 4.4) indicates that most reports involving schizophrenic and autistic children have serious methodological deficiencies, making the results difficult to interpret. The exceptions are the more recent studies of Campbell et al. involving studies of haloperidol and an earlier study by Fish et al. (1966) of trifluoperazine in young autistic children, and the *with Schizophrenic Disorder Age Range 5–22 Years*

Fluphenazine (.75–12.0)	Haloperidol (.75–16.0)	Loxapine (M=87.5, maximum 200)	Pimozide (1.0–9.0)	Thioridazine (91–228)	Thiothixene (4.8–60.0)
Parkinsonian extrapyramidal reactions	Parkinsonian extrapyramidal reactions	Parkinsonian extrapyramidal reactions		Excessive sedation Parkinsonian extrapyramidal reactions	Excessive sedation Parkinsonian extrapyramidal reactions
				Dizziness	
				Orthostatic hypotension	
Akathisia	Akathisia	Dizziness	Excessive sedation		
Excessive sedation	Acute dystonic reactions			Orthostatic hypotension	Acute dystonic reactions
Skin rash	Excessive sedation				Akathisia
	Skin rash				Weight gain
					Vomiting, nausea
					Constipation
					Elevated temperature
					Enuresis

143

clinical trial of Pool et al. (1976) of schizophrenic adolescents. Most other reports involve very small and/or heterogeneous patient samples. A minimum of 20 subjects is considered adequate. Especially in the earlier studies patient samples were diagnostically heterogeneous (schizophrenics, autistics, and mentally retarded with behavioral problems were studied together) and/or diagnostic criteria were not specified. Different diagnostic categories may respond differently to the same drug and have untoward effects at different dose levels. In some studies, even though the subjects were diagnostically homogeneous, the age range is excessive (ranging from preschool-age to young adulthood). The patient's status (inpatient vs. outpatient) can also influence the outcome (Christensen, 1973) and/or the level of therapeutic dose required. For example, in two studies comparing haloperidol to fluphenazine in comparable populations (autistics, age 5–12 years), markedly different doses were used. In the inpatient sample, the daily dosage ranged from .75–3.75 mg (Faretra et al., 1970) while in outpatients, surprisingly, it ranged from 2–16 mg, mean 10.4 (Engelhardt et al., 1973). This large discrepancy could be due to variables other than the status of subjects: noncompliance (expected to be, but not necessarily higher in outpatients) and criteria for or method of rating untoward effects. Level of intellectual functioning or degree of associated mental retardation also will affect outcome. Random assignment should eliminate or diminish these differences; however, in small samples these characteristics may not be equally distributed across groups. In addition to psychiatric diagnosis, patients should be defined by various demographic parameters (e.g., presence or absence of seizures, pre and perinatal complications, duration of illness).

Prior to enrollment of a subject into a clinical trial, a drug-washout period of adequate length is necessary. A baseline placebo period of 2–3 weeks is required in order to carry out the baseline assessments, to achieve a stable baseline, and to eliminate the placebo responders. In very disturbed and/or retarded young children, this placebo period also accustoms the child to taking medication.

In psychiatric subjects where the intersubject variability is great, and particularly in children, where such variables as maturation, IQ, and psychosocial environment may be compounding and/or powerful factors influencing outcome, it is particularly important to assess critically treatment effects and to reduce bias. This is specially true in cases of schizophrenic and autistic children, in whom changes produced by any type of therapeutic intervention are at best modest. Bias can be reduced by randomization, double-blind procedures, and by use of placebo as control. Because the young child's behavior may vary a great deal over time, and the symptoms are frequently influenced by ecological factors, it is important to achieve a stable baseline and rate the child under a variety of conditions. Assessments should be carried out independently by trained raters. Clearly, the results will be influenced by the choice of measurement approaches and instruments. Rating instruments should be sensitive to drug-induced changes and appropriate for the population under study. Preferably widely used instruments should be chosen to facilitate communication among investigators. A special issue of the Psychopharmacology Bulletin (1973) is recommended for additional reading.

In recent years our studies of autistic children utilize a combination of intensive or longitudinal within-subjects design (Chassan, 1979), for example ABAB or ABA, and extensive or between-groups (Turner et al., 1974) design (Campbell et al., 1982; Anderson et al., 1984). This is an appropriate design in a chronic condition. It is an economic design in a condition that is as rare as infantile autism, because each child serves as his or her own control. The problem of matching is thus eliminated; actually, we know very little about the variables one should match for.

For a review of methodological issues in studies of disturbed children the reader is referred to a chapter by Conners in this book, and a chapter by Campbell and Deutsch (in press), by Fish (1968) and a paper by Fish et al. (1966).

REFERENCES

American Psychiatric Association. (1952). *Diagnostic and statistical manual of Mental Disorders.* Washington, DC: American Psychiatric Association.

American Psychiatric Asociation. *Diagnostic and statistical manual of mental disorders* (1968). (2nd ed.). Washington, DC.: American Psychiatric Association.

American Psychiatric Association. 1980 (3rd ed.). *Diagnostic and statistical manual of mental disorders.* Washington DC.: American Psychiatric Association.

Apter, A., Dickerman, Z., Gonen, N., Assa, S., Prager-Lewin, R., Kaufman, H., Tyano, S., & Laron, Z. (1983). Effect of chlorpromazine on hypothalamic-pituitary-gonadal function in 10 adolescent schizophrenic boys. *American Journal of Psychiatry, 140,* 1588–1591.

Anderson, L. T., Campbell, M., Grega, D. M., Perry, R., Small, A. M., & Green, W. H. (1984). Haloperidol in infantile autism: Effects on learning and behavioral symptoms. *American Journal of Psychiatry, 141,* 1195–1202.

Bender, L. (1942). Schizophrenia in childhood. *Nervous Child, 1,* 138–140

Campbell, M., Anderson, L. T., Meier, M., Cohen, I. L., Small, A. M., Samit, C., & Sachar, E. J. (1978). A comparison of haloperidol, behavior therapy and their interaction in autistic children. *Journal of the American Academy of Child Psychiatry, 17,* 640–655.

Campbell, M., Anderson, L. T., Small, A. M., Perry, R., Green, W. H., & Caplan, R. (1982).

The effects of haloperidol and learning and behavior in autistic children. *Journal of Autism and Developmental Disorders, 12,* 167–175.

Campbell M., Cohen, I. L., & Anderson, L. T. (1981). Pharmacotherapy for autistic children: A summary of research. *Canadian Journal of Psychiatry, 26,* 265–273.

Campbell, M., & Deutsch, S. I. (in press). Neuroleptics in children. In G. D. Burrows, T. Norman, & B. Davis (Eds), *Drugs in Psychiatry: Vol. 3, Antipsychotics.* Amsterdam: Amsterdam-Elsevier Biomedical Press.

Campbell, M., Fish, B., David, R., Shapiro, T., Collins, P., & Koh, C. (1972a). Response to triiodothyronine and dextroamphetamine: A study of preschool schizophrenic children. *Journal of Autism and Childhood Schizophrenia, 2,* 343–358.

Campbell, M., Fish, B., Korein, J., Shapiro, T., Collins, P., & Koh, C. (1972b). Lithium and chlorpromazine: A controlled crossover study of hyperactive severely disturbed young children. *Journal of Autism and Childhood Schizophrenia, 2,* 234–263.

Campbell, M., Fish, B., Shapiro, T., & Floyd, A., Jr. (1970). Thiothixene in young disturbed children: A pilot study. *Archives of General Psychiatry, 23,* 70–72.

Campbell, M., Fish, B., Shapiro, T., & Floyd, A., Jr. (1971). Study of Molindone in disturbed preschool children. *Current Therapeutic Research, 13,* 28–33.

Campbell, M., Fish, B., Shapiro, T., & Floyd, A., Jr. (1972c). Acute responses of schizophrenic children to a sedative and a "stimulating" neuroleptic: A pharmacologic yardstick. *Current Therapeutic Research, 14,* 759–766.

Campbell, M., Geller, B., & Cohen, I. L. (1977). Current status of drug research and treatment with autistic children. *Journal of Pediatric Psychology, 2,* 153–161.

Campbell, M., & Green, W. H. (1985). Pervasive developmental disorders of childhood. In H. I. Kaplan and B. J. Sadock (Eds.), *Comprehensive Textbook of Psychiatry/IV* (4th ed.). Baltimore: Williams & Wilkins. pp. 1672–1683.

Campbell, M., Grega, D. M., Green, W. H., & Bennett, W. G. (1983a). Neuroleptic-induced dyskinesias in children. *Clinical Neuropharmacology, 6,* 207–222.

Campbell, M., Green, W. H., Anderson, L. T., & Deutsch, S. I. (1985). *Childhood Pharmacology.* Beverly Hills: Sage Publications.

Campbell, M., Perry, R., Bennett, W. G., Small, A. M., Green, W. H., Grega, D. M., Schwartz, V., & Anderson, L. (1983b). Long term therapeutic efficacy and drug related abnormal movements: A prospective study of haloperidol in autistic children. *Psychopharmacology Bulletin, 19*(1), 80–82.

Campbell, M., Petti, T. A., Green, W.H., Cohen, I. L., Genieser, N. B., & David, R. (1980). Some physical parameters of young autistic children. *Journal of the American Academy of Child Psychiatry, 19,* 193–212.

Campbell, M., Small, A. M., Green, W. H., Jennings, S. J., Perry, R., Bennett, W. G., & Anderson, L. (1984). A comparison of haloperidol and lithium in hospitalized aggressive conduct disorder children. *Archives of General Psychiatry, 41,* 650–656.

Campbell, M., Small, A. M., Collins, P. J., Friedman, E., David, R., & Genieser, N. B. (1976). Levodopa and levoamphetamine: A crossover study in schizophrenic children. *Current Therapeutic Research, 18,* 70–86.

Chassan, J. B. (1979). *Research design in clinical psychology and psychiatry* (2nd ed.). New York: Irvington Publishers.

Chouinard, G., & Jones, B. D. (1980). Neuroleptic-induced supersensitivity psychosis: Clinical and pharmacologic characteristics. *American Journal of Psychiatry, 137,* 16–21.

Christensen, D. E. (1973). Combined effects of methylphenidate (Ritalin) and a classroom behavior modification program in reducing the hyperkinetic behaviors of institutionalized mental retardates. Thesis submitted for the degree of doctor of philosophy in psychology, University of Illinois at Urbana-Champaign.

Cohen, I. L., Campbell, M., Posner, D., Small, A.M., Triebel, D., & Anderson, L. T. (1980). Behavioral effects of haloperidol in young autistic children: An objective analysis using a within-subjects reversal design. *Journal of the American Academy of Child Psychiatry, 19,* 665–677.

Creak, M. (1964). Schizophrenic syndrome in childhood. Further progress report of a working party. *Developmental Medicine and Child Neurology, 6,* 530–535.

Deutsch, S. I., Campbell, M., Perry, R., Green, W. H., Poland, R. E., & Rubin, R. T. (1985). Plasma growth hormone response to insulin-induced hypoglycemia in infantile autism: A pilot study. *Journal of Autism and Developmental Disorders, 15.*

Die Trill, M. L., Wolsky, B. B., Shell, J., Green, W. H., Perry, R., & Campbell, M. (1984). Effects of long term haloperidol treatment on intellectual functioning in autistic children: A pilot study. Paper presented at the 31st Annual Meeting of the American Academy of Child Psychiatry, Toronto, Canada, October 10–14, 1984.

DiMascio, H., & Shader, R. I. (1970). Behavioral toxicity, Part I: Definition and Part II: Psychomotor functions. In R. I. Shader and A. DiMascio (Eds.), *Psychotropic drug side effects* (pp. 124–131). Baltimore: Williams & Wilkins.

DiMascio, A., Soltys, J. J., & Shader, R. I. (1970). Psychotropic drug side effects in children. In R. I. Shader & A. DiMascio (Eds.), *Psychotropic drug side effects* (pp. 235–260). Baltimore: Williams & Wilkins.

Ebert, M. E., & Shader, R. I. (1970a). Hemotological effects. In R. I. Shader & A. DiMascio (Eds.), *Psychotropic drug side effects*(pp. 164–174). Baltimore: Williams & Wilkins.

Ebert, M. E., & Shader, R. I. (1970b). Hepatic effects. In R. I. Shader & A. DiMascio (Eds.), *Psychotropic drug side effects* (pp. 175–197). Baltimore: Williams & Wilkins.

Eggins, L., Barker, P., & Walker, R. J. (1975). A study of the heights and weights of different groups of disturbed children. *Child Psychiatry and Human Development, 5*(4), 203–208.

Engelhardt, D. M., & Polizos, P. (1978). Adverse effects of pharmacotherapy in childhood psychosis. In M. A. Lipton, A. DiMascio, & K. F. Killam (Eds.), *Psychopharmacology: A generation of progress* (pp. 1463–1469). New York: Raven Press.

Engelhardt, D. M., & Polizos, P. (1980). Dyskinetic and neurological complications in children treated with psychotropic medication. In W. E. Fann, R. C. Smith, J. M. Davis, & E. F. Domino (Eds.), *Tardive dyskinesia. Research and treatment* (pp. 193–199). Jamaica, New York: Spectrum Publications.

Engelhardt, D. M., Polizos, P., Waizer, J., & Hoffman, S. P. (1973). A double-blind comparison of fluphenazine and haloperidol in outpatient schizophrenic children. *Journal of Autism and Childhood Schizophrenia, 3,* 128–137.

Faretra, G., Dooher, L., & Dowling, J. (1970). Comparison of haloperidol and fluphenazine in disturbed children. *American Journal of Psychiatry, 126,* 1670–1673.

Fish, B. (1960). Drug therapy in child psychiatry: Pharmacological aspects. *Comprehensive Psychiatry, 1,* 212–227.

Fish, B. (1968). Methodology in child psychopharmacology. In D. H. Efron, J. O. Cole, J. Levine, & J. R. Wittenborn (Eds.), *Psychopharmacology, A Review of Progress, 1957–1967.*

Washington, DC.: Public Health Service Publication No. 1836, U. S. Government Printing Office, pp. 989–1001.

Fish, B. (1970). Psychopharmacologic response of chronic schizophrenic adults as predictors of responses in young schizophrenic children. *Psychopharmacology Bulletin, 6,* 12–15.

Fish, B. (1975). Biological antecedents of psychosis in children. In D. X. Freedman (Ed.), *The biology of the major psychoses: A comparative analysis.* (Association for Research in Nervous and Mental Disease, vol. 50), New York: Raven Press.

Fish, B., Shapiro, T., & Campbell, M. (1966). Long-term prognosis and the response of schizophrenic children to drug therapy: A controlled study of trifluoperazine. *American Journal of Psychiatry, 123,* 32–39.

Gardos, G. (1981). Dystonic reaction during maintenance antipsychotic therapy. *American Journal of Psychiatry, 138,* 114–115.

Gardos, G., & Cole, J. O. (1980). Problems in the assessment of tardive dyskinesia. In W. E. Fann, R. C. Smith, J. M. Davis, & E. F. Domino (Eds.), *Tardive dyskinesia, research and treatment* (pp. 201–214). Jamaica, New York: Spectrum Publications.

Gardos, G., Cole, J. O., & La Brie, R. (1977). The assessment of tardive dyskinesia. *Archives of General Psychiatry, 34,* 1206–1212.

Geller, B., Guttmacher, L. B., & Bleeg, M. (1981). Coexistence of childhood onset pervasive developmental disorder and attention deficit disorder with hyperactivity. *American Journal of Psychiatry, 138,* 388–389.

Geller, E., Ritvo, E. R., Freeman, B. J., & Yuwiler, A. (1982). Preliminary observations on the effect of fenfluramine on blood serotonin and symptoms in three autistic boys. *New England Journal of Medicine, 307,* 165–169.

Gershon, S. (1973). Clinical standards in pediatric psychopharmacology. *Psychopharmacology Bulletin, Special Issue, Pharmacotherapy of Children.*

Green, W. H., Campbell, M., Wolsky, B. B., Deutsch, S. I., Golden, R. R., & Cicero, S. D. (1984). Effects of short and long term haloperidol administration on growth in young autistic children. Paper presented at the 31st Annual Meeting of the American Academy of Child Psychiatry, Toronto, Canada, October 10–14, 1984.

Green, W. H., Campbell, M., Hardesty, A. S., Grega, D. M., Padron-Gayol, M., Shell, J., & Erlenmeyer-Kimling, L. (1984). A comparison of schizophrenic and autistic children. *Journal of the American Academy of Child Psychiatry, 23,* 399–409.

Group for the Advancement of Psychiatry (GAP). (1975). *Pharmacotherapy and psychotherapy: Paradoxes, problems and progress* (Vol. IX, Report No. 93).

Gualtieri, C. T., Barnhill, J., McGimsey, J., & Schell, D. (1980). Tardive dyskinesia and other movement disorders in children treated with psychotropic drugs. *Journal of the American Academy of Child Psychiatry, 19,* 491–510.

Gualtieri, C. T., Breuning, S. E., Schroeder, S. R., & Quade, D. (1982). Tardive dyskinesia in mentally retarded children, adolescents and young adults: North Carolina and Michigan Studies. *Psychopharmacology Bulletin, 18*(1), 62–65.

Himwich, H. E. (1960). Biochemical and neurophysiological action of psychoactive drugs. In L. Uhr & J. G. Miller (Eds.), *Drugs and behavior* (pp. 41–48). New York: Wiley.

Irwin, S. (1968). A rational framework for the development, evaluation, and use of psychoactive drugs. *American Journal of Psychiatry, 124,* 1–19 (Supplement).

Kanner, L. (1943). Autistic disturbances of affective contact. *Nervous Child, 2,* 217–250.

Klein, D. F., Gittelman, R., Quitkin, F., & Rifkin, A. (1980). *Diagnosis and drug treatment of psychiatric disorders: Adults and childrens* (2nd ed). Baltimore: Williams & Wilkins.

van der Kolk, B. A., Shader, R. I., & Greenblatt, D. J. (1978). Autonomic effects of psychotropic drugs. In M. A. Lipton, A. DiMascio, & E. F. Killam (Eds.), *Psychopharmacology: A generation of progress* (pp. 1009–1020). New York: Raven Press.

Kolko, D. J., Anderson, L. T., & Campbell, M. (1980). Sensory preference and overselective responding in autistic children. *Journal of Autism and Developmental Disorders, 10*(3), 259–271.

Kolvin, I. (1971). Psychoses in childhood—a comparative study. In M. Rutter (Ed.), *Infantile autism: Concepts, characteristics, and treatment* (pp. 7–26). Edinburgh: Churchill Livingstone.

Kydd, R. R., & Werry, J. S. (1982). Schizophrenia in children under 16 years. *Journal of Autism and Developmental Disorders, 12,* 343–358.

LeVann, L. J. (1969). Haloperidol in the treatment of behavioural disorders in children and adolescents. *Canadian Psychiatric Association Journal, 14*(2), 217–220.

Lovaas, O. I., & Newsom, C.D. (1976). Behavior modification with psychotic children. In H. Leitenberg (Ed.), *Handbook of behavior modification and behavior therapy* (pp. 303–360) Englewood Cliffs, N. J.: Prentice-Hall.

McGlashan, T. H., & Cleary, P. (1976). Clinical laboratory test standards for schizophrenic research subjects. *ECDEU Assessment Manual,* DHEW Publication No. (ADM) 76–338, pp. 379–382.

McGlashan, T. H., & Cleary, P. (1975). Clinical laboratory test standards for a sample of schizophrenics. *Psychopharmacologia, 44*(3), 281–285.

Naruse, H., Nagahata, Y., Nakane, K., Shirahashi, M., Takesada, M., Yamazaki, K. (1982). A multi-center double-blind trial of pimozide (Orap), haloperidol and placebo in children with behavioral disorders, using crossover design. *Acta Paedopsychiatrica, 48,* 173–184.

Pangalila-Ratulangi, E. A. (1973). Pilot evaluation of Orap® (Pimozide, R6238) in child psychiatry. *Psychiatria, Neurologia, Neurochirurgia, 76,* 17–27.

Paulson, G. W., Rizvi, C. A., & Crane, G. E. (1975). Tardive dyskinesia as a possible sequel of long-term therapy with phenothiazines. *Clinical Pediatrics, 14,* 953–955.

Platt, J. E., Campbell, M., Green, W. H., and Grega, D. M. (1984). Cognitive effects of lithium carbonate and haloperidol in treatment resistant aggressive children. *Archives of General Psychiatry, 41,* 657–662.

Poland, R. E., Campbell, M., Rubin, R. T., Perry, R., & Anderson, L. (1982). Relationship of serum haloperidol levels and clinical response in autistic children. 13th CINP Congress, Abstracts, Vol. II, p. 591.

Pool, D., Bloom, W. Mielke, D. H., Roniger, J. J., & Gallant, D. M. (1976). A controlled evaluation of loxitane in seventy-five adolescent schizophrenic patients. *Current Therapeutic Research, 19,* 99–104.

Psychopharmacology Bulletin. (1973). Pharmacotherapy of children, Special Issue.

Rapoport, J. L., and Ismond, D. R. (1983). *DSM-III training guide in child psychiatry.* New York: Brunner/Mazel.

Realmuto, G. N., Erickson, W. D., Yellin, A. M., Hopwood, J. H., & Greenberg, L. M. (1984). *American Journal of Psychiatry, 141,* 440–442.

Ritvo, E. R., Freeman, B. J., Geller, E., & Yuwiler, A. (1983). Effects of fenfluramine on 14 outpatients with the syndrome of autism. *Journal of the American Academy of Child Psychiatry, 22,* 549–558.

Ritvo, E. R., Yuwiler, A., Geller, E., Kales, A., Rashkis, S., Schicor, A., Plotkin, S., Axelrod, R., & Howard, C. (1971). *Journal of Autism and Childhood Schizophrenia, 1,* 190–205.

Rivera-Calimlim, L., Nasrallah, H., Strauss, J., & Lasagna, L. (1976). Clinical response and plasma levels: Effect of dose, dosage, schedules, and drug interactions on plasma chlorpromazine levels. *American Journal of Psychiatry, 133,* 646–652.

Roche, A. F., Lipman, R. S., Overall, J. E., & Hung, W. (1979). The effects of stimulant medication on the growth of hyperkinetic children. *Pediatrics, 63*(6), 847–850.

Rogeness, G. A., & Macedo, C. A. (1983). Therapeutic response of a schizophrenic boy to a methylphenidate-chlorpromazine combination. *American Journal of Psychiatry, 140,* 932–933.

Simeon, J., Gross, M., & Mueller, J. (1977). Neuroleptic drug effects on children's body weight and height. *Psychopharmacology Bulletin, 13*(2), 50–53.

Simeon, J., Saletu, B., Saletu, M., Itil, T. M., & Da Silva, J. (1973). Thiothixene in childhood psychoses. Paper presented at the Third International Symposium on Phenothiazines. Rockville, Maryland.

Simon, G. B., & Gillies, S. M. (1964). Some physical characteristics of a group of psychotic children. *British Journal of Psychiatry, 110,* 104–107.

Simpson, G.M., Lee, J.H., Zoubok, B., & Gardos, G. (1979). A rating scale for tardive dyskinesia. *Psychopharmacology* (Berlin), *64,* 171–179.

Sprague, R. L. (1972). Psychopharmacology and learning disabilities. *Journal of Operational Psychiatry, 3,* 56–67.

Tarjan, G., Loery, V. E., & Wright, S. W. (1957). Use of chlorpromazine in two hundred seventy-eight mentally deficient patients. *Journal of Diseases of Children, 94,* 294–300.

Thompson, T., & Schuster, C. R. (1968). *Behavioral pharmacology.* Englewood Cliffs, N. J.: Prentice-Hall.

Turner, D. A., Purchatzke, G., Gift, T., Farmer, C., & Uhlenhuth, E. H. (1974). Intensive design in evaluating anxiolytic agents. In J. Levine, B. C. Schiele, & W. J. R. Taylor (Eds.). *Principles and techniques of human research and therapeutics.* (Vol. 8) Mt. Kisco, NY: Futura Publishing.

Villeneuve, A. (1972). The rabbit syndrome: A peculiar extrapyramidal reaction. *Canadian Psychiatric Association Journal, 17,* 69–72.

Waizer, J., Polizos, P., Hoffman, S. P., Engelhardt, D. M., & Margolis, R. A. (1972). A single-blind evaluation of thiothixene with outpatient schizophrenic children. *Journal of Autism and Childhood Schizophrenia, 2,* 378–386.

Werry, J. S., & Aman, M. G. (1975). Methylphenidate and haloperidol in children. *Archives of General Psychiatry, 32,* 790–795.

Winsberg, B. G., & Yepes, L. E. (1978). Antipsychotics. In J. S. Werry(Ed.), *Pediatric Psychopharmacology* (pp. 234–273). New York: Brunner/Mazel.

Wolpert, A., Hagamen, M. B., & Merlis, S. (1967). A comparative study of thiothixene and trifluoperazine in childhood schizophrenia. *Current Therapeutic Research, 9,* 482–485.

World Health Organization (WHO) (1967). *Scientific group on psychopharmacology: research in psychopharmacology.* Tech. Rep. Series No. 371. Geneva: World Health Organization.

Young, J. G., Kavanagh, M. E., Anderson, G. M., Shaywitz, B. A., & Cohen, D. J. (1982). Clinical neurochemistry of autism and associated disorders. *Journal of Autism and Developmental Disorders, 12,* 147–165.

Affective Disorders in Childhood and Adolescence

JOAQUIM PUIG-ANTICH M.D., NEAL D. RYAN M.D.,
and HARRIS RABINOVICH M.D.

The existence of affective disorders in children and adolescents gained increasing acceptance during the last decade, although accurate clinical descriptions had been published as far back as the 1960s (Puig-Antich, 1980). Concurrently, clinicians are increasingly aware of the use of semi-structured interview techniques and DSM-III diagnostic criteria (1980) for the assessment of affective symptoms in youngsters. This new clinical awareness, like the body of existing research on these conditions, is more extensive in regard to prepubertal children than adolescents, and attends almost exclusively to depressive disorders rather than different types of bipolar illness. The latter may be much more prevalent than generally thought, especially in adolescence, as we will note later. These subtypes may be crucial to proper psychopharmacological treatment of these conditions.

The most difficult aspects of this evolution in child psychiatric nosology have been the reestablishment of the importance of phenomenological analysis, as opposed to a purely psychodynamic viewpoint that dominated the field until recently, and the ongoing integration of biological and psychodynamic viewpoints. Both phenomenology and psychobiology are crucial to solid advances in psychopharmacology. Attribution of etiology to interpersonal events (within or outside the family) when there is evidence only of temporal association for the onset or course of psychiatric disorders looms very large in the case of children and youth. Their psychological immaturity, the availability and readiness of environmental influences, and the general adult reluctance to recognize psychological suffering in children, all make this temptation very strong. Thus, a significant tendency still exists to overestimate the role of environmental variables and underestimate biological determinants. The use of psychopharmacological agents is strongly associated, in the minds of many lay and mental health professionals, with an implicit recognition of biological determinism for mental phenomena, eliciting strong emotional reactions to what should be simply a set of scientific questions and their answers, arrived at by systematic clinical research.

One persistent reaction to a phenomenological approach was an overestimation of the importance of developmental differences in affective symptoms and diagnoses between adults and youngsters. The use of diagnostic criteria for affective disorders in adults was challenged as inappropriate for younger samples. The claim was made (Phillips, 1979) that such an approach was not suitable because it was not developmentally based, but no alternative proposal was put forth, other than the ill-fated concept of masked depression (Kovacs & Beck, 1977; Carlson & Cantwell, 1980; Cytryn et al., 1980; Puig-Antich, 1982a). The passage of time led to the current consensus on the use of DSM-III criteria for school-aged children and, implicitly, to an acceptance that the variability between children and adults in affective symptoms can in great part be subsumed by the necessary adaptations in interview techniques. Although the frequency of some symptoms do vary with age and can be convincingly related to developmental patterns, the nature of some symptoms does not vary with age. Thus, the use of DSM-III criteria are now standard for clinical practice.

DEVELOPMENTAL TRENDS IN AFFECTIVE DISORDER TYPOLOGY

Understanding the phenomenological complexity of the affective disorders in children and adolescents is crucial for an understanding of psychopharmacological treatment. Partly because of progress in systematic assessment there have been four recent nosological developments in the area of juvenile affective disorders: (1) The demise of the concept of masked depression; (2) the demonstration of the existence of endogenous and psychotic forms of affective disorders (Strober et al., 1982, Carlson and Strober, 1979); (3) the initial validation of the diagnosis of dysthymic disorder (Kovacs et al., 1984a; Kovacs et al., 1984b); and (4) the recognition of psychosocial and relationship deficits that accompany major depression in children (Puig-Antich, et al., in press).

Although the theoretical construct of "masked depression" was reasonable (Rutter, 1972), no systematic criteria were ever proposed that could reliably distinguish children in whom "depressive equivalent" symptoms masked a depressive disorder from those in whom it did not. Thus the diagnosis could be made on no evidence other than clinical intuition, carrying with it the risk of overprescription of powerful psychopharmacological agents. The concept of "masked depression" did not withstand careful examination. Depressive "equivalents" were not found to be associated with depressive mood or syndrome (Pearce, 1977; Kuperman & Stewart, 1979). It became quite clear that the so-called "masking" symptoms were either presenting complaints (Carlson & Cantwell, 1980; Kovacs & Beck, 1977) or associated features (Puig-Antich, 1982a) of major depression.

But developmental differences in clinical presentation of affective disorders do exist. For example, the recent findings that a proportion of children (Chambers & Puig-Antich, 1982) and adolescents (Strober et al., 1982) with a major depressive disorder, evidence psychotic symptoms (depressive hallucinations and delusions) have implications for developmental nosology. Depressive delusions are very rare in prepubertal children; almost all such psychotically depressed youngsters present only hallucinations. Depressive delusions are more frequent in adolescence, although hallucinations also occur. In contrast, in psychotically depressed adults, delusions predominate. This apparent age effect suggests that the younger child's cognitive immaturity makes the development of a depressive delusional system unlikely. In adults, psychotic depressions are less likely to respond to standard tricyclic antidepressants (TCAs), (Spiker et al., in press; Glassman et al., 1975). Unfortunately, most recent psychopharmacological studies of severely depressed youngsters have not taken psychotic subtype into account (Kramer & Feiguine, 1983; Preskorn et al., 1982; Geller et al., 1983).

A third recent nosologic development has been the description and validation of a chronic, relatively low-grade protracted depressive picture among school-aged children and early adolescents (Kovacs et al., 1984a and b). In DSM-III (1980), this phenomenon is labeled dysthymic disorder. The prognostic importance of dysthymia in children is similar to that for the same disorder in adults (Keller et al., 1982a and b). Furthermore, by virtue of its association with major depression, and its potential to induce long term psychosocial disability (Puig-Antich et al., in press, a and b), the recognition of juvenile dysthymia is clinically very important. In addition, its recognition in association with episodes of major depression in psychopharmacological studies targeting children with major depressive disorder has not been standard method until now, but should be done routinely in the future, as it may have significance for both short and long term outcome.

The demonstration of psychosocial deficits and impairments in relationships that are associated with major depression in prepuberty (Puig-Antich et al., in press) and their lack of full resolution in spite of pharmacologically induced affective recovery, echo the well known findings concerning the social functioning of adult depressives (Weissman et al., 1971, 1974). These findings also may serve to delimit the goals of psychopharmacological treatment, provide guidelines as to the variables that should be assessed in future treatment studies, and inform recommendations about optimal timing and sequence of psychotherapeutic and psychopharmacological interventions.

Another important phenomenological aspect of affective illness in youngsters is the extent of bipolar clinical pictures or outcomes in this age group. Frank manic-depressive illness, including full depressive and manic episodes, has been convincingly described in adolescents for many years (Campbell, 1952; Carlson & Strober, 1978, 1979). But this presentation is exceedingly rare in prepuberty (Anthony & Scott, 1960) and should be applied to preschoolers only with great caution. Also, it should be appreciated that mixed disorders, rapid cycling, hypomania, and cyclothymia can and do occur in adolescents, either spontaneously or pharmacologically triggered by antidepressants. (Descriptions and discussions of these difficult-to-recognize bipolar presentations can be found in Akiskal & Puzantian, 1979; Himmelhoch, 1979; Dunner, 1979). In fact, extrapolating from these data in young adults, it is likely that over half of adolescents with bipolar disorder do not show typical full-fledged mania, but instead display less easily diagnosable forms of the disorder. It should be mentioned at this point that unipolar depression is a very heterogeneous depressive subtype in adolescence, and in all likelihood includes many patients who later in life will turn out to be bipolar I or II (or unipolar II) (Akiskal, 1983).

Mixed states are diagnosed in patients who simultaneously present significant symptoms of depression and mania. Mixed disorders or states should be suspected in adolescents where irritability and anger constitute a major component of the clinical picture of a major depressive disorder. They should also be considered in any adolescent with a primary diagnosis of major depression and a secondary diagnosis of conduct disorder, since a prolonged mixed state with high irritability may be associated with deviant behaviors that are mistaken for conduct disorder. Mixed states are very important for treatment purposes as TCAs are likely to fail or to aggravate the condition, and these forms of bipolar illness in youngsters can be rather resistant to other treatments. Mixed states may present spontaneously or may be precipitated by drug and alcohol abuse (Himmelhoch, 1979). Either way, it is not an uncommon initial presentation of bipolar illness.

The justification of any treatment lies in its risk—benefit ratio compared to the risks inherent in the natural history of the disorder. Prospective follow-up studies of carefully selected and uniformly diagnosed samples of depressed children and adolescents were initiated only in the last five to six years. Therefore, the long-term outcome of juvenile depressive illness is not yet known, although it is strongly suspected to be continuous with adult affective disorders. Intriguingly, convergent findings have been reported by several projects in progress that apply similar assessment and diagnostic strategies to depressed children (Kovacs et al., 1984a and b), adolescents (Strober, 1983) and adults (Keller et al, 1982a and b). The evidence is quite strong that the rates of recovery from major depression and the risk of relapse or recurrence are similar across these three age groups. These studies indicate that the course is frequently chronic, persistent, and recurrent, with accumulating widespread functional and psychosocial deficits (Puig-Antich et al., in press, a and b). They provide the most convincing argument for the systematic exploration of pharmacological and psychotherapeutic treatment techniques.

DEVELOPMENTAL TRENDS IN DRUG-RELATED VARIABLES

Besides age-related changes in typology, the effect of age on pharmacokinetics should be considered in assessing drug effects in affective disorders in children (Rane & Wilson, 1983). Although there is no evidence of drug absorption differences between adults and school-aged children, there are major age-related differences in body composition, liver mass to body mass ration, metabolic pace, and renal excretion, influencing drug distribution, metabolism, and elimination. In this age group in general there is a higher rate of elimination of drugs from plasma, lower half-lives and lower plasma level to dose ratios than in adults (Rane & Wilson, 1983). As a result, merely fractionating (according to weight) the adult dose of a medication for the equivalent disorder in children is always unwarranted, underscoring the need for separate drug efficacy studies in children and the fallacy of extrapolating from adult data.

These considerations have direct bearing to the pharmacological treatment of affective disorders in youngsters. Imipramine (IMI), a prototypic TCA, and its main active metabolite desmethylimipramine (DMI), have a shorter half-life in children than in adults (Perel, 1974). Faster metabolic rate, increased relative liver mass, and lower relative adipose mass are likely to be at least partly responsible for this effect. Little is known regarding any possible child—adult differences in metabolite production or renal excretion. There is evidence in children that a lower percentage of IMI is bound to plasma proteins, resulting in a much higher proportion of free IMI and DMI (Pruitt & Dayton, 1971; Winsberg et al., 1974) in plasma. The latter's role in either therapeutic or side effects in children is not known. In general, children are relatively more susceptible to cardiotoxic effects of tricyclic antidepressants than are adults (Weinberg et al., 1973; Saraf et al., 1974; Preskorn et al., 1983). They are also likely to need a higher weight corrected IMI dose than do adults when used for the same indication (i.e., major depression).

Lithium poses another type of problem in children. Lithium excretion occurs mainly through the kidney, and renal function in most children is more efficient than later in life. As a result children usually tolerate lithium quite well and frequently will require higher doses for their body weight than do adults in order to achieve plasma levels in the therapeutic range (Schou, 1972).

The above instances exemplify the age-dependent pharmacokinetic variability of some psychoactive drugs, which can affect treatment response in children and adolescents. Usually, but not always, school-aged children will need somewhat higher weight corrected dosages than adults. In addition, the possibility of developmental variations in pharmacodynamics may also affect treatment response in youngsters. The clearest example is the lack of euphoria in response to dextroamphetamine in normal children (Rapoport et al., 1980) which, together with the rarity of mania in prepuberty, suggests that puberty-induced (or associated) neuroregulatory changes are necessary to produce or sustain elation.

ANTIDEPRESSANT DRUGS IN CHILDHOOD AFFECTIVE DISORDERS

Early Trials with Antidepressant Drugs

The use of antidepressants in children for the treatment of "depression" began prior to nosological consensus. Results from open trials reported uniformly high response rates (Frommer, 1968, Connell, 1972; Kuhn & Kuhn, 1972; Lucas et al., 1965). For a variety of fundamental methodological limitations including lack of controls, unstandardized assessment methods and diagnostic criteria, low drug dosage, and variable length of therapeutic trial, these studies were quite difficult to interpret.

In two studies, diagnostic criteria were used (Weinberg et al., 1973; Puig-Antich et al., 1978). In the first, 19 children fitting Weinberg's criteria were treated with imipramine or amitriptyline. There was no clear rationale nor randomness in the choice of drug assignment. The trial lasted from 3–7 months. Dosage was not reported. Although the measure(s) of improvement was not reported, the authors indicated that all but one of the children treated improved, while only six of those youngsters not receiving TCAs showed improvement.

In the other (pilot) study, eight prepubertal children who fit RDC criteria for major depressive disorder were treated with IMI up to 4.5 mg/kg/day in an open design for 6–8 weeks. Semistructured symptom-oriented interviews and electrocardiographic (EKG) monitoring were used. Six patients responded. The other two received lower IMI dosages because of conservative handling of side effects. One of these patients responded when the dose was adjusted upwards to 5 mg/kg/day after the trial.

These studies suggested that TCAs may be effective in depressive disorders in childhood and adolescence. Together with the advances in assessment and diagnosis (Orvaschel et al., 1980), two different and complementary methodologies have been employed: (1) The classical double-blind placebo controlled study and (2) studies exploring the relationship between drug and metabolite plasma levels and clinical response. Probably because of IMI's use in children with enuresis, aggressive–hyperactive behavior, and separation anxiety disorder, most studies in depressed children have used IMI. The results will be presented separately for pre and postpubertal children.

Double-Blind Placebo Controlled Studies in Prepubertal Children

Frommer (1967) was the first to conduct a controlled double-blind study with crossover design of antidepressant medication in children diagnosed as depressed. She compared the combination of phenelzine and chlordiazepoxide for two weeks to phenobarbital for two weeks in 32 children. Only half of the children improved on phenobarbital, compared to 78 percent who improved on the combination. Besides the assessment and diagnostic problems inherent to the time this study was performed, which would limit generalization to other samples, the design of the study does not allow for firm conclusions regarding its own sample. The effect found may be due to the therapeutic action of phenelzine alone, of chlordiazepoxide alone, or of the combination. Two weeks are frequently not enough time to obtain antidepressant effects of phenelzine in adult studies, and barely enough time for full MAO inhibition to be established with proper dosage of this drug (Robinson et al., 1978a and b). Furthermore, this study used a relatively low dose of phenelzine. The short time period makes a specific antidepressant action an unlikely explanation for the results.

Puig-Antich et al. (in press) studied the efficacy of IMI in prepubertal major depression using a five week double-blind placebo controlled design after a diagnostic protocol including two independent K-SADS-P evaluations blind to each other done two weeks apart. Patients had to fit RDC criteria for major depression both times. Thirty-eight mostly outpatient children completed protocol, 22 had received placebo, and 16 IMI. Dosages went up to 5 mg/kg/day, although in half the sample dose was lower, mostly because of overly restrictive EKG safety criteria. No significant differences were found between the two groups in any of the measures utilized. Response rates were 56 percent for the IMI groups and 68 percent for the placebo. This study was done conjointly with a plasma level to clinical response design that is discussed below.

Kashani et al. (1984) compared amitriptyline (AMI) and placebo in a randomized double-blind crossover design in nine prepubertal depressed children. Each phase lasted four weeks. The study was preceded by a three to four week inpatient drug-free baseline period. Dosage was low: 1.5 mg/kg/day. As a group, children showed a trend toward greater improvement during the drug phase than during the placebo phase, but this was not significant. Because of the small sample size, the results are inconclusive. It is not clear in the report if any children were excluded because of spontaneous improvement in the inpatient service during the baseline phase. Outcome of each phase was measured with the Bellevue Depression Index. The possibility of carryover effects was not taken into account at the time the data were analyzed.

In summary, there is as yet no evidence that any antidepressant is better than placebo in treating prepubertal major depressives, especially because of the unexpectedly high placebo response rate in the largest study. Another reason, low IMI dosages, will become apparent as we discuss the evidence relating pharmacokinetic factors to clinical outcome.

TCA Plasma Levels and Clinical Response in Prepubertal Major Depressive Disorder

At the time of this writing, only three studies have addressed this question. Preskorn et al. (1982) demonstrated a relationship between plasma levels of IMI and DMI and clinical response in 20 prepubertal inpatient children diagnosed as major depressive disorder. The study lasted 6 weeks divided into two consecutive three week periods. At a fixed dose of 75 mg/day, for three weeks only four children responded. Their plasma levels were between 125 and 225 ng/ml. None of the 15 children above 225 ng/ml, or below 125 ng/ml, responded. Dose adjustments were carried out at the onset of the second three week period. At the end of the sixth treatment week, 11 of the 12 children whose plasma levels fell within the 125–225 ng/ml range had responded, while there was only one responder among the four children who had completed protocol and were outside the range.

The data in this study suggest that three weeks is an insufficient time interval to assess antidepressant response to IMI in children. By limiting the chances for clinical response, the first part of this study was biased against finding a relationship with pharmacokinetic variables. The conclusion of a curvilinear relationship proposed by the authors should be taken very cautiously. In the upper side of plasma level range this relationship is based only on four cases at three weeks and two cases at six weeks. This finding needs confirmation. If replicated, the pharmacokinetics of IMI would have different implications for clinical response in different age groups. (Friedel et al., 1979; Glassman et al., 1977; Reisby et al., 1977).

A curvilinear plasma level–clinical response relationship in the treatment of depressive illness has been demonstrated for nortriptyline in adults (Asberg et al., 1971, Kragh-Sorensen et al., 1973, 1976). Preliminary findings in a small sample size of children with major depression are consistent with a similar relationship in this age group (Geller et al., 1983), although the evidence is not yet sufficient to support a firm conclusion.

Puig-Antich et al. (in press) studied IMI + DMI plasma level–clinical response relationship in 30 prepubertal children with major depressive disorder, a sample that overlapped with that in the placebo contrast. The IMI dose was up to 5 mg/kg/day, and the protocol lasted five weeks. The outcome measure was the K-SADS (last week), which integrates information from the mother's interview about the child and from the child's interview about himself. There were two main findings: maintenance plasma levels of IMI plus DMI were positively related to clinical response, so that plasma levels in the responders were significantly higher than in the nonresponders $(p. < .01)$. In addition, pretreatment severity was negatively associated to clinical response $(p < .01)$, and psychotic subtype was associated with a lower response rate $(p < .05)$. In summary, it appears that when prepubertal children receive IMI as treatment for an episode of major depression, clinical response is more likely to lower the severity of the symptoms and the higher the plasma levels of the drug and its main metabolite.

When the results from this plasma level study were combined with those of the placebo contrast, two trends emerged: Children with major depression who were maintained on a low IMI plus DMI plasma level showed a response rate much lower than placebo, while of those maintained at a plasma level over 150 ng/ml, almost all responded. The possibility that low plasma levels inhibit placebo response has to be considered further, and we will come back to it. There was no evidence in this study of a curvilinear relationship between IMI and DMI plasma levels and clinical response.

At the present time, there is more evidence supporting the effectiveness of IMI in prepubertal major depression than a few years ago. The results from the plasma level–clinical response studies of IMI suggest its effectiveness as an antidepressant in this age group. They also suggest that antidepressant response to IMI in prepubertal children can be optimized by titrating the dose of IMI to achieve a plasma level in the range most likely to be associated with clinical response. But all the studies so far have failed the final test: significantly better antidepressant effects than placebo in the double-blind random antidepressant design. Further studies are necessary to evaluate this question. They could incorporate in their design dose titration to optimal plasma level range, higher absolute dose limit (with proper monitoring) and selecting out early placebo responders by an initial placebo washout phase.

TCA Treatment of Adolescent Major Depression

To date only two studies have addressed the question of effectiveness of these drugs in major depression in adolescents. In a double-blind, six week, placebo controlled study, Kramer et al. (1983) found no significant advantage of AMI 200 mg/day over placebo in adolescent inpatients with major depression. The design did not involve a crossover, and 10 patients were included in each group. Both groups showed significant improvement, thus repeating an unexpectedly high placebo response. Nevertheless, the small sample size precludes any conclusions.

In another study, Ryan and co-workers (unpublished manuscript) attempted to ascertain the relationship between IMI plus DMI maintenance plasma level and antidepressant response at six weeks in 34 adolescents with major depressive disorder. Contrary to expectations, only 44 percent of the patients responded and no relationship was found between plasma level and clinical response. Mean dose was 243 mg/day, and mean total plasma level was 284 ng/ml. No strong predictors of clinical response were found.

In summary, most of the available evidence does not support the general expectation that TCAs are effective in adolescent major depression. Although future double-blind placebo controlled studies selecting out initial placebo responders are probably indicated, it also would make sense at this point to include another type of antidepressant medication.

The Possibility of Age Influences on Antidepressant Effects of IMI

The effectiveness of IMI and other TCAs in adult depression is firmly established, albeit with considerable variability. As reviewed by Morris and Beck (1974), only 65 percent of all the double-blind placebo controlled studies in TCAs in adult depressives found a significant drug effect. As most of these are studies done during the 1950s and 1960s, the reports are incomplete by today's standards. No doubt, methodological shortcomings and compliance problems affected these results. Nevertheless, several modern studies and observations have shown convincingly that a variety of factors negatively affect the responsivity of major depression to TCAs (Wehr & Goodwin, 1979; Quitkin et al., 1983; Leibowitz et al., 1984; Matuzas et al., 1982; Spiker et al., in press; Nelson & Bowers, 1978). Bipolarity, "atypicality," psychotic symptoms, and plasma levels outside the therapeutic range are all associated with poor clinical response to TCAs in adults. It is interesting to note that plasma levels and psychotic symptoms have been also shown to influence clinical response to IMI in prepubertal major depression. Puig-Antich et al., (in press).

Age also is reported to affect TCA effectiveness in some (Raskin, 1975) but not all (Deykin & DiMascio, 1972) double-blind studies of adult depression. Patients over 40 years of age are reported to respond better than younger adults. The recent findings of a low response rate of atypical depression to 150 mg/day of IMI is also consistent with an age effect (Quitkin et al., 1983, Liebowitz et al., 1984). The studies that support a plasma level–clinical response relationship among adult depressives treated with IMI tend to concern samples of older patients. In Glassman et al.'s study (1977) the mean age was 59 years. In Reisby et al. (1977) the mean age was 51 years. These authors indicate that the older patients had higher plasma levels than their younger counterparts. Nevertheless, they also reported that the effect of plasma level in the endogenous group persisted when patients over and under 50 years were analyzed separately. But the analyses did not address possible interactions of affective typology, age, and plasma levels on clinical response.

The age range expands considerably when the above studies are contrasted with those in younger age groups. Then the possibility of strong effects of age and/or of the secretory status of sex hormones (during puberty and young adulthood) on IMI's antidepressant potency appears even more likely. From the data summarized above and that on children and adolescents, it would appear that TCA plasma level/antidepressant response correlations are much clearer in prepubertal children and older adults, the age groups outside the reproductive range. In contrast, the period of highest sex hormone secretion, adolescence and young adulthood, seem to be characterized by a poorer antidepressant response to IMI and, at least in adolescence, little relationship between plasma level and clinical outcome. Given the range of plasma levels observed by us in adolescents, it is unlikely that pharmacokinetic variables account for the lower response rate. Instead, the pharmacodynamics of IMI in this age group are more likely to be implicated. As indicated before, this may be in part due to the frequency of mixed bipolar patients in adolescent affective disorders. It may also be due to the possible effects of estrogen on imipramine antidepressant action, bearing in mind that estrogen concentrations are high in young males as well as females.

The Issue of Placebo Response

Response to placebo treatment is a baffling phenomenon, especially if placebo response is thought to indicate the absence of the disorder. By all accounts, placebo responses in major depression are not infrequent. The majority of adult studies today are preceded by a prerandomization 10-day placebo period during which 15–20 percent of patients will respond and are excluded from the study. In addition, of the patients who initially did not respond to placebo, another 15–20 percent will respond to placebo during the protocol. This placebo response may be even more frequent among severely depressed adolescents and children (Kramer, 1983; Puig-Antich et al., in press). Placebo response rates of about two-thirds have been reported. High responsivity to placebo is not characteristic of all psychiatric disorders of childhood and adolescence. For example, placebos are not very effective in attention deficit disorder with hyperactivity (Gittelman-Klein et al., 1975). Thus it may not necessarily be a question of age alone, but age within the depressive disorders.

In order to offset high placebo response rates, many investigators adopted an initial placebo washout phase. By the elimination of initial placebo responders, the placebo response rate in the controlled study is kept low. The disadvantage is that the results cannot be generalized to all the patients with depressive disorder; only to those who do not respond to an initial placebo trial. It can be argued that observation of a depressed patient one week to ten days before treatment is good clinical practice and, therefore, the placebo washout period parallels the best clinical practice. Nevertheless, placebos are rarely used clinically, and the above argument assumes that spontaneous recovery and recovery during placebo treatment are one and the same phenomenon. This assumption may not be warranted. Its consideration brings up the question of the nature of antidepressant response during placebo administration.

The high placebo response rate in youngsters with major depression contrasts with the long duration and stability of these disorders, even when such children are engaged in nonpharmacological treatments (Kovacs et al., 1984). Therefore antidepressant response to placebo in this age group may not represent just a cluster of spontaneous recoveries in a highly variable condition. Alternatively, those patients who respond to placebo may constitute phenocopies. To test this hypothesis we compared placebo responders and nonresponders for familial aggregation of depressive illness among first degree relatives. We found no significant differences or trends, suggesting that placebo responders among depressed children do not constitute phenocopies of the disorder.

A full consideration of placebo responsivity may be informative as to CNS mechanisms involved in pychological functions relevant to depression. Levine et al. (1978) studied the response of postoperative dental pain to placebo. On the average placebo produced a 50 percent reduction in pain. This effect was completely reversed by subsequent intravenous administration of naloxone, an opiate receptor blocker. This result suggests that the analgesic response to placebo was mediated by endorphins. Thus placebo effects, at least in acute pain, may have a neurobiological basis.

The phenomenology and possible mechanisms of placebo response in depressed youngsters should be investigated further. Without solid knowledge of the patterns and stability of placebo response in depression, informed decisions on treatment cannot be made. Thus currently there is no answer to the following question: Should we use placebo before active drug in prepubertal or adolescent depression? Certainly a 68 percent response rate without any risks or side effects is a very enticing possibility for any clinician. However, the main issue may be that of long term stability of antidepressant response to placebo. Thus, in our study (in press), all patients who responded to placebo at five weeks had these pills discontinued. Of these, 60 percent relapsed in less than one month. In contrast, patients who responded to imipramine had their treatment continued for three more months after the last pill. Less than one-fifth relapsed in one month. These differences in short term oucome may have been due as much to treatment duration (total of five weeks for placebo; four months for IMI patients) as to drug–placebo differences. This could not be teased out in this design.

Obviously, if it were shown that placebo response is almost certainly followed by relapse and that most patients will end up with active drug, the value of placebo treatment would be minimal. At present the long-term stability of placebo responses in depressed youngsters is not known. Further, no predictors of depression response to placebo are known in this age group. There is some evidence of differences in temporal pattern of response to antidepressant drugs and to placebo from controlled studies of adult depression (Quitkin et al., 1984), but it is not known if these are also true in depressed children and adolescents. In summary, the phenomenology of placebo response in depressed youngsters requires further study, including placebo maintenance of depressed children who respond to the initial trial, in order to elucidate the stability of this response. In future studies, the question of differential patterns and types of drug–placebo response in depressed youngsters should also be addressed.

Side Effects of TCAs in Children and Adolescents

The major side effects are cardiovascular. TCAs cardiotoxic action is similar to that of quinidine. In addition, other noncardiovascular "nuisance" side effects can occur but are much less serious. All TCAs are cardiotoxic and overdoses can result in death due to cardiac arrest, circulatory collapse, or coma (Saraf et al., 1974; Vohra et al., 1975). A case of death has been reported in a six-year-old girl who was prescribed 300 mg at bedtime, a dose equivalent to over 15 mg/kg/day (Saraf et al., 1974), but, by far, most lethal TCA overdoses in children are due to the child's accidental ingestion of the mother's antidepressant pills. In therapeutic doses, TCAs do produce small changes in EKG patterns. In fact these changes are so common that their complete absence suggests lack of compliance. The question is not if such changes should occur but up to which point should they be allowed. The most common EKG changes are a slight increase in resting heart rate (which should not be greater than 130/min), lengthening of the PR interval (to no more than .22 second), and widening of the QRS (to no more than 30 percent increase over baseline). Blood pressure and ECG should be routinely measured at baseline, before every dosage increase, and less frequently during maintenance. Dosage is increased every fourth day from 1.5 to 3, to 4, and to 5 mg/kg/day. Faster increases usually induce marked "nuisance" side effects like tiredness, sleepiness, and drowsiness, which can be easily avoided in most cases by slower titration upwards.

The blood pressure effects of TCAs in children and adolescents are most often a slight rise in both systolic and diastolic pressure, with orthostatic changes generally rare in this age group (in contrast to adults with the same drugs). An infrequent side effect seen with larger doses is forgetfulness and learning difficulties. This usually requires discontinuation of that particular tricyclic antidepressant. Children rarely exhibit the myoclonic jerks, midriasis, and increased body temperature caused by cholinergic blockade from TCAs. Seizures have been reported but they tend to occur only in children with preexisting CNS pathology (Petti & Campbell, 1975).

Because of the toxic potential of tricyclic antidepressant medication in children and adolescents, the dose should not be increased further if at any point EKG safety limits are exceeded. The maximum dosage of

AMI, IMI, or DMI is 5 mg/kg/day. Lower doses are needed where nortriptyline is used, but safety limits apply the same. Because of the risk of suicide or accidental overdose, the parent or guardian should obtain the medication and keep it in a secure place. They should be administered by the parent except in nonsuicidal older adolescents where this is not feasible.

Children and adolescents can be very sensitive to withdrawal effects. In some, if TCAs are stopped suddenly they develop an afebrile picture with symptoms of nausea, vomiting, diarrhea, abdominal pain and a flulike general myalgia, which develops between 24 and 48 hours from the last pill. All symptoms disappear one or two hours after renewal of the TCA. The most frequent cause of withdrawal effects is lack of compliance. If the physician is unaware of the latter, withdrawal effects may be interpreted as side effects. Thus, sudden onset of an acute picture with the characteristics described above in an otherwise uneventful maintenance TCA treatment should raise the question of lack of compliance. The return to baseline of the EKG measures is confirmatory. In prepubertal patients who are very sensitive to withdrawal effects we have seen them appear in the afternoon when IMI is administered as a single dose at bedtime. Redistribution of drug administration to twice or three times a day resolves this problem (frequently interpreted as a side effect).

LITHIUM IN CHILDHOOD AFFECTIVE DISORDERS

There are only limited noncontrolled experimental data on the efficacy of lithium for childhood affective disorders. Controlled adult studies demonstrating the efficacy of lithium in the prophylaxis and treatment of mania and depression (Schou et al., 1954; Bunney et al., 1968; Goodwin et al., 1969; Fieve et al., 1968; Goodwin et al., 1972; and Baron et al., 1975) suggest that lithium may be used for the same indications in childhood and adolescence. Although there is no controlled evidence, when clinicians have used lithium in the treatment of child and adolescent disorders, therapeutic and side effects seem very similar to those in adults with the same diagnosis.

Reviewing the literature of lithium use in childhood and adolescence, Youngerman and Canino (1978) found two childhood and 18 adolescent cases of typical manic depressive illness (DSM-II) successfully treated with lithium carbonate. All cases had alternating mania and depression. Some had other organic disorders including mental retardation, seizure disorders, and EEG abnormalities. There were 58 cases of lithium carbonate responsiveness in youngsters without clear alternating manic depressive symptomatology, but only 15 (2 children and 13 adolescents) were described in sufficient detail to further classify. These cases did not meet criteria for manic depressive illness, but had mood disturbances with and without mood swings, and had other concomitant psychiatric symptoms including anorexia, enuresis, epilepsy, and auditory hallucinations. This review concluded that children and adolescents who responded successfully to lithium carbonate therapy suffer major mood disturbances with an irregular cyclic pattern that may be expressed as typical bipolar disease or as recurrent stupors, frequent outbursts, or multiple suicide attempts. Children with aggressivity or hyperactivity did not in general improve with lithium unless they had concurrent periodic mood disturbances. In the better documented studies, most lithium-responsive children had a positive family history for affective disorders and frequently had a lithium-responsive parent.

Another strategy has been to study the offspring of lithium responsive, bipolar adults regardless of the child's diagnosis (McKnew et al., 1981; Dyson & Barcai, 1970). Dyson and Barcai report favorable lithium response in two hyperactive children whose parents were lithium responders. This contrasted with two controlled studies of lithium in hyperactive children (regardless of parental diagnoses) that showed no therapeutic effect (Whitehead et al., 1970; Greenhill et al., 1973). The study by McKnew et al. (1981) provides a controlled study of lithium use in affective disorders in prepubertal children and adolescents. In this study six psychiatrically ill offspring (ages 6–12) of lithium responsive manic-depressives were given lithium in a double-blind crossover study lasting 16–18 weeks. Dosage was adjusted to achieve a blood level of .8– 1.2 mEq/l while on active medication. The two children diagnosed as DSM-III bipolar, mixed disorder (girls aged 6 and 12 years) were both lithium responsive. Of the other four children (each of whom had multiple DSM-III diagnoses including major depressive disorder, cyclothymic disorder, overanxious disorder, attention deficit disorder, and encopresis but who did not have bipolar disorder), three did not show significant improvement with lithium and one (an 11-year-old boy) showed improvement of his major depressive disorder, overanxious disorder, and attention deficit disorder. The two children with bipolar disorder, both of whom were lithium responsive, were also strong augmenters on the evoked potential test, which correlates highly with lithium responsiveness in adult bipolar disorder (Schou et al., 1954). There is little question that more systematic research is needed in this age group, especially regarding therapeutic and prophylactic effect in affective disorders and aggressive behavior.

Side Effects of Lithium in Children and Adolescents

In general, children tolerate lithium treatment well and seem to be less prone to side effects than adults (Youngerman & Canino, 1978; Schou, 1972).

Lithium in therapeutic concentrations decreases free thyroxine (T_4) and triiodothyronine (T_3) during the first four months of administration. In euthyroid patients thyroid releasing hormone (TRH) increases in compensation, increasing thyroid stimulating hormone (TSH) and normalizing thyroid hormone levels. Patients on long term lithium therapy (but not short term therapy) with a known history of thyroiditis and low thyroid reserves based on thyroid antibodies may then develop transient or occasionally permanent hypothyroidism (Bakker, 1977). Among adults, lithium-related thyroid disorders occur only in patients with previous clinical or subclinical thyroid disorders and only after long term lithium treatment (Shopsin & Gershon, 1973), unless the patient is given iodides together with lithium, a combination that may produce goiter. Therefore, if lithium is to be used in youngsters baseline and maintenance monitoring of thyroid hormone levels is mandatory and iodides are to be avoided.

The renal side effects of lithium include sodium diuresis, polyuria, and polydypsia, which are reversible after decreasing or discontinuing lithium (Baldessarini, 1976). Diabetes insipidus and decreased renal function have been reported only after many years of lithium treatment. It is usually reversible, but there are some reports of irreversible decreased renal function with chronic tubular necrosis, fibrosis, and nephron atrophy (Lindop & Padfield 1975; Hestbech et al., 1977). Schou and Vestegaard (1981), in summarizing the evidence of lithium-induced renal damage, state that there is significantly more nephropathy in patients given lithium than in normal controls, but that similar nonspecific changes occur at almost the same rate in patients with long-standing affective illness never treated with lithium, that lithium-induced nephropathy does not share the serious prognosis of the nephropathies caused by phenacetin and the heavy metals, and that the risk of renal insufficiency and terminal azotemia is remote even in patients given lithium for many years. They advise "the observation that lithium may produce, or accentuate, nonspecific morphologic changes in the kidneys and that lithium treatment may lead to impairment of renal water reabsorption, not always fully reversible, does not seem to justify radical changes in the use of lithium on proper psychiatric indications."

In a study of four adolescents (2 boys and 2 girls ages 13–15) who received lithium carbonate for 3–5 years with serum levels maintained at

.5—1.0 mEq/l (Khandelwal, 1984) and where renal function was tested before initiation of treatment and after 3—5 years, there was no impairment of either tubular or glomerular function as assessed by 24-hour urine volume, urine osmolality, creatinine clearance, 24-hour urinary protein levels, serum electrolytes, serum creatinine, blood urea nitrogen, and microscopic urine examination. All children tolerated the medication well with minimal transient side effects.

Diuretics will decrease renal clearance of lithium and lead to increased plasma concentration. Youngsters on lithium should be advised against their unauthorized use especially if they also have associated eating disorders and are concerned about weight. Strict dietary measures, by decreasing sodium intake, also can lead to lithium toxicity.

Animal studies implicate lithium in effects on bone size (Birch, 1980), various endocrine functions (Mannistro, 1980), and on growth hormone secretion (Smythe et al., 1979). There is no information about growth hormone changes with lithium treatment in children, but studies in adults find no change in growth hormone (Merwin & Abuzzahab, 1971; Lal et al., 1978).

In normal adult volunteers lithium causes a slight but significant impairment of mental concentration, comprehension, and memory (Judd et al., 1977), but in therapeutic doses adult bipolar patients do not appear to present such side effects. Lithium may aggravate preexisting ventricular arrhythmias (Tilkian, 1976) and induce a nonallergic folliculitis (Rifkin et al., 1973; Callaway et al., 1968).

Lithium Usage in Childhood

Despite a lack of controlled trials, a course of lithium is advisable for the treatment of mania in children and adolescents. Short term use of neuroleptics also may be added for the acute control of manic symptomatology. The potentially problematic renal, thyroid, and bone effects of lithium are sufficient reasons to avoid long term lithium use unless the demonstrated risk of withholding lithium is very high. Lithium is indicated for longer term prophylaxis only after recurrent episodes of childhood bipolar illness. Because of a lack of studies of side effects in childhood, a conservative approach should be taken in the child with a single manic episode who responds well to the acute use of lithium carbonate. Lithium should be discontinued after 3—6 months while observing for the earliest signs of a recurrence of manic symptomatology. As is always the case with pharmacological interventions in children and adolescents, the assessment of the risk—benefit ratio must include the possibility of as yet unknown adverse effects and the potentially greater vulnerability of developing organisms to such risks.

In pharmacologically precipitated mania in childhood (i.e., precipitated by tricyclic antidepressants or MAOIs) the first treatment should be a decrease or change in the medication, with or without brief use of neuroleptics for acute symptom control. In this group one should be especially reluctant to commit the child to chronic lithium treatment unless nonpharmacologically triggered manic episodes ensue.

Clinical experience suggests a group of lithium responsive children and adults who do not present typical bipolar symptomatology, but rather have an affective disorder with episodic irritability, outbursts, or behavioral symptomatology that is relatively independent of environmental stimuli. These youngsters frequently have a family history of bipolar disorder or lithium responsiveness. Because of the lack of systematic studies, the decision to try lithium carbonate in these adolescents should be made based on individual and family history and on responsiveness to nonpharmacological interventions. Nevertheless, since most of the serious lithium side effects occur after chronic use, a brief trial is probably warranted in many youngsters with these symptoms.

Prior to beginning lithium, the child should have a physical and laboratory examination including serum creatinine, thyroid indices, urinalysis, and EKG. Twenty-four hour urinary creatinine for the calculation of glomerular filtration rate is advisable. The usual starting dose for lithium carbonate is 150 mg/day in younger children and 300 mg/day in older children and adolescents, given in divided doses. Steady state is achieved after about five days on a constant dose (Prien et al., 1972). Blood for lithium levels should be obtained in the morning 10–12 hours after the last dose, and the dose of lithium increased by 150 mg (or 300 mg in adolescents) every 5–7 days until a favorable response is obtained, further increases are limited by side effects, or blood levels reach .8–1.2 mEq/l. Side effects of nausea and diarrhea, which are closely related to a sudden increase in lithium blood level, may be minimized by a slow upward titration of dosage. Other common side effects are weakness, tremor, polyuria, blurred vision, and excessive thirst. Nausea, vomiting, slurring, and drowsiness should always make the clinician think of lithium toxicity, which will be confirmed if the plasma level is over 1.5 mEq/l. When lithium levels have stabilized in a constant therapeutic lithium dose, levels need only be checked every month. Yearly checks of thyroid function and glomerular filtration rate are advisable, as well as monitoring of growth. Because of decreased lithium excretion by the kidneys during salt depleted states, the family should be instructed to hold the lithium dose and contact the physician if the child has decreased food intake or diarrhea (e.g., with the flu) or goes on a severe diet.

THE PSYCHOPHARMACOLOGICALLY NONRESPONSIVE CHILD

Several groups of children present particularly complicated psychopharmacological decisions. These include children with typical unipolar or bipolar disorder who fail to respond to standard pharmacological treatment, children with psychotic depression, children who have a complicated psychiatric syndromal pattern with affective symptomatology but where the affective symptoms are not the most pronounced manifestation, and children whose affective symptoms worsen on antidepressant medication.

For children who present typical unipolar or bipolar affective disorder and who fail to respond to adult standard pharmacological treatment, the psychiatrist is justified in using other pharmacological approaches that have been proven useful in adults with similar disorders. This always requires that the parents and child be fully informed of the rationale and risks associated with each clinical approach, and that the psychiatrist has considered appropriate nonpharmacological treatments. The risks of treatment must be balanced by the risks of withholding possibly effective treatment. We have found in our own practice that monoamine oxidase inhibitors (MAOIs—both phenelzine and tranylcypromine) are well tolerated and appear to be effective in children both alone or in combination with tricyclic antidepressants. We have also found that in some bipolar children and adolescents in whom lithium prophylaxis is ineffective, carbamazepine alone or with lithium may be effective. Electroconvulsive therapy has been used successfully for childhood mania (Carr et al., 1983). Thyroid hormone is probably useful in combination with TCAs in adult depression and should be considered in refractory childhood depression. Levothyroxine, T_4, is clearly useful in some adults with rapid-cycling manic depressive disorder and should be considered for children for the same indication (Stancer & Persad, 1982). Pyridoxine (vitamin B_6) may be useful in women on the birth control pill, a possibility to consider in adolescent girls (Klein et al., 1980).

It is our clinical impression that like their adult counterparts adolescents with psychotic depression frequently respond to a combination of tricyclic antidepressant and neuroleptic. After the psychosis resolves, the neuroleptic may be slowly discontinued.

The child with a complicated syndromal pattern including affective symptomatology who also meets criteria for other psychiatric diagnoses and where the affective symptomatology does not predominate is a frequent presentation. In these children both nonpharmacological methods and the full range of pharmacological treatment for affective disorder should be considered. Specifically, some children in this group will respond well to TCAs, MAOIs, or lithium depending on the type of affective disorder they present. One of us has described that in children with primary depressive and secondary conduct disorder, the later remits after affective recovery (Puig-Antich, 1982a).

In our experience, the few children who clinically worsen on antidepressant medication (paradoxical effect) frequently have a history of organic brain damage (e.g., seizures and past encephalitis).

Systematic research in the treatment of child and adolescent affective disorders has barely begun. Because of the many leads from adult studies, it is likely to proceed rapidly. Now that the question of the existence of such disorders in youngsters is pretty much answered, pediatric psychopharmacological research should rapidly develop a fuller body of knowledge.

REFERENCES

Akiskal, H. S. (1983). The bipolar spectrum: New concepts in classification and diagnosis. In L. Grinspoon, (Ed.), *Psychiatry Update, 2,* 271–293.

Akiskal, H. S., & Puzantian, V. R. (1979). Psychotic forms of depression and mania. *Psychiatric Clinic North America, 2,* 419–440.

American Psychiatric Association. (1980). *Diagnostic and statistical manual of mental disorders* (3rd ed.). American Psychiatric Association: Washington, DC.

Anthony, E. J., & Scott, P. (1960), Manic depressive psychosis in in childhood. *Journal Child Psychology and Psychiatry, 1,* 52–72.

Asberg, M., Cronholm, B., Sjoqvist, F., & Tuck, D. (1971). Relationship between plasma level and therapeutic effect of nortriptyline. *British Medical Journal, 3,* 331–334.

Bakker K. (1977). The influence of lithium carbonate on the hypothalamic-pituitary-thyroid asix. Doctoral thesis. University of Gronigen, Holland.

Baldessarini, R. (1976). Lithium Salts 1970–1975. In D. F. Kleim, R. Gittleman-Kline (Eds.), *Psychiatric drug treatment* (Vol. 2). Brunner/Mazel: New York.

Baron, M., Gershon, E., Rudy, V., Jonas, W., & Buchsbaum, M. (1975). Lithium carbonate response in depression. *Archives of General Psychiatry, 32,* 1107–1111.

Birch, N. J. (1980). Bone side-effect of lithium. In F. N. Johnson (Ed.), *Lithium therapy* (pp. 365–371). Lancaster: MTP Press.

Bunney, W. E., Goodwin, F. K., Davis, J. M., & Fawcett, J. S. (1968). A behavioral-biochemical study of lithium in therapy. *American Journal of Psychiatry, 125,* 499–512.

Callaway, C. L., Hendrie, H. C., & Luby, E. D. (1968). Cutaneous conditions observed in patients during treatment with lithium. *American Journal of Psychiatry, 124,* 1124–1125.

Campbell, J. D. (1952). Manic-depressive psychosis in children; report of 18 cases. *Journal Nervous and Mental Diseases, 116,* 424–439.

Carlson, G., & Cantwell, D. (1980). Unmasking masked depression in children and adolescents. *American Journal of Psychiatry, 137,* 445–449.

Carlson, G., & Strober, M. (1978). Manic-depressive illness in early adolescence, *Journal American Academy of Child Psychiattry, 12,* 138–153.

Carlson, G., & Strober, M. (1979). Affective disorders in adolescence. *Psychiatric Clinics North America, 2,* 511–525.

Carr, V., Dorrington, C., Schrader, G., & Wale, J. (1983). The use of ECT for mania in childhood bipolar disorder. *British Journal of Psychiatry, 143,* 411–415.

Chambers, W. J., & Puig-Antich, J. (1982). Psychotic symptoms in prepubertal major depressive disorder. *Archives General Psychiatry, 39,* 921–927.

Connell, H. M. (1972). Depression in childhood. *Child Psychiatry and Human Development, 4,* 71–85.

Cytryn, L., McKnew, D., & Bunney, W. (1980). Diagnosis of depression in children: A reassessment. *American Journal of Psychiatry, 137,* 22–25.

Deykin, E. Y., & Dimascio, A. (1972). Relationship of patient background characteristics to efficacy of pharmacotherapy in depression. *Journal Nervous and Mental Diseases, 155,* 209–215.

Dunner, D. L. (1979). Rapid cycling bipolar manic depressive illness. *Psychiatric Clinics North America, 2,* 461–468.

Dyson, L., & Barcai, A. (1970). Treatment of children of lithium-responding parents. *Current Therapeutic Research, 12,* 286–290.

Fieve, R. R., Platman, S. R., & Plutchik, R. R. (1968). The use of lithium in affective disorders. II. Prophylaxis of depression in chronic recurrent affective disorders. *American Journal Psychiatry, 125,* 492–498.

Friedel, R. O., Veith, R. C., Bloom, V., & Bielski, R. J., (1979). Desipramine plasma levels and clinical response in depressed outpatients. *Communications in Psychopharmacology, 3,* 81–88.

Frommer, E. A. (1967). Treatment of childhood depression with antidepressant drugs. *British Medical Journal, 1,* 729–732.

Frommer, E. A. (1968). Depressive disorders in childhood. *British Journal of Psychiatry,* Special Publication, no. 2 London, R.M.P.A., pp. 117–136.

Geller, B., Perel, J. M., Knitter, E. F., et al. (1983). Nortriptyline in major depressive disorder in children: Response steady state plasma levels, predictive kinetics and pharmacokinetics. *Psychopharmacology Bulletin, 19,* 62–65.

Gittelman-Klein, R. (1975). Review of clinical pharmacological treatment of hyperkinesis. In D. F. Klein and R. Gittelman-Klein (Eds.), *Progress in Psychiatric Drug Treatment* (pp. 661–681). Brunner/Mazel: New York.

Glassman, A. H., Kantor, S. J., & Shostak, M. (1975). Depression, delusions, and drug response. *American Journal of Psychiatry, 132,* 716–719.

Glassman, A. H., Perel, J. M., Shostak, M., Kanton, S. J., & Fleiss, J. L. (1977). Clinical implications of imipramine plasma levels for depressive illness. *Archives of General Psychiatry, 34,* 197–204.

Goodwin, F. K., Murphy, D. L., & Bunney, W. E. (1969). Lithium carbonate treatment in depression and mania. *Archives of General Psychiatry, 21,* 486–496.

Goodwin, F. K., Murphy, D. L., Dunner, D. & Bunney, W. E. (1972). Lithium response of unipolar versus bipolar depression. *American Journal of Psychiatry, 129,* 44–47.

Greenhill, L. L., Rieder, R., Wender, P., Buchsbaum, M., & Zahn, T. (1973). Lithium carbonate in the treatment of hyperactive children. *Archives of General Psychiatry, 28,* 636–640.

Hestbech, J., Hansen, H. E., Amdisen, A., & Olseon, S., (1977). Chronic lesions following long-term treatment with lithium. *Kidney International, 12*: 205.

Himmelhoch, J. M. (1979). Mixed states, manic depressive illness and the nature of mood. *Psychiatric Clinics North America, 2,* 449–460.

Judd, L. L., Hubbard, B., Janowsky, D. S. et al. (1977). The effect of lithium on the cognitive functions of normal subjects. *Archives General Psychiatry, 34,* 352–357.

Kashani, J., Shekin, W. O., & Reid, J. C. (1984). Amitriptyline in children with major depressive disorder: A double blind cross over pilot study. *Journal of the American Academy of Child Psychiatry. 23,* 348–351.

Keller, M. B., Shapiro, R. W., Lavori, P. W. et al. (1982a). Recovery in major depressive disorder. *Archives of General Psychiatry, 39,* 905–910.

Keller, M. B., Shapiro, R. W., Lavori, P. W., et al. (1982b). Relapse in major depressive disorder. *Archives of General Psychiatry, 39,* 911–915.

Khandelwal, S. K., Vijoy, K. V., & Murthy, R. S. (1984). Renal function in children receiving long-term lithium prophylaxis. *American Journal of Psychiatry, 141,* 278–279.

Klein, D. F., Gittelman, R., Quitkin, F. & Rifkin, A. (1980). *Diagnosis and drug treatment of psychiatric disorders: Adults and children.* (2nd ed.) (pp. 343–370). Waverly Press: Baltimore.

Kovacs, M., & Beck, A. T. (1977). An empirical clinical approach towards a definition of childhood depression. In J. G. Schulterbrandt & A. Raskin (Eds.), *Depression in children: Diagnosis, treatment and conceptual models* (pp. 1–25). Raven Press: New York.

Kovacs, M., Feinberg, T. L., Crouse, M. A., Paulaskas, S., & Finkelstein, R. (1984a). Depressive disorders in childhood. *Archives of General Psychiatry, 41,* 229–237.

Kovacs, M. Feinberg, T. L., Crouse, M. A., Paulaskas, S., Pollock, M., & Finkelstein, R. (1984b). Depressive disorders in childhood II. Risk of a subsequent major depression. *Archives of General Psychiatry. 41,* 643–649.

Kragh-Sovensen, P., Hansen, C. E., & Asberg, M. (1973). Plasma levels of nortriptyline in the treatment of endogenous depression. *Acta Psychiatrica Scandinavia, 49,* 444–456.

Kragh-Sovensen, P., Hansen, C. E., Gaastrup, T. et al. (1976). Self inhibiting action of nortriptyline to antidepressant effects at high plasma levels. Psychopharmacologia *45,* 305–312.

Kramer, E., & Feiguine, R. (1983). Clinical effects of amitryptiline in adolescent depression. *Journal of the American Academy of Child Psychiatry, 20,* 636–644.

Kuhn, B., & Kuhn, R. (1972). Drug therapy for depression in children. In A. L. Annel (Ed.), *Depressive states in childhood and adolescence* (pp. 163–203). Stockholm: Almqvist and Wkksell.

Kuperman, S., & Steward, M. A. (1979). The diagnosis of depression in children. *Journal of Affective Disease, 1,* 213–217.

Lal, S., Nair, N. P. V., & Guyda, H. (1978). Effect of lithium on hypothalamic-pituitary dopaminergic function. *Acta Psychiatrica Scandinavia, 57,* 91–96.

Levine, J. D., Gordon, N. C., & Fields, H. L. (1978). The mechanism of placebo analgesia. *Lancet,* 654–657.

Liebowitz, M. R., Quitkin, F. M., Stewart, J. W., et al. (1984). Phenelzine vs. imipramine in atypical depression. *Archives of General Psychiatry, 41,* 669–677.

Lindop, G. B. M., & Padfield, P. L. (1975). The renal pathology in a case of lithium-induced diabetes insipidus. *Journal of Clinical Pathology, 24,* 472.

Lucas, A. R., Locket, H. J., & Grimm, F. (1965). Amitriptyline in childhood depressions. *Diseases of the Nervous System, 26,* 105–110.

McKnew D. H., Cytryn, L., Buchsbaum, M. S., Hamovit, J., Lamour, M., Rappoport, J. L., & Gershon, E. S. (1981). Lithium in children of lithium-responding parents. *Psychiatry Research, 4,* 171–180.

Mannistro, P. T. (1980). Endocrine side-effects of lithium. In F. N. Johnson (Ed.), *Handbook of Lithium Therapy.* Lancaster: MTP.

Matuzas, W., Javaid, J. I., Glass, R., Davis, J. M., Ross, J. A., & Uhlenhuth, E. H. (1982). Plasma concentrations of imipramine and clinical response among depressed outpatients. *Journal of Clinical Psychopharmacology, 2,* 140–142.

Merwin, G. E., & Abuzzahab, F. S. (1971). The effects of lithium carbonate on glucose, human growth hormone and insulin in manic-depressive patients. *Pharmacologist, 13,* 631.

Morris, J. B., & Beck, A. T. (1974). The efficacy of antidepressant drugs. *Archives of General Psychiatry, 30,* 667–674.

Nelson, J. C., & Bowers, M. B. (1978). Antidepressant drug treatment. *Archives of General Psychiatry, 35,* 1321–1328.

Orvaschel, H., Sholomkhas, D., & Weissman, M. M. (1980). The assessment of psychopathology and behavioral problems in children: A review of scales suitable for epidemiological and clinical research, (1959–1979). *Monograph for NIMH,* series AN No. 1, DDHS Publication #(ADM) AD-1037, Superintendant of Documents, U. S. Governent Printing Office, Washington, DC.

Pearce, J. B. (1977). Childhood depression. M. Rutter and L. Hersov (Eds.), *Child Psychiatry: Modern Approaches.* London: Blackwell, 448.

Perel, J. M. (1974). Review of pediatric and adult pharmacology of imipramine and other drugs. In O. S. Robinson (Ed.), Report of Chairman. Ad Hoc Committee on Tricyclic Antidepressant Cardiotoxicity, Federal Drug Administration, 1–4.

Petti, T., & Campbell, M. (1975). Imimpramine and seizures. *American Journal of Psychiatry, 132,* 538–540.

Phillips, I. (1979). Childhood depression: Interpersonal interactions and depressive phenomena. *American Journal of Psychiatry, 136,* 511–515.

Preskorn, S., Weller, E., & Weller, R. (1982). Childhood depression: Imipramine levels and response. *Journal of Clinical Psychiatry, 43,* 450–453.

Preskorn, S., Weller, E., Weller, R., & Glotzbach, E. (1983). Plasma levels of imipramine and adverse effects on children. *American Journal of Psychiatry, 140,* 1332–1335.

Prien, R. F., Caffey, E. M., & Klett, C. J. (1972). The relationship between serum lithium level and clinical response in acute manics treated with lithium carbonate. *British Journal of Psychiatry, 120,* 409–412.

Pruitt, A., & Dayton, P. A. (1971). A comparison of the binding of drugs to adult and cord plasma. *European Journal Clinical Pharmacology, 4,* 59–62.

Puig-Antich, J. (1980). Affective disorders in childhood: A review and perspective. *Psychiatric Clinics North America, 3,* 403–424.

Puig-Antich, J. (1982a). Major depression and conduct disorder in prepuberty. *Journal of the American Academy of Child Psychiatry, 21,* 118–128.

Puig-Antich, J. (1982b) The use of RD criteria for major depressive disorder for children and adolescence. (Editorial) *Journal of the American Academy of Child Psychiatry, 21,* 291–293.

Puig-Antich, J., Blau, S., Marx, N., Greenhill, L. L., & Chambers, W. J. (1978). Prepubertal major depressive disorder: A pilot study, *Journal of the American Academy of Child Psychiatry, 17,* 659–707.

Puig-Antich, J., Lukens, E., Davies, M., Goetz, D., Quattrock, J., & Todak, G. (in press, a). Controlled studies of psychosocial functioning in prepubertal major depressive disorders. I: Interpersonal relationships during the depressive episode. *Archives of General Psychiatry.*

Puig-Antich, J., Lukens, E., Davies, M., Goetz, D., Quattrock, J., & Todak, G. (in press, b). Controlled studies of psychosocial functioning in prepubertal major depressive disorders: II. Interpersonal relationships after sustained recovery from the affective episode. *Archives of General Psychiatry.*

Puig-Antich, J., Perel, J. M., Lupatkin, W. et al. Imipramine in prepubertal major depression. *Archives of General Psychiatry* (in press).

Quitkin, F. M., Rabkin J. G., Ross, D., & McGrath, P. J. (1984). Duration of antidepressant drug treatment. *Archives of General Psychiatry, 41,* 238–245.

Quitkin, F. M., Schwartz, D., Liebowitz, M. R., Stewart, J. R., McGrawth, P. J., Harrison, W., Halpers, F., Puit-Antich, K., Tricamo, E., Sachar, E. J., & Klein, D. F. (1983). Atypical depressives: A preliminary report of antidepressant response, sleep patterns, and cortisol secretion. In P. J. Clayton & J. E. Barrett (Eds.), *Treatment of Depression: Old Controversies and New Approaches* (pp. 253–263). Raven Press: New York.

Rane, A., & Wilson, J. T. (1983). Clinical pharmacokinetics in infants and children. In M. Gibaldi, L. Prescott (Eds), *Handbook of Clinical Pharmacokinetics* (pp. 142–168). Adis Health Science Press, New York.

Rapoport, J., Buchsbaum, M. S., Weingartner, H. et al. (1980). Dextroamphetamine: Its cognitive and behavioral effects in normal and hyperactive boys and normal men. *Archives of General Psychiatry, 37,* 933–943.

Raskin, A. (1975). Age-sex differences in response to antidepressant drugs. *Journal of Nervous and Mental Diseases, 159,* 120–130.

Reisby, N., Gram, L. F., Bech, P., Nagy, A., Peterson, G. O., Ortman, J., Ibsen, I, Dencker, S. J., Jocobsen, O. Krautwald, O., Sondergaard, I., & Christiansen, J. (1977). Imipramine: Clinical effects and pharmacokinetic variability. *Psychopharmacology, 54,* 263–272.

Rifkin, A., Kurtin, S., Quitkin, F., & Klein, D. F. (1973). Lithium-induced folliculitis. *American Journal of Psychiatry, 130,* 1081–1019.

Robinson, D. S., Nies, A., Ravaris, C. L., Ives, J., & Barlett, D. (1978a). Clinical pharmacology of phenelzine. *Archives of General Psychiatry, 35,* 629–638.

Robinson, D. S., Nies, A., Ravaris, C. L., Ives. J. O., & Barlett, D. (1978b). Clinical psychopharmacology of phenelzine: Mao activity and clinical response. In M. Lipson, A. DiMascio, & K. F. Kitlam (Eds.), *Psychopharmacology: A generation of progress* (pp. 961–974). Raven Press: New York.

Rutter, M. (1972). Relationships between child and adult psychiatric disorders. *Acta Psychiatrica Scandinavia, 48,* 3–21.

Saraf, K. R., Klein, D. F., Gittelman-Klein, R. et al. (1974). Imipramine side effects in children. *Psychopharmacologia* (Berlin), *37,* 265–274.

Schou, M. (1972). Lithium in psychiatric therapy and prophylaxis. A review with special regard to its use in children. In A. L. Arnell (Ed.), *Depressive states in childhood and adolescence.* Halsted Press: New York.

Schou, M., Joel-Nielsen, N., Stromgren, E., & Voldby, H. (1954). The treatment of manic psychosis by the administration of lithium salts. *Journal of Neurology, Neurosurgery, and Psychiatry, 17,* 250–260.

Schou, M., & Vestergaard, P. (1981) Lithium and the kidney scare. *Psychosomatics, 22,* 93–94.

Shopsin, B., & Gershon, S. (1973). Toxicology of the lithium ion. In S. Gershon and B. Shopsin (Eds.), *:Lithium ion: Its role in psychiatric treatment and research* (p. 107). Plenum Press: New York.

Smythe, G. A., Brandstater, J. F., & Lazarus, L. (1979). Acute effect of lithium on central dopamine serotonin activity reflected by inhibition of prolactin and growth hormone secretion in the rat. *Australian Journal of Biological Science, 32,* 329–334.

Spiker, D., Cofsky-Weiss, J., Dealy, R. F., Griffin, S. J., Hanin, I., Neil, J. F., Perel, J., Rossi, A. J., & Soloff, P. H. (in press). Pharmacological treatment of delusions in depression. *American Journal of Psychiatry.*

Stancer, H. & Persad, E. (1982). Treatment of intractable rapid-cycling manic-depressive disorder with levothyroxine. *Archives of General Psychiatry, 39,* 311–312.

Strober, M. (1983). Natural history of major depressive disorder in adolescence. Presented at the Annual Meeting of the American Psychiatric Association, New York City, May.

Strober, M., Green, J., & Carlson, G. (1982). Phenomenology and subtypes of major depressive disorder in adolescents. *Journal of Affective Disease, 3,* 281–290.

Tilkian, A. G., Schroeder, J. S., Kao, J., & Hultgren, H. (1976). Effect of lithium on cardiovascular performance: Report on extended ambulatory monitoring and exercise testing before and during lithium therapy. *American Journal of Cardiology, 38,* 701–708.

Vohra, L., Burrows, G., Hunt, D., & Sloman, G. (1975). The effect of toxic and therapeutic doses of tricyclic antidepressant drugs on intracardiac conduction. *European Journal of Cardiology, 3*(3), 219–227.

Wehr, T. A., & Goodwin, F. K. (1979). Rapid cycling in manic-depressives induced by tricyclic antidepressants. *Archives of General Psychiatry, 36,* 555–559.

Weinberg, W. A., Rutman, J., & Sullivan, L. (1973). Depression in children referred to an educational diagnostic center: Diagnosis and treatment. *Journal of Pediatrics, 83,* 1065–1072.

Weissmann, M. M., Klerman, G. L., Paykel, E. S., et al. (1974). Treatment effects of the social adjustment of depressed patients. *Archives of General Psychiatry, 30,* 771–778.

Weissmann, M. M., Paykel, E. S., Siegel, R., et al. (1971). Social role performance of depressed women: Comparisons with a normal group. *American Journal of Orthopsychiatry, 41,* 391–405.

Whitehead, P., & Clerk, L., (1970). Effect of lithium carbonate, placebo, and thioridazine on hyperactive children. *American Journal of Psychiatry, 127,* 824–825.

Winsberg, B. G., Goldstein, S., Yepes, L., & Perel, J. M. (1972). Imipramine and electrocardiographic abnormalities in hyperactive children. *American Journal of Psychiatry, 132,* 542–545.

Winsberg, B. G., Perel, J. M., Hurwic, M., & Klutch, A. (1974). Imipramine protein binding and pharmacokinetics in children. In I. S. Forest, C. J. Carr, & E. Usdin (Eds.), *The phenothiazines and structurally related compounds* (pp. 425–431). Raven Press: New York.

Youngerman, J., & Canino, I. A. (1978). Lithium carbonate use in children and adolescents: A survey of the literature. *Archives of General Psychiatry, 35,* 216–224.

Attention Deficit Disorders

MAUREEN DONNELLY, M.D. and
JUDITH L. RAPOPORT, M.D.

DEFINITION

Attention Deficit Disorder, as now classified in the American Psychiatric Association *Diagnostic and Statistical Manual III*, refers to three behavioral syndromes characterized by: (1) developmentally inappropriate inattention (failure to complete activities, distractibility, difficulty concentrating on tasks and sticking to play, the appearance of not listening); (2) impulsivity (difficulty with organizing and with waiting for turns, shifting from activity to activity, acting before thinking, often calling out in class, and needing much supervision); (3) and hyperactivity (excessive running, climbing, and moving, awake and asleep, difficulty staying still and staying seated, fidgeting). The subdivisions are Attention Deficit Disorder with Hyperactivity (ADDH) (314.01), Attention Deficit Disorder without Hyperactivity (ADD) (314.00), and Attention Deficit Disorder, Residual Type (ADD, RT) (314.80), the latter referring to individuals having once met criteria for ADDH, but retaining only symptoms of inattention and impulsivity. ADDH corresponds to the International Classification of Disease—9 Hyperkinetic Syndrome of Childhood (American Psychiatric Association, 1980; Rutter et al., 1979).

Onset must be before age seven, with a duration of at least six months, and without evidence of schizophrenia, affective disorder, severe or profound mental retardation, and in adults, without schizotypal or borderline personality disorder. Associated with the disorders are poor social functioning, low self-esteem, conduct problems, lack of response to discipline, specific developmental disorders, and academic difficulties (American Psychiatric Association, 1980; Rutter & Garmezy, 1983).

DIAGNOSTIC CONSIDERATIONS AND VARIATIONS

Prior to the DSM-III designation as Attention Deficit Disorder, this syndrome (or syndromes) was popularly referred to as Minimal Brain Damage (Gesell & Amatruda, 1949), Minimal Brain Dysfunction (Clements, 1966; Wender, 1971), the Hyperactive Child Syndrome (Stewart et al., 1966), the Hyperkinetic Child Syndrome (Cantwell, 1977), and by the DSM-II label of Hyperkinetic Reaction of Childhood (308.0) (American Psychiatric Association, 1968). These groupings of behavioral difficulties and abnormal clinical signs are similar to each other and ADD, but not necessarily in all aspects. The change in terminology resulted from a belief that attention deficit is invariably present and is the core symptom, while motor restlessness is not. Although never part of official terminology, the term "Minimal Brain Damage/Dysfunction" was deliberately avoided. As numerous authors (e.g., Cantwell, 1977; Klein et al., 1980; Nichols & Chen, 1980) have pointed out, the majority of children with these problems do not have demonstrable brain damage and many do not evidence subtle neurological signs; most brain damaged children do not exhibit hyperactivity; there are no variables to quantify as "minimal"; there is no validation of a single syndrome that groups neurologic, academic, and behavioral characteristics or demonstrates a common etiology, biology, treatment, course, or prognosis. In addition, the term ADD reflects the belief that problems in attention are central to the other behaviors of the syndrome (Douglas & Peters, 1979). Finally, a population of adolescents and adults with a prior history of hyperactivity was identified (Weiss, 1983; Wender et al., 1981).

It should be noted, however, that the entity of ADD is controversial and raises many questions (see Rutter & Garmezy, 1983). There are problems in defining and measuring attention and hyperactivity. It is unclear whether the disorder should be demonstrated across multiple situations. There are large variations in diagnostic practice, as shown especially by the differences in the frequency of its diagnosis in the United States (often) and in the United Kingdom (rarely), probably in part because the British do not differentiate ADD from conduct disorders. There is also evidence that hyperactivity is a central variable and not secondary to inattention (Porrino et al., 1983a and b), suggesting that Hyperkinetic Disorder might be equally as appropriate a label.

Therefore, several points should be kept in mind: most studies have not used the diagnosis of ADD to define the research populations; though many subjects would probably fit this classification, not all would. Research has heretofore been hampered by a lack of precision in defining the subject populations, yet surprisingly consistent results have been obtained in psychopharmacologic investigations of ADD-like behaviors. Finally, the concept and diagnosis of ADD continue to change.

PHARMACOLOGICAL TREATMENT OF ATTENTION DEFICIT DISORDER

Pharmacological treatments for the behaviors included in ADDH have been well documented over the past 25 years. Drug treatment for ADD and ADD,RT will be discussed separately at the end of this section since these classifications and their treatments are not well established.

The major class of drugs indicated for ADDH is the central nervous system stimulants, especially dextroamphetamine and methylphenidate

(MP). This chapter will also discuss antidepressants, antipsychotics, and other agents that are of some clinical value and/or research interest.

Stimulants

Pharmacology.   Stimulants are drugs that have significant CNS excitatory actions, in addition to other central and peripheral effects. They are generally divided into two major groups, the sympathomimetics (amphetamine, MP, and magnesium pemoline) and the xanthines (caffeine). Deanol is a stimulant that differs somewhat in structure and function from the others.

Amphetamines, which are similar in structure to norepinephrine, come in three forms, dextroamphetamine (Dexedrine), levoamphetamine (no longer marketed), and racemic amphetamine (Benzedrine), an equal mixture of the two isomers. They have CNS stimulant and peripheral $\propto$ and β sympathomimetic actions. The D-isomer is three to four times more potent than the L-isomer in terms of CNS effects, but has less potent cardiovascular effects (Weiner, 1980).

The amphetamines are well absorbed when taken orally, achieve peak plasma levels in children in two to three hours, easily cross the blood brain barrier, and have a half-life in children of 4–6 hours (with large interindividual variation) (Modell et al., 1976; Brown et al., 1977; Cantwell & Carlson, 1978). Subjective clinical effects seem to peak earlier than plasma levels, at approximately 1–3 hours (Ebert et al., 1976). Chronic use for six or more months yields a steady state half-life of about 10 hours (Greenhill et al., 1984). These drugs are mainly metabolized via oxidative deamination to benzoic acid and hippuric acid (which are inactive). Given an acid urine and normal renal function, about one-third to one-half of the drugs is excreted unchanged (Saunders, 1974; Ebert et al., 1976; Cantwell & Carlson, 1978).

Methylphenidate (MP) is a piperidine derivative with structural and pharmocological properties similar to amphetamines. Its actions are mainly central. In children, it is easily absorbed after oral administration, is poorly bound to plasma proteins, readily crosses the blood brain barrier, reaches peak plasma levels in 1–2 hours and has a half-life of 2–3 hours. Its clearance also shows large interindividual and intraindividual variability (Cantwell & Carlson, 1978; Franz, 1980; Gualtieri et al., 1982; Shaywitz et al., 1982; Chan et al., 1983; Greenhill et al., 1984). Serum levels seem to correspond to the time course of clinical effects (Gualtieri et al., 1982; Swanson et al., 1983). It is chiefly deesterified to ritalinic acid, which accounts for about 80 percent of the oral dose. The remainder is metabolized to parahydroymethylphenidate, which is potent, and to oxoritaelinic acid and oxomethylphenidate, which are weakly active. Essentially none of the drug appears unchanged in the urine (Cantwell & Carlson, 1978; Franz, 1980).

Magnesium pemoline is like amphetamine and MP in function, though it has minimal sympathomimetic effects. It is dissimilar in structure. It reaches peak serum level in children in 2–4 hours; its half-life is 12 hours. Clinical improvement can take up to 3 or 4 weeks (Cantwell & Carlson, 1978; Weiner, 1980; Friedman, 1981).

Amphetamines and related drugs enhance catecholamine actions through release of amines from storage sites, blockage of re-uptake, and monoamine oxidase inhibition, although this latter action is weak (Cantwell & Carlson, 1978; Weiner, 1980; Creese, 1983).

Deanol, an organic salt of 2-dimethyl amino-ethanol, is not covered here, as it is not in general use and its pharmacology in children is not well described.

Caffeine is a methylated xanthine resembling uric acid. In adults, it is rapidly absorbed, achieves maximum concentration within 1 hour and peak effect within 2 hours, and has a half-life of about 4 hours. Important among its actions are its competitive inhibition of the benzodiazepine receptor and its affinity for the adenosine receptor (Cantwell & Carlson, 1978; Rall, 1980; Elkins et al., 1981).

Physiological and Psychophysiological Effects. Centrally, stimulants excite the medullary respiratory center, though without significant effects on respiratory rate. They stimulate the reticular activating system, sometimes resulting in insomnia, and perhaps by this mechanism, improving attention and task performance (Barkley, 1977; Cantwell & Carlson, 1978; Weiner, 1980). Sleep physiology and EEG architecture may be altered, though specific research findings have not been consistent (Busby et al., 1981; Chatoor et al., 1983; Greenhill et al., 1983, Greenhill et al., 1984). There is depression of appetite, perhaps secondary to effects on the lateral hypothalmic center (Cantwell & Carlson, 1978). In addition, methylphenidate and amphetamine have been shown to have differential neuroendocrine effects. Acutely MP increases growth hormone and minimally decreases prolactin. Chronic use yields increased growth hormone and unchanged prolactin levels. Chronic amphetamine is associated with decreased prolactin and unchanged growth hormone (Shaywitz et al., 1982; Greenhill et al., 1984).

Peripherally, stimulants mildly elevate systolic and diastolic blood pressure, as well as heart rate, though the clinical significance of this is not clear. They also relax bronchial smooth muscle, cause some contraction of the urinary bladder sphincter, and have unpredictable gastrointestinal effects (Weiner, 1980).

A variety of laboratory measures, such as EEG, Averaged Evoked Responses (AER), skin conductance, and electropupillograms have been studied in children with ADD, both on and off medication. Results have been inconsistent. These studies are of research interest, especially to elucidate pathophysiological mechanisms of the disorder and mechanisms of drug action (Barkley, 1977; Conners & Werry, 1979; Klein et al., 1980).

Behavioral Effects. There are many careful studies that demonstrate that dextroamphetamine and MP consistently, readily, and sometimes quite dramatically improve the behaviors of ADDH. This clinical effect occurs even when subject groups are *not* strictly defined, the sample sizes are small, and the drug dosages span a wide range. Most likely to improve are hyperactive, restless, impulsive, disruptive, aggressive, socially inappropriate behaviors (Conners & Werry, 1979; Klein et al., 1980). A large number of studies show improvement on global impression, on parent, and on teacher scales (Conners et al., 1967; Finnerty et al., 1971; Rapoport et al., 1971; Weiss et al., 1971; Rapoport et al., 1974; Werry & Aman, 1975; Gittelman-Klein et al., 1976; Arnold et al., 1978; Firestone et al., 1978). Investigators have also reported positive changes with drug treatment in mother-child and teacher-child interactions, as well as normalization of social behavior (making hyperactive children indistinguishable from their peers) (Whalen & Henker, 1976; Cunningham & Barkley, 1978; Humphries et al., 1978, Whalen et al., 1978; Whalen et al., 1980a and b; Whalen et al., 1981). Dextroamphetamine and MP seem to be equally effective in achieving these results.

Magnesium pemoline also is clinically effective, though generally thought to be less so than these other stimulants (which have had better outcome in some studies) (Conners et al., 1972; Dykman et al., 1976; Gittelman-Klein et al., 1976; Firestone et al., 1978).

Deanol treatment, of which there has been a limited amount of research, has yielded some positive clinical findings, though much less than those for the other drugs (Coleman et al., 1976; Lewis & Young, 1975).

Caffeine studies, which are few, generally have demonstrated no significant improvement in children with ADDH. However, there might be weak positive effects, particularly in certain subgroups who crave caffeine (Elkins et al., 1981; Gittelman, 1983; Rapoport, 1983).

In addition to research on the general or global clinical effects of stimulants, there has been much work on treatment of particular behaviors, such as cognition, academic achievement, mood, and motor behavior. Dextroamphetamine and MP have been the drugs most frequently employed. Stimulants improve performance on many cognitive tests of attention, vigilance, reaction time, visual and verbal learning, and short term memory (Aman, 1978; Fisher, 1978; Sostek et al., 1980; Gittelman, 1983). There is some evidence that the improvement is due to increased concentration or vigilance, through both more focused attention and less distraction by extraneous stimuli (Thurston et al., 1979). However, in spite of better performance on particular measures, children's overall academic performance and achievement have not been shown to be enhanced. Another research and clinical issue related to cognition is whether stimulants are associated with a state dependent effect on learning (Swanson & Kinsbourne, 1976); however, most studies have not substantiated this finding (Stenhausen & Kreuser, 1981; Becker-Mattes, 1982; Weingartner et al., 1982).

Stimulant effect on mood is of interest, also. Much further research is needed in this area. Stimulants have been thought not to induce euphoria in children (Office of Child Development, 1971; Safer & Allen, 1976), but there have been reports of positive and, to a lesser extent, negative, mood changes (Bender & Cottington, 1942; Ounstead, 1955; Connors, et al., 1965; Barkley, 1977).

Motor activity is another important variable in the study of ADDH. Generally, stimulants have been found to decrease activity levels in structured settings, while yielding inconsistent results for less restricted situations. A recent study in a naturalistic setting, using 24 hour activity monitors, showed that dextroamphetamine significantly decreased activity in the structured classroom and significantly increased activity during physical recreation times. The overall decrease lasted about 8 hours and was followed by a slight "rebound" increase in motor activity (Porrino et al., 1983a and b).

Of note is the fact that stimulant actions are not specific for the population of children with ADDH. They have been shown to have similar cognitive and behavioral effects on "normal" children and adults (Rapoport et al., 1978; Rapoport et al., 1980).

Clinical Usage. Stimulants are indicated for the treatment of ADDH. Not all children with ADDH, however, need to take medication.

A careful psychiatric and physical diagnostic evaluation is made. The decision to employ medication follows and is a clinical one, based on consideration of such factors as severity of symptoms, preferences of the child and parents, ability of the child, parents, and school to cope with the problem behaviors, and success and failure of previous treatment.

Contraindications to drug use are the presence of psychosis or a thought disorder. Relative contraindications are presence of tics, extreme anxiety, or any medical condition precluding the use of sympathomimetics. Use with the child who has mental retardation, tics, and anxiety is controversial (Cantwell & Carlson, 1978; Connors & Werry, 1979; Shapiro et al., 1978). Use in preschool-age children and adolescents has not been routine, though there is recent work which suggests that stimulants are clinically effective in these groups (Connors, 1975; Schleifer, 1975; Varley, 1983).

In spite of much research (Klein et al., 1980), there is no reliable method to predict which children will respond to or benefit from medication, perhaps related to the nonspecificity of the effect. There is a paucity of information on issues of compliance, but recent studies suggest that this may be a significant problem with maintenance medication (Firestone, 1982; Sleator, 1982).

MP and dextroamphetamine are the drugs of choice, followed by pemoline. Children may respond to one, but not the others. There may be infrequent indications for treatment with more than one psychotropic medication at a time, related to application of the finding that the effects of MP and thioridazine may be additive (Gittelman-Klein, 1976; Klein et al., 1980).

Dosages for the stimulants are given in Table 6.1. The usual beginning dose of dextroamphetamine is 5 mg q.d. or b.i.d. (for ages six or older), of MP is 5 mg b.i.d., and of pemoline is 37.5 mg q.d. The medication is increased gradually every three to five days (weekly for pemoline) until therapeutic effect or adverse effects occur. Different dosages may be optimum for different behaviors (lower for cognitive improvement versus higher for overall clinical improvement, but with decrement on cognitive variables) (Sprague & Sleator, 1977), but this is controversial and much research is still needed before practical application of those findings (Charles et al., 1981). Dosage must be reevaluated as the child grows. The timing of doses is based on duration of drug action, which is relatively short for dextroamphetamine and MP and longer for pemoline. There are sustained release preparations of dextroamphetamine and MP, but no systematic studies have demonstrated their superiority. Alternatively, some practitioners have successfully used the short-acting preparations on a once a day regimen, though this is not usual.

The general recommendation has been to administer stimulants before meals (which assumed favored absorption on an empty stomach), though some have suggested use with meals to avoid the anorexia associated with the drug. There is some recent evidence (Chan et al., 1983;

Table 6.1.   Dosage of Stimulants

Drug	Starting Dose	Maximum Dose	Daily Dose Range (mg/kg)
Dextroamphetamine	5 mg q.d. or b.i.d. (age 6 or older) 2.5 mg q.d. (ages 3–5)	40 mg	.15–0.5
Methylphenidate	5 mg b.i.d.	60 mg	.3–1.0
Pemoline	37.5 mg q.d.	112.5 mg	.5–2.0

Swanson et al., 1983) that drug effects are similar when stimulants are taken in a fasting or fed state, with absorption actually faster in the latter.

The development of tolerance in children to stimulants is extremely rare, and dependence and abuse have been almost nonexistent (Cantwell & Carlson, 1978; Goyer et al., 1979; Gittelman, 1983).

Combining medication with other treatments is usual. Parent counseling and modification of the school milieu are often indicated. In most research investigations, however, stimulants alone have been more effective than other treatments alone. There are some data which suggest that combination of stimulant with behavior therapy gives an insignificantly better outcome than drug alone (Christensen & Sprague, 1973; Christensen, 1975; Firestone et al., 1978; O'Leary & Pelham, 1978; Gittelman et al., 1979; Gittelman-Klein et al., 1980; Wolraich et al., 1980).

The decision of when to discontinue stimulants is a clinical one, also. Lack of improvement after two weeks at maximum dosage of dextroamphetamine and MP or five weeks of pemoline is indication to stop. Dosage can usually be lowered for most side effects, though more severe adverse effects might necessitate ending treatment. Weekend "drug holidays" for dextroamphetamine and MP are routine, but exceptions must be made on an individual basis, that is, where home problems are prominent and dramatically improve on drug. The drug should be discontinued at least once a year to assess continued need for treatment. Studies indicate that a fairly high percentage of children do not need to resume treatment when this is done (Sleator et al., 1974). At the present time, drugs have not been shown to produce long term benefits, in terms of factors such as better life adjustment or better jobs (Weiss et al., 1975; Riddle & Rapoport, 1976; Weiss et al., 1979).

Adverse Effects. The most common short term adverse effects are anorexia and insomnia. Less common are weight loss, abdominal pain, and headache. These are generally short-lived and rarely require the stopping of medication. Drowsiness, dizziness, mood changes, dyskinesias, and toxic psychosis are rare (Cantwell & Carlson, 1978; Connors & Werry, 1979; Weiner, 1980; Gualtieri et al., 1984). Idiosyncratic responses do occur, such as the development of a blood dyscrasia. Relatively few side effects occur with dosages below .5 mg/kg of dextroamphetamine or 1 mg/kg of MP.

Suppression of weight and height has been found in short term treatment with dextroamphetamine, MP, and pemoline (Safer et al., 1972; Gross, 1976; Friedman, 1981; Gualtieri et al., 1982). Though many investigators have found that growth suppression is temporary, there are recent reports of small, but significant decreases in height and weight percentiles with chronic treatment with dextroamphetamine and MP, which might prove important for specific individuals (Mattes & Gittelman, 1983; Greenhill et al., 1984).

Antidepressants: Behavioral Effects of Clinical Usage

This discussion is limited to the effects of antidepressants in ADDH. The other aspects of antidepressants are presented elsewhere in this volume (Chapter 5).

Tricyclic antidepressants have shown clinical efficacy in several studies (Rapoport et al., 1974; Quinn & Rapoport, 1975; Greenberg, 1975; Connors & Werry, 1979; Klein et al., 1980). Improvement is as rapid and sometimes as striking as with the stimulants. However, the effects seem to be short-lived for many subjects. All reports show that effects are elicited in dosages less than those used for depression. Side effects seem to become a limiting factor in continued treatment. Antidepressants are therefore considered second line drugs for ADDH.

There is clinical and research interest in the monoamine oxidase inhibitors, especially because they have stimulant effects. There are rare studies of MAOI treatment in adults with ADD, RT (Wender et al., 1983) that show some behavioral improvement. Investigation of MAOI effects in children with ADDH are currently in progress and indicate beneficial effects (Zametkin, personal communication).

Antipsychotics: Behavioral Effects of Clinical Usage

Antipsychotic medications are discussed in more detail elsewhere in this volume (Chapter 4).

Several studies, using different classes of antipsychotics, have shown improvement in various symptoms of ADDH. However, overall clinical efficacy is not as striking as with stimulants (Rapoport et al., 1971; Gittelman-Klein et al., 1976; Werry et al., 1976; Connors & Werry, 1979; Klein et al., 1980). Use of antipsychotics is usually limited because of adverse effects. A decrease in cognitive functions has been demonstrated with their use. In addition, there is possible development of tardive dyskinesia, though this is unlikely to occur with low doses and relatively short term use (Gualtieri et al., 1984).

Other Drugs

Lithium carbonate (Whitehead & Clark, 1970; Greenhill et al., 1973), diphenhydramine (Fish, 1975), phenobarbital (Connors, 1972), and benzodiazepines (Millichap, 1973) have all been employed in the treatment of ADD-like behaviors. They have not been found to be effective and are of mostly historical interest.

Attention Deficit Disorder Without Hyperactivity

This diagnosis has not been well documented. Treatment has not been systematically studied. It is possible that children with this disorder are not readily identified or might not have symptoms severe enough for drug treatment. One would speculate that stimulants might be valuable in this population for their effects on increasing attention, particularly if academic failure stems chiefly from inattention.

Attention Deficit Disorder, Residual Type

This diagnosis is not yet well documented. There is current research attempting to define and validate the disorder, as well as to evaluate treatments. Stimulants and MAOIs appear to be of some benefit (Shelly & Reister, 1972; Mann & Greenspan, 1976; Wood et al., 1976; Packer, 1978; Wender et al., 1981).

ASSESSMENT

Assessment of treatment begins with careful diagnostic evaluation, which is necessary for obtaining adequate information and making accurate observations. The latter aid in the establishment of overall treatment goals and in specifying target behaviors for the focus of drug treatment.

It is often helpful to use objective measures (such as rating scales) to assess drug effects, including side effects and behavioral changes. The various Conners Rating Scales (Conners, 1969, 1972, 1976) and the Subject's Treatment Emergent Symptoms Scale or the Dosage Record and Treatment Emergent Symptoms Scale are several such measures for behavioral response and adverse effects, respectively (Early Clinical Drug Evaluation Unit, 1976). It is helpful to obtain ratings from parents, teachers, or other significant people in the child's life. Some measures of academic achievement are useful in evaluating, planning, and measuring progress in that important area of function.

Careful attention to assessment is required in the treatment of such complicated problems. This is especially true in the case of ADDH, where major treatment decisions are made chiefly on clinical grounds.

SUMMARY

1.   Attention Deficit Disorders are new and still changing conceptual and diagnostic entities. Validation of the syndromes, as well as clarification of the underlying variables, are major outstanding issues.

2.   The pharmacologic treatment of ADDH is one of the best described and researched treatments in child psychiatry. Stimulants, in particular dextroamphetamine and methylphenidate, are the current drugs of choice. Their short-term benefits are well documented. Long-term benefits from drug, or any other, treatment are unclear.

3.   Much remains to be learned about the clinical use of pharmacologic agents in ADD. However, enough is known presently to make use safe and effective. Short term adverse effects are rarely of major clinical significance. Long term adverse effects on growth and learning are still of interest.

4.   Important treatment decisions—such as when to initiate or discontinue medication—continue to be chiefly clinical decisions.

5.   ADD remains a topic of much active research, in almost all areas that have been discussed in this chapter.

REFERENCES

American Psychiatric Association (1968). *Diagnostic and Statistical Manual of Mental Disorders* (2nd ed.). Washington, DC: American Psychiatric Association.

American Psychiatric Association (1980). *Diagnostic and Statistical Manual of Mental Disorders* (3rd ed.). Washington, DC: American Psychiatric Association.

Aman, G. (1978). Drugs, learning and the psychotherapies. In J. S. Werry (Ed.), *Pediatric psychopharmacology: The use of behavior modifying drugs in children* (pp. 79–108). New York: Brunner/Mazel.

Arnold. L. F., Christopher, J., Huestis, R., & Smeltzer, D. J. (1978). Methylphenidate vs. dextroamphetamine vs. caffeine in minimal brain dysfunction: Controlled comparison by placebo washout design with Bayes analysis. *Archives of General Psychiatry, 35,* 463–473.

Barkley, R. (1977). A review of stimulant drug research with hyperactive children. *Journal of Child Psychology and Psychiatry, 18,* 137–165.

Becker-Mattes, A. (1982). A study of state-dependent learning in hyperactive children on Ritalin. Doctoral dissertation. Department of Psychology, George Washington University, Washington DC.

Bender, L., & Cottington, F. (1942). The use of amphetamine sulfate (benzedrine) in child psychiatry. *American Journal of Psychiatry, 99,* 116–121.

Brown, G. L., Ebert, M. H., Hunt, R. D., & Bunney, W. E. (1977). Amphetamine blood levels, behavior and activity in minimal brain dysfunction. Presented at the Annual Meeting of the American Psychiatric Association, Toronto.

Busby, K., Firestone, P., & Pivik, R. T. (1981). Sleep patterns in hyperkinetic and normal children. *Sleep, 4,* 366–383.

Cantwell, D. P. (1977). Psychopharmacologic treatment of the minimal brain dysfunction syndrome. In J. M. Wiener (Ed.), *Psychopharmacology in childhood and adolescence* (pp. 119–148). New York: Basic Books.

Cantwell, D. P., & Carlson, G. A. (1978). Stimulants. In J. S. Werry (Ed.), *Pediatric psychopharmacology: The use of behavior modifying drugs in children* (pp. 171–207). New York: Brunner/Mazel.

Chan, Y. P., Swanson, J. M., Soldin, S. S., Thiessen, J. J., Macleod, S. M., & Logan, W. (1983). Methylphenidate hydrochloride given with or before breakfast: II. Effects on plasma concentration of methylphenidate and ritalinic acid. *Pediatrics, 72,* 56–59.

Chatoor, I., Wells, K., Conners, C. K., Seidel, W. T., & Shaw, D. (1983). The effects of nocturnally administered stimulant medication on EEG, sleep and behavior in hyperactive children. *Journal of the American Academy of Child Psychiatry, 22,* 343–348.

Christensen, D. E. (1975). Effects of combining methylphenidate and a classroom token system in modifying hyperactive behavior. *American Journal of Mental Deficiency, 80,* 266–276.

Christensen, D. E., & Sprague, R. L. (1973). Reduction of hyperactive behvior by conditioning procedures alone and combined with methylphenidate (Ritalin). *Behavior Research and Therapy, 11,* 331–334.

Clements, S. (1966). Minimal brain dysfunction in children. NINDB Monograph No. 3. Washington, DC: U. S. Public Health Service.

Coleman, N., Dexheimer, P., DiMascio, A., Redman, W., & Finnerty, R. (1976). Deanol in the treatment of hyperkinetic children. *Psychosomatics, 17,* 68–72.

Conners, C. K. (1969). A teacher rating scale for use in drug studies with children. *American Journal of Psychiatry, 126,* 152–156.

Conners, C. K. (1972). Pharmacotherapy of psychopathology in children. In H. Quay &

J. Werry (Eds.), *Psychopathological disorders of childhood* (pp. 316–348). New York: Wiley.

Conners, C. K. (1975). A placebo-crossover study of caffeine treatment of hyperkinetic children. In R. Gittelman-Klein (Ed.), *Recent advances in child psychopharmacology* (pp. 136–147). New York: Human Sciences Press.

Conners, C. K. (1976). Rating scales for use in drug studies with children. In *Assessment manual*. Rockville, Md.: Early Clinical Drug Evaluation Unit, National Institute of Mental Health.

Conners, C. K., & Werry, J. S. (1979). Pharmacotherapy. In H. C. Quay and J. S. Werry (Eds.), *Psychopathological disorders of childhood* (2nd ed.) (pp. 336–386). New York: Wiley.

Conners, C. K., Eisenberg, L., & Sharpe, L. A. (1965). A controlled study of the differential application of outpatient psychiatric treatment for children. *Japanese Journal of Child Psychiatry, 6,* 125–132.

Conners, C. K., Eisenberg, L., & Barcai, A. (1967). Effect of dextroamphetamine on children. *Archives of General Psychiatry, 17,* 478–485.

Conners, C. K., Taylor, E., Meo, G., Kurtz, M. A., & Fournier, M. (1972). Magnesium pemoline and dextroamphetamine: A controlled study in children with minimal brain dysfunction. *Psyhopharmacologia, 26,* 321–336.

Charles, L., Schain, R., & Zelniker, T. (1981). Optimal dosages of methylphenidate for improving the learning and behavior of hyperactive children. *Journal of Developmental and Behavioral Pediatrics, 2,* 78–81.

Creese, I. (Ed.) (1983). *Stimulants: Neurochemical, behavioral, and clinical perspectives.* New York: Raven Press.

Cunningham, C. E., & Barkley, R. A. (1978). The interactions of hyperactive and normal children with their mothers in free play and structured task. *Child Development, 50,* 217–224.

Douglas, V. I., & Peters, K. G. (1979). Toward a clearer definition of the attentional deficit of hyperactive children. In G. A. Hale & M. Lewis (Ed.), *Attention and cognitive development.* New York: Plenum.

Dykman, R. A., McGrew, J., Harris, T. S., Peters, J. F., & Ackerman, P. (1976). Two blinded studies of the effects of stimulant drugs on children: Pemoline, methylphenidate, and placebo. In R. P. Anderson & C. G. Halcomb (Eds.), *Learning disability/minimal brain dysfunction syndrome.* Springfield, IL: Charles C. Thomas.

Early Clinical Drug Evaluation Unit (1976). *Assessment Manual.* Rockville, Md. : National Institute of Mental Health.

Ebert, M. H., Van Kammen, D. P., & Murphy, D. L. (1976). Plasma levels of amphetamine and behavioral response. In L. A. Gottschalk & S. Merlis (Eds.), *Pharmacokinetics of psychoactive drugs.* New York: Spectrum Publications.

Elkins, R., Rapoport, J., Zahn, T., Buchsbaum, M., Weingartner, H., Kopin, I., Langer, D., & Johnson, C. (1981). Acute effects of caffeine in normal and prepubertal boys. *American Journal of Psychiatry, 138,* 178–183.

Finnerty, R. J., Soltys, J. J., & Cole, J. O. (1971). The use of D-amphetamine with hyperkinetic children. *Psychopharmacologia, 21,* 302–308.

Firestone, P. (1982). Factors associated with children's adherence to stimulant medication. *American Journal of Orthopsychiatry, 52,* 447–457.

Firestone, P., Kelly, M. J., Goodman, J. T., & Peters, S. (1978). The effects of caffeine and methylphenidate on hyperactive children. *Journal of the American Academy of Child Psychiatry, 17,* 445–456.

Fish, B. (1975). Drug treatment of the hyperactive child. In D. Cantwell (Ed.), *The hyperactive child: Diagnosis, management, and current research.* New York: Spectrum Publications.

Fisher, M. A. (1978). Dextroamphetamine and placebo practice effects on selective attention in hyperactive children. *Journal of Abnormal Child Psychology, 6,* 25–32.

Franz, D. (1980). Central nervous system stimulants. In L. Goodman & A. Gilman (Eds.), *The pharmacologic basis of therapeutics* (6th ed.) (pp. 585–591). New York: Macmillan.

Friedman, N., Thomas, J., Carr, R., Elders, J., Ringdahl, I., & Roche, A. (1981). Effect on growth in pemoline-treated children with attention deficit disorder. *American Journal of Diseases of Children, 135,* 329–332.

Gesell, A., & Amatruda, C. S. (1949). *Developmental diagnosis* (2nd ed.). New York: Hoeber.

Gittelman, R. (1983). Experimental and clinical studies of stimulant use in hyperactive children and children with other behavioral disorders. In I. Creese (Ed.), *Stimulants: Neurochemical, behavioral, and clinical perspectives* (pp. 205–225). New York: Raven Press.

Gittelman, R., Abikoff, H., Mattes, J., & Klein, D. (1979). A controlled trial of behavior modification and methylphenidate in hyperactive children. Presented at the Annual Meeting of the American Academy of Child Psychiatry, Atlanta.

Gittelman-Klein, R., Klein, D., Katz, S., Saraf, K., & Pollack, E. (1976). Comparative effects of methylphenidate and thioridazine in hyperactive children. *Archives of General Psychiatry, 33,* 1217–1231.

Gittelman-Klein, R., Abikoff, H., Pollack, E., Klein, D., Katz, S., & Mattes, J. (1980). A controlled trial of behavior modification and methylphenidate in hyperactive children. In C. Whalen & B. Henker (Eds.), *Hyperactive children: The social ecology of identification and treatment.* New York: Academic Press.

Goyer, P., Davis, G., & Rapoport, J. (1979). Abuse of prescribed stimulant medication by a 13-year-old hyperactive boy. *Journal of the American Academy of Child Psychiatry, 18,* 170–175.

Greenberg, L., Yellin, A., Spring, C., & Metcalf, M. (1975). Clinical effects of imipramine and methylphenidate in hyperactive children. In R. Gittelman-Klein (Ed.), *Recent advances in child psychopharmacology.* New York: Human Sciences Press.

Greenhill, L., Puig-Antich, J., Novacenko, H., Solomon, M., Anghern, C., Florea, J., Goetz, R., Fiscina, B., & Sachar, E. (1984). Prolactin, growth hormone, and growth responses in boys with attention deficit disorder. *Journal of the American Academy of Child Psychiatry, 23,* 58–67.

Greenhill, L., Puig-Antich, J., Goetz, R., Hanlon, C., & Davies, R. (1983). Sleep architecture and REM sleep measures in perpubertal children with attention deficit disorder with hyperactivity. *Sleep, 6,* 91–101.

Greenhill, L., Rieder, R., Wender, P., Buchsbaum, M., & Zahn, T. (1973). Lithium carbonate in the treatment of hyperactive children. *Archives of General Psychiatry, 28,* 636–640.

Gross, M. (1976). Growth of hyperkinetic children taking methylphenidate, dextroamphetamine, or imipramine, desipramine. *Pediatrics, 58,* 423–431.

Gualtieri, C., Quade, D., Hicke, R., Mayo, J., & Schroeder, S. (1984). Tardive dyskinesia and other clinical consequences of neuroleptic treatment in childhood and adolescence. *American Journal of Psychiatry, 141,* 20–23.

Gualtieri, C., Wargin, W., Kanoy, R., Patrick, K., Shen, C., Youngblood, W., Mueller, R., & Breese, G. (1982). Clinical studies of methylphenidate serum levels in children and adults. *Journal of the American Academy of Child Psychiatry, 21,* 19–26.

Humphries, T., Kinsbourne, M., & Swanson, J. (1978). Stimulant effects on cooperation and social interaction between hyperactive children and their mothers. *Journal of Child Psychology and Psychiatry, 19,* 13–22.

Klein, D., Gittelman, R., Quitkin, F., & Rifkin, A. (1980). Diagnosis and drug treatment of childhood disorders. In *diagnosis and drug treatment of psychiatric disorders: Adults and children* (2nd ed.) (pp. 590–756). Baltimore: Williams & Wilkins.

Lewis, J., & Young, R. (1975). Deanol and methylphenidate in minimal brain dysfunction. *Clinical Pharmacology and Therapeutics, 17,* 534–540.

Mann, H., & Greenspan, S. (1976). The identification and treatment of adult brain dysfunction. *American Journal of Psychiatry, 133,* 1013.

Mattes, J., & Gittelman, R. (1983). Growth of hyperactive children on a maintenance regimen of methylphenidate. *Archives of General Psychiatry, 40,* 317–321.

Millichap, J. (1973). Drugs in management of minimal brain dysfunction. *Annals of the New York Academy of Science, 205,* 321–334.

Modell, W., Schild, H., & Wilson, A. (1976). *Applied pharmacology.* Philadelphia: Saunders

Nichols, P., & Chen, T. (1980). *Minimal brain dysfunction: A prospective study.* Hillsdale, NJ: Erlbaum.

Office of Child Development (1971). Report of the conference on the use of stimulant drugs in the treatment of behaviorally disturbed young school children. Washington, D. C.: Department of Health, Education and Welfare.

O'Leary, S., & Pelham, W. (1978). Behavior therapy and withdrawal of stimulant medication in hyperactive children. *Pediatrics, 61,* 211–217.

Ounstead, C. (1955). The hyperkinetic syndrome in epileptic children *The Lancet, 2,* 303–311.

Packer, S. (1978). Treatment of minimal brain dysfunction in a young adult. *Canadian Psychiatric Association Journal, 23,* 501.

Porrino, L., Rapoport, J., Behar, D., Ismond, D., & Bunney, W. (1983a). A naturalistic assessment of the motor activity of hyperactive boys. I. Comparison with normal controls. *Archives of General Psychiatry, 40,* 681–687.

Porrino, L., Rapoport, J., Behar, D., Ismond, D., & Bunney, W. (1983b). A naturalistic assessment of the motor activity of hyperactive boys. II. Stimulant drug effects. *Archives of General Psychiatry, 40,* 688–693.

Quinn, P., & Rapoport, J. (1975). One year follow-up of hyperactive boys treated with imipramine or methylphenidate. *American Journal of Psychiatry, 132,* 241–245.

Rall, T. (1980). Central nervous system stimulants—the xanthines. In L. Goodman & A. Gilman (Eds.), *The Pharmacologic Basis of Therapeutics* (6th ed.) (pp. 592–607). New York: Macmillan.

Rapoport, J. (1983). Methodology for assessing effects of dietary substances in grade-school children. *Journal of Psychiatric Research,* in press.

Rapoport, J., Abramson, A., Alexander, D., & Lott, I. (1971). Playroom observations of hyperactive children on medication. *Journal of the American Academy of Child Psychiatry, 10,* 524–534.

Rapoport, J., Quinn, P., Bradbard, G., Riddle, D., & Brooks, E. (1974). Imipramine and methylphenidate treatments of hyperactive boys. *Archives of General Psychiatry, 30*, 789–793.

Rapoport, J., Buchsbaum, M., Zahn, T., Weingartner, H., Ludlow, C., & Mikkelson, E. (1978). Dextroamphetamine: Cognitive and behavioral effects in normal prepubertal boys. *Science, 199*, 560–563.

Rapoport, J., Buchsbaum, M., Weingartner, H., Zahn, T., Ludlow, C., Bartko, J., Mikkelson, E., Langer, D., & Bunney, W. (1980). Dextroamphetamine: Cognitive and behvioral effects in normal and hyperactive boys and normal adult males. *Archives of General Psychiatry, 37*, 933–946.

Riddle, K., & Rapoport, J. (1976). A two-year follow-up of hyperactive boys. *Journal of Nervous and Mental Disease, 162*, 126–134.

Rutter, M., & Garmezy, N. (1983). Developmental psychopathology. In P. Mussen (Ed.), *Handbook of child psychology* (4th ed.), (Vol. IV, pp. 775–912). New York: Wiley.

Rutter, M., Shaffer, D., & Sturge, C. (1979). *A guide to a multi-axial classification scheme for psychiatric disorders in childhood and adolescence.* London: Institute of Psychiatry.

Safer, D., & Allen, R. (1976). *Hyperactive children: diagnosis and management.* Baltimore: University Park Press.

Safer, D., Allen, R., & Barr, E. (1972). Depression of growth in hyperactive children on stimulant drugs. *New England Journal of Medicine, 287*, 217–220.

Saunders, L. (1974). *The absorption and distribution of drugs (pp. 132–153).* London: Bailliere Tindall.

Schleifer, N., Weiss, G., Cohen, N., Elman, M., Cvejic, H., & Kruger. (1975). Hyperactivity in preschoolers and the effect of methylphenidate. *American Journal of Orthopsychiatry, 45*, 38–50.

Shapiro, A., Shapiro, E., Bruun, R., & Sweet, R. (1978). Current treatment of Tourette Syndrome. In *Gilles de la Tourette Syndrome.* New York: Raven Press.

Shaywitz, S., Hunt, R., Jatlow, P., Cohen, D., Young, J., Pierce, R., Anderson, G., & Shaywitz, B. (1982). Psychopharmacology of attention deficit disorder: Pharmacokinetic, neuroendocrine, and behavioral measures following acute and chronic treatment with methylphenidate. *Pediatrics, 69*, 688–694.

Shelly, E., & Reister, F. (1972). Syndrome of MBD in young adults. *Diseases of the Nervous System, 33*, 335.

Sleator, E. (1982). How do hyperactive children feel about taking stimulants and will they tell the doctor? *Clinical Pediatrics (Philadelphia), 21*, 474–479.

Sleator, E., vonNeumann, A., & Sprague, R. (1974). Hyperactive children: A continuous long-term placebo-controlled follow-up. *Journal of the American Medical Association, 229*, 316–317.

Sostek, A., Buchsbaum, M., & Rapoport, J. (1980). Effects of amphetamine on vigilance performance in normal and hyperactive children. *Journal of Abnormal Child Psychology, 8*, 491–500.

Sprague, R., & Sleator, E. (1977). Methylphenidate in hyperkinetic children: Differences in dose effects on learning and social behavior. *Science, 198*, 1274–1276.

Stenhausen, H., & Kreuzer, E. (1971). Learning in hyperactive children: Are three stimulant-related and state-dependent effects? *Psychopharmacology, 74*, 384–390.

Stewart, M., Pitts, F., Craig, A., & Dieruf, W. (1966). The hyperactive child syndrome. *American Journal of Orthopsychiatry, 36*, 861–867.

Swanson, J., & Kinsbourne, M. (1976). Stimulant-related state-dependent learning in hyperactive children. *Science, 192,* 1354–1357.

Swanson, J., Sandman, C., Deutsch, C. & Baren, M. (1983). Methylphenidate hydrochloride given with or before breakfast: I. behavioral, cognitive, and electrophysiologic effects. *Pediatrics, 72,* 49–55.

Thurston, C., Sobol, M., Swanson, J., & Kinsbourne, M. (1979). Effects of methylphenidate (Ritalin) on selective attention in hyperactive children. *Journal of Abnormal Child Psychology, 7,* 471–481.

Varley, C. (1983). Effects of methylphenidate in adolescents with attention deficit disorder. *Journal of the American Academy of Child Psychiatry, 22,* 351–354.

Weiner, N. (1980). Norepinephrine, epinephrine, and sympathomimetics. In L. Goodman & A. Gilman (Eds.), *The pharmacologic basis of therapeutics* (6th ed.) (pp. 138–175). New York: Macmillan.

Weingartner, H., Langer, D., Grice, J., & Rapoport, J. (1982). Acquisition and retrieval of information in amphetamine treated hyperactive children. *Psychiatric Research, 6,* 21–29.

Weiss, G. (1983). Long-term outcome: Findings, concepts, and practical implications. In M. Rutter (Ed.), *Developmental neuropsychiatry.* New York: Guilford Press.

Weiss, G., Minde, K., Douglas, V., Werry, J., & Sykes, D. (1971). Comparison of the effects of chlorpromazine, dextroamphetamine, and methylphenidate on the behavior and intellectual functioning of hyperactive children. *Canadian Medical Association Journal, 104,* 20–25.

Weiss, G., Kruger, E., Danielson, V., & Elman, M. (1975). Effects of long-term treatment of hyperactive children with methylphenidate. *Canadian Medical Association Journal, 112,* 159–165.

Weiss, G., Hechtman, L., Perlman, T., Hopkins, J., & Wener, A. (1979). Hyperactive children as young adults: A controlled prospective ten-year follow-up of 75 children. *Archives of General Psychiatry, 36,* 675–681.

Wender, P. (1971). *Minimal brain dysfunction in children.* New York: Wiley-Interscience.

Wender, P., Reimherr, F., & Wood, D. (1981). Attention deficit disorder ("minimal brain dysfunction") in adults. *Archives of General Psychiatry, 38,* 449.

Wender, P., Wood, D. Reimherr, F., & Ward, M. (1983). An open trial of pargyline in the treatment of attention deficit disorder, residual type. *Psychiatry Research, 9,* 329–336.

Werry, J., & Aman, M. (1975). Methylphenidate and haloperidol in children: effects on attention, memory, and activity. *Archives of General Psychiatry, 32,* 790–795.

Werry, J., Aman, M., & Lampen, E. (1976). Haloperidol and methylphenidate in hyperactive children. *Acta Paedopsychiatrica* (Basel), *42,* 26–40.

Whalen, C., & Henker, B. (1976). Psychostimulants and children: A review and analysis. *Psychology Bulletin, 83,* 1113–1130.

Whalen, C., Collins, B., Henker, B., Alkus, S., Adams, D., & Stapp, J. (1978). Behavior observations of hyperactive children and methylphenidate effects in systematically structured classroom environments: Now you see them, now you don't. *Journal of Pediatric Psychology, 3,* 177–187.

Whalen, C., Henker, B., & Dotemoto, S. (1980a). Methylphenidate and hyperactivity: effects on teacher behaviors. *Science, 208,* 1280–1282.

Whalen, C., Henker, B., & Finck, D. (1980b). Medication effects in the classroom: Three naturalistic indicators. *Journal of Abnormal Child Psychology, 9,* 419–433.

Whalen, C., Henker, B., & Dotemoto, S. (1981). Teacher response to the methylphenidate (Ritalin) versus placebo status of hyperactive boys in the classroom. *Child Development, 52,* 1005–1014.

Whitehead, P., & Clark, L. (1970). Effect of lithium carbonate, placebo and thioridazine on hyperactive children. *American Journal of Psychiatry, 127,* 824–825.

Wolraich, M., Drummond, T., Salomon, M., O'Brien, M., & Sivage, C. (1978). Effects of methylphenidate alone and in combination with behavior modification procedures on the behavior and academic performance of hyperactive children. *Journal of Abnormal Child Psychology, 6,* 149–161.

Wood, D., Reimherr, F., Wender, P., & Johnson, G. (1976). Diagnosis and treatment of minimal brain dysfunction in adults. *Archives of General Psychiatry, 33,* 1453.

Zametkin, A. (1983). Personal communication.

Anxiety Disorders

STEVEN L. JAFFE, M.D. and J. VERNON MAGNUSON, M.D.

Anxiety is a basic human emotion that in mild and transient forms is a part of everyone's daily experience. In a more intense form, it may be part of all psychiatric disorders, and within the DSM III (1980) section of child and adolescent disorders, it is the predominant clinical feature of the group labeled Anxiety Disorders. Mild to moderately intense anxiety also is experienced as a normal part of the developmental process. Although not addressed by DSM III, these "developmental" anxieties are an important aspect of the clinical evaluation of anxiety in children and adolescents. In this chapter, we outline a classification of anxiety related primarily to adult disorders, and also consider anxiety states related to normal growth and development. Anxiety Disorders as classified in DSM III are discussed, and under this group, Overanxious Disorder and Separation Anxiety Disorder are presented. Because Obsessive-Compulsive Disorder has anxiety as a significant symptom, it also is included. Lastly, the pharmacodynamics and clinical studies of antihistamines and benzodiazepines are reviewed because these are the medications that have most frequently been used for developmental and other anxiety symptoms.

DEFINITION AND CLASSIFICATION OF ANXIETY

Anxiety is defined as a "normal inborn response either to a threat to one's person, attitudes, or self-esteem or to the absence of people or objects that assure and signal safety" (Kandel, 1983). Anxiety has both subjective and objective features. The subjective features are identical to fear experienced under conditions of actual danger (Klein, 1964). They range from a heightened sense of awareness and uneasiness to a deep fear of impending tragedy and disaster. Objective features include verbalized worries and anticipated fears, heightened responsiveness with irritability and distractibility, signs of motor tension (being shaky, tremulous), and autonomic hyperactivity (sweating, clammy hands, dry mouth, increased heart rate, intestinal cramps and diarrhea, and hyperventilation with light-headedness and paresthesias).

Kandel (1983) classifies anxiety into actual (automatic) anxiety and acquired (signal) anxiety: actual anxiety is an in-born response to external or internal danger; acquired anxiety is subdivided into panic attacks, anticipatory anxiety, and chronic anxiety. Panic attacks are spontaneous episodes of terror with accompanying sympathetic crisis. These often respond to tricyclic antidepressants. Anticipatory anxiety refers to brief anxiety periods that are related to real or imagined signals. It tends to respond to benzodiazepines. Chronic anxiety is a persistent feeling of apprehension unrelated to external dangers, and may be responsive to benzodiazepines.

ANXIETY DISORDERS

DSM III (American Psychiatric Association 1980) describes three diagnostic groups within the Anxiety Disorder category: Avoidant, Overanxious, and Separation Anxiety Disorders. There are no controlled studies of medication treatment of children with the diagnoses of Avoidant or Overanxious Disorders. Only Separation Anxiety Disorder (school phobia variant) has been studied. This is partly reflective of the recency of these diagnostic categories. Even prior to DSM III, however, Gittelman (1980) found no controlled studies of the effectiveness of antianxiety medication in children selected specifically for anxiety symptoms. Reasons proposed for this lack of methodologicaly good studies include imprecision of psychodiagnosis, the transience and reactivity of symptoms, and the tendency for children to be evaluated because of others' concerns and not the child's subjective distress. Hershberg et al. (1982) demonstrated the feasibility of such studies by identifying anxiety disorders by DSM III criteria in 14 of 102 randomly selected outpatient children and adolescents. These children and adolescents reported a large number and variety of fears, ruminations, and compulsions as well as observable behavior reflective of anxiety. Seven were diagnosed as Overanxious Disorder, one as Avoidant Disorder, three as simple phobia or obsessive-compulsive, and three as Separation Anxiety Disorder.

Separation Anxiety Disorder

Making the diagnostic distinction between expected anxiety in the context of actual separation and pathological separation anxiety is not always easy. The former is related to separation from significant attachment figures, has temporal limits, and does not prohibit necessary productive action. Pathological separation anxiety is diagnosed Separation Anxiety Disorder in children and Agoraphobia in adults. Although not related to each other for purposes of classification, the histories of agoraphobic adults often include symptoms of separation anxiety as children (Klein, 1964). The response of some adult agoraphobic patients to imipramine led to the study of its efficacy in the school phobia variant of separation anxiety disorder in children (Gittelman-Klein & Klein, 1971, 1973), as will be discussed below.

Diagnostic Considerations. DSM III lists two inclusionary and two exclusionary criteria for the diagnosis of Separation Anxiety Disorder. The first criterion defines by nine behaviors the excessive anxiety when the child is separated from a significant attachment figure; the presence of three of the nine is sufficient. Two of the nine have to do with school-avoidant behaviors, covering those cases labeled "school phobia" in the literature and in common parlance.

The second criterion requires manifest excessive anxiety for a minimum of two weeks. The exclusionary criteria require that the symptoms not be due to a psychotic condition and that the individual not meet the criteria for Agoraphobia if 18 years old or older.

The incidence and prevalence of this disorder are not known, but it is not uncommon. There is no sex predominance. While there are statements in the literature that school phobia is a disorder of middle-and-upper class children, Separation Anxiety Disorder is not unusual in lower socioeconomic class children. Onset is most common in school-age children, but may occur in preschoolers or adolescents.

School avoidance due to separation anxiety must be distinguished from truancy. Truant children do not avoid school in order to be at home or to sustain the presence of an attachment figure and do not experience excessive anxiety when entering the school building. It is important to establish that the child is not avoiding school because of some real threat to personal safety. In the same way, care must be taken not to overlook actual physical illness in the face of somatic complaints that appear to legitimize staying home.

While school avoidant behavior (i.e., school phobia) is the best known form of this disorder, a not uncommon presentation involves sleep avoidance, nightmares depicting separation themes, and unrealistic worry about the safety of major attachment figures, or somatic complaints in anticipation of being left alone or with a baby sitter. Temper tantrums may replace or accompany the somatic complaints.

In early childhood, the distinction between normal separation anxiety and Separation Anxiety Disorder requires clinical judgment. Normal separation anxiety usually fluctuates in intensity and by situation. Furthermore, the ambivalent attitude of the major attachment figure regarding separation from the child is absent.

It is possible for a child who has experienced the death of a loved one to meet the criteria for Separation Anxiety Disorder with or without school avoidant symptoms. This group of children deserves further investigation with a view toward diagnostic refinement and definition of possible therapeutic needs.

Drugs of Choice. Gittelman-Klein and Klein (1971) established the efficacy of imipramine hydrochloride at doses of 100–200 mg/day in the treatment of school phobic children. In this study, children unresponsive to initial efforts at encouraging return to school were placed in a double-blind placebo controlled study, combining drug and placebo with individual and family psychotherapy. The drug group returned to school significantly sooner than the placebo group (Gittelman-Klein, 1973). Although the methodology and results of this study are convincing, a replication study is not yet reported. No other drug is reported effective by methodologically acceptable studies in the treatment of school phobia. An earlier report of chlordiazepoxide efficacy (D'Amato, 1962) is from an open and uncontrolled study, not yet confirmed. In addition, Eisenberg (1958, 1959) reports efficacy with psychosocial treatment essentially comparable to the Gittleman-Klein imipramine group, but taking a longer time. Clomipramine is reported ineffective in the treatment of school phobia (Berney et al., 1981).

Currently, imipramine in dosages of 1.0–5.0 mg/kg/day is recommended for the treatment of school phobic children in conjunction with other established psychosocial approaches in the hands of experienced clinicians and reserved for cases unresponsive to psychosocial therapies. Imipramine efficacy is not established for any variant of separation anxiety disorder other than school phobia. The nonschool avoidant variants of separation anxiety disorder deserve systematic investigation and their relationship to childhood grief reactions need clarification. No specific drug therapy for these variants can be recommended at present.

Adverse Effects. The adverse effects of imipramine are the same as those for other tricyclic drugs (Chapters 1 and 5).

Imipramine, at dosages of 5 mg/kg/day produces EKG abnormalities that reflect conduction defects (Winsberg et al., 1975). At a single bedtime dosage of up 2–3 mg/kg/day, no EKG abnormalities were measurable the following day (Martin & Zang, 1975). Even though the EKG findings at the high end of the dosage range do not reflect life-threatening cardiac dysfunction, the lower doses are preferable. Hayes et. al (1975) advises EKG monitoring when imipramine is administered to children and that imipramine use be regarded as investigational.

Overanxious Disorder

This diagnostic group consists of children with generalized and persistent anxiety or worry about future events and performance, not related to concerns about separation, not focused on a specific situation or object, and not due to a recent psychosocial stress. DSM III requires at least four of the following seven clinical features must be present for the diagnosis: (1) Unrealistic worry about future events. (2) Preoccupation with the appropriateness of past behavior. (3) Overconcern about competence in such areas as academic, athletic, and social performance. (4) Excessive need for reassurance about a variety of worries. (5) Somatic complaints such as headaches or stomach aches for which no physical basis can be established. (6) Marked self-consciousness or susceptibility to embarrassment or humiliation. And (7) marked feelings of tension or inability to relax. These symptoms must have been persistent for at least six months. Children with Attention Deficit Disorders (ADD) do not have the worries about the future and performance, and children with Overanxious Disorder do not have the impulsivity of ADD. A child may have both diagnoses if the criteria for each are met. Antihistamines, benzodiazepines, and even low doses of major tranquilizers are in clinical use for these children, but there are no controlled studies of efficacy. Hershberg et al. (1982) find 7 percent of an outpatient population to have Overanxious Disorder.

Obsessive-Compulsive Disorder

Obsessive thinking and compulsive behavior are common experiences. Both are the stuff from which are made bedtime and waking rituals; policies and procedures of industry, commerce, and education; grief and separation reactions; and superstitions. Beginning around the age of two or three years and continuing into latency, obsessive and compulsive phenomena are expectable features of normal psychological development. Under all these circumstances the activities are experienced as being under voluntary control and useful to the individual, referred to as "ego syntonic."

In Obsessive-Compulsive Disorder, the thoughts and actions are "ego dystonic," experienced as intrusive, involuntary and unwanted. Obsessions are recurrent thoughts, images, or impulses invading consciousness, regarded as irrational and/or out of character (Lewis, 1935). Likewise, compulsions are repetitive, often stereotyped behaviors that are carried out as magical guarantors or prohibitors of some future situation, occurring in association with obsessions. Compulsions typically are established to afford temporary relief from the anxiety that accompanies obsessions (Anthony, 1975).

From a psychodynamic point of view, obsessive-compulsive symptoms are understood as an attempt on the part of ego mechanisms to satisfy anal-sadistic id impulses while complying with rigid, moralistic superego prohibitions (A. Freud, 1966; S. Freud, 1913). Furthermore, the individual has insight with respect to the irrationality and disruptiveness, but is unable to utilize that insight to change. Elkins, Rapoport, and Lipsky (1980) reviewed data from twin studies, Giles de la Tourette Syndrome, neuropsychological testing, neurology/neurosurgery, and psychopharmacology. They find evidence suggestive of a neurobiological substrate. Behavioral theorists propose a learning model to explain obsessive-compulsive symptoms (Salzman & Thaler, 1981).

Further research is clearly needed since none of the current etiological hypotheses leads to consistently effective treatment. Follow-up studies (Judd, 1965; Hollingsworth et al., 1980) establish that Obsessive-Compulsive Disorder is a relatively stable illness which persists through childhood into adulthood. Treatment of various types yields improvement in about half of cases, but complete recovery is rare (Hollingsworth et al., 1980).

Diagnostic Considerations and Variations. According to DSM-III (1980) three criteria are necessary to establish the diagnosis: (1) The presence of obsessions or compulsions that are ego dystonic and resisted by the sufferer. (2) The symptoms are a source of significant distress for the individual and an interference with social or role functioning. (3) The exclusion of another mental disorder to which the symptoms are secondary.

These criteria are the same for children and adults. The disorder is rare among children, occurring in 1.2 percent of child psychiatric inpatients studied by Judd (1965) and 0.2 percent of inpatients and outpatients reviewed by Hollingsworth et al., (1980). However, it is common to learn from adult sufferers that they were symptomatic as children. Some controversy surrounds the issue of age of onset. The disorder has been found in children as young as three years, and onset appears to average between seven and nine years of age. Children for whom this diagnosis is made are typically of average to above average intelligence and perform well in school. There is no gender preference. An overattachment to the mother is often observed.

In one study, the families of children with Obsessive-Compulsive Disorder feature serious mental illness in up to 80 percent of cases although the prevalence of obsessive-compulsive disorder is not prominent (Hollingsworth et al., 1980). Rapoport et al., (1981) report minimal disturbance among the families of their patients.

There are features in children that initially may obscure the diagnosis. In younger children, fear may be a prominent accompaniment of obsessions and may be more distressing to patient and family than compulsions. Thus a phobic reaction may be considered until the obsessive-compulsive complex is fully recognized. Some patients with tic disorders and Tourette's Syndrome display obsessions and/or compulsions (Shapiro et al., 1978); if tic disorder or Tourette's Syndrom is established, obsessive-compulsive disorder is excluded (American Psychiatric Association, 1980).

In older children and adolescents affective symptoms, especially depression, may be present along with obsessions–compulsions (Rapoport et al., 1981). A judgment is required as to which disorder is primary, since diagnosis has important treatment and prognostic implications. If a decision cannot be made with confidence, it may be judicious to treat for affective illness since this disorder is usually more responsive, and a therapeutic trial may clarify the diagnosis. In view of new evidence from Rapoport (personal communication, see below), clomipramine may be the rational drug choice because of its beneficial effect on depression and some cases of obsessive-compulsive disorder.

Drugs and Treatment. Clomipramine hydrocholoride, a tricyclic antidepressant, results in marked improvement-to-resolution of obsessive and compulsive symptoms in about 50 percent of adult patients with the disorder (Thoren et al., 1980a and b). In adults, clomipramine is significantly better than other tricyclic antidepressants and its effect is sustained when a benefited patient remains on the drug (Thoren et al., 1980a). In a pilot study by Rapoport et al. (1980), clomipramine had little beneficial effect upon a group of a children with Obsessive-Compulsive Disorder. Further investigation (personal communication from Dr. Rapoport, manuscript in preparation) reports clomipramine significantly better than placebo in relieving Obsessive-Compulsive Disorder in children. As with adults, approximately 50 percent of drug-treated children improve.

Any of the anxiolytic agents may be used in children with Obsessive-Compulsive Disorder to provide relief from anxiety. There are no indications for or benefits from the anxiolytic drugs unique to this disorder. It is important to use the anxiolytics for relief of anxiety and not for the dysphoria or dissatisfaction that focuses on the obsessions or compulsions, since they have no effect upon the latter.

There is a recent increased clinical and research interest in Obsessive-Compulsive Disorder in childhood. It is likely that new information regarding the psychobiology of this disorder will be forthcoming and, in particular, further data on the efficacy of clomipramine.

Summary. Obsessive-Compulsive Disorder is a pervasive, disabling, rather stable mental disorder that is rare in children. Ths disorder has essentially the same clinical presentation in children as in adults, and childhood sufferers often manifest the same symptoms into adulthood. Multimodal psychotherapy has been found to effect improvement in children, but complete recovery is rare. New evidence indicates that clomipramine is efficacious in some children with the disorder. Anxiolytic tranquilizers may be used selectively to provide relief from the anxiety that accompanies the disorder.

ANXIETY RELATED TO DEVELOPMENTAL STAGES

Psychoanalytic theory introduced the concepts of anxiety as ubiquitously experienced in relationship to stages in development, and of anxiety itself as undergoing a developmental progression based on cognitive maturation, sequences of attachment, separation-individuation, and object relations. In addition there are constitutional temperamental differences among infants, characterized by varying capacities to tolerate internal and external stress and adapt to the environment (Chess et al., 1967). These differences in temperament may variously predispose or modulate the individual's experience of anxiety throughout the developmental process.

In development itself "signal" rather than "automatic" anxiety is identified first in connection with the reaction to strangers ("stranger anxiety") at 5–7 months. True separation anxiety is experienced beginning during the second year, expressed by protesting, angry, and clinging behavior, and often accompanied by sleep disturbances.

Specific fears and simple phobias begin during the third year; for example, of animals, the dark, and a bit later of bodily injury, dentists, and doctors. The school-age child must begin to deal with more internalized sources of anxiety centering around issues of performance, peer relationships, athletic ability and impulse control. Obsessive worries and compulsive behaviors tend to occur at this time.

The early adolescent must cope with the changes attendant to puberty-biological, cognitive, psychological, and sociocultural. Struggling to maintain mastery and control in the face of many competing, conflicting, and regressive pressures, the pubertal child tends to deny anxieties and express conflicts in terms of behavior, attitudes, and moods. The older adolescent may feel more comfortable with these developmental pressures and able to allow more access to the subjective aspects of anxiety states around changes in the body, peer relationships, sexuality, and self-definition.

This brief review of anxiety related to developmental pressures highlights the importance of distinguishing the normal, necessary, and positive role of anxiety from pathological anxiety states during childhood and adolescence. The former both reflects and stimulates the developmental process. The latter reflect major difficulties in the capacity of the individual to sustain developmental progress, and further adversely influence the capacity for mastery and sustained maturation in object relations and defenses, and often result in regression and/or distortions in character development.

It is critical for the clinician to be able to identify pathological anxiety states that are overwhelming, persistent and disruptive, even if not yet crystallized into a definable DSM III clinical disorder. While medication (such as the antianxiety and antihistamic agents discussed below) may be a helpful adjunctive treatment, such anxiety states are also responsive to emphathic understanding varying from support and reassurance to specific therapies such as individual psychodynamic psychotherapy, family therapy, behavior modification, or cognitively oriented approaches. Depending on many variables, medication may provide more rapid symptom relief when the anxiety is intense and function significantly impaired. Risks to consider with medication include adverse effects and the possibility that an opportunity for mastery and growth is circumvented.

Pharmacological Agents Used for Developmental and Other Anxiety Symptoms

Two classes of medication are used frequently for mild to moderate anxiety states. Only when these conditions are intense and appear overwhelming should medication be considered. These medications have not been studied in developmental anxieties, but have been studied in clinical trials, primarily on hospitalized children with severe psychopathology.

Antihistamines. Diphenhydramine (Benadryl®) is an H-1 histamine receptor antagonist as its peripheral effect, and is used frequently in the treatment of allergic reactions. It regularly produces central nervous system sedation as a central effect. There is no abuse potential and no physical dependence. It is rapidly absorbed from the gastro-intestinal tract and is frequently effective within 30 minutes. It has a relatively short serum half-life of about 6 hours, and the duration of the sedative effect is from 3–6 hours. It is then degraded in the liver and excreted within a 24 hour period. Effects are biphasic and dose dependent so that central nervous system sedation is produced within a therapeutic dosage range. Because it lowers the seizure threshold, toxic doses will act as a central nervous system stimulant and may precipitate seizures. Stimulatory effects are very rare. White (1977) states that other than occasional dizziness and oversedation, antihistamines are "virtually without significant adverse reactions." Ocassionally there may be incoordination, blurred vision, or stimulation. Dry moutn, nausea and abdominal cramping are anticholenergic effects. Leukopenia and agranulocytosis are extremely rare. Children may become tolerant to the sedative effects over time. Because of the drying action on the mucous membranes, diphenhydramine should not be used with bronchial asthma, and because of anticholenergic effects, it should not be used in children who have glaucoma or bladder neck obstruction. Recommended dosages range between 50–500 mg. Hydroxyzine (Atarax® or Vistaril®), is also an H-1 blocking antihistamine and has similar pharmacodynamics.

Clinical studies of diphenhydramine are reported over a number of years from the Bellevue Medical Center. Effron and Freedman (1953) described diphenhydramine (Benadryl) as effective in reducing anxiety in an uncontrolled study of a mixed hospitalized group of children. A later placebo controlled study on a similar hospital population reported diphenhydramine to be efficacious in the therapy of primary behavior disorders, especially in those with considerable manifest anxiety (Freedman et al., 1955). Fish (1968) described diphenhydramine to be effective in disorders associated with hyperactivity, especially to decrease anxiety in young children. Diphenhydramine decreass in effectiveness at puberty. Prior to puberty there is less sedative effect in comparison to anti-anxiety effect, while after puberty it frequently produces drowsiness and is more helpful for bedtime sedation. In comparison to these positive clinical reports, Korein et al. (1971) studied a similar Bellevue Hospital population in a comparison of diphenhydramine, chlorpromazine, and placebo. The 15 children on diphenhydramine showed no significant behavioral improvement in comparison to placebo. Diphenlhydramine is frequently used for transient sleep disorders, and there is a placebo controlled study by Russo et al. (1976) that demonstrates diphenlhydramine to be significantly superior to placebo in decreasing time before onset of sleep and decreasing number of awakenings over a period of one week. Greenberg (1972) reports an eight week double-blind study of 61 hyperactive school-age boys in which chlorpromazine and dextroamphetamine were significantly more effective than hydroxyzine or placebo. While only these few studies are available, the antihistamines apparently are used extensively by physicians treating children for anxiety relief. Adams (1979) describes that hydroxzine is "the great subduer of childhood neurosis in North America." The antihistamines are frequently used for sedation and anxiety relief especially in young children. Werry (1978) laments that the information available on antihistamines "when used as sedatives is so inadequate that it is not possible to state whether or not disinhibition occurs." Campbell (1983) relates that chronic antihistaminic administration may be associated with tardive dyskinesia. While acute dystonic reactions may occur in young people, the rare case reports of tardive dyskinesia are in patients over 55 years of age (Smith & Domino, 1980), and irreversible tardive dyskinesia induced by antihistamines has not been reported in children (Gualtieri, personal communication).

Benzodiazepines. The benzodiazepines are the second group of drugs in use for anxiety in children and adolescents. Common examples include diazepam, chlordiazepoxide, and oxazepam. Diazepam and chlordiazepoxide are rapidly and completely absorbed. Oxazepam is rather poorly absorbed. The benzodiazepines are highly bound to plasma proteins and are highly lipid-soluble and therefore rapidly distributed to brain tissue. Diazepam has a peak concentration in one hour, and its elimination kinetics are best described by a two compartment model (Coffey et al., 1983). The distributive (alpha) half-life is about 2½ hours, which is followed by an elimination (beta) phase in which the half-life is about 1½ to three days. One of diazepam's primary metabolic products, desmethyldiazepam, appears to have a half-life of 51–120 hours. Oxazepam has a slow absorption and therefore a more delayed onset. It has no active metabolites and has a relatively short half-life of 5–15 hours. Chlordiazepoxide has an intermediate absorption speed and half-life of 5–30 hours. Coffey et al. (1983) describe that children will metabolize diazepam faster than adults after age five months when liver maturation occurs. The central nervous system effects of the benzodiazepines are sedation and disinhibition, slowing of psychomotor function, and muscle relation occurring largely on a central basis. Tyrer (1982) emphasizes the selective antianxiety effects in the limbic system. Benzodiazepine receptors were discovered in the central nervous system in 1976, and benzodiazepines have been demonstrated to facilitate GABA transmission in the central nervous system. Tyrer (1982) describes benzodiazepines specifically binding to a special recognition site on the GABA receptor that itself is functionally linked to the benzodiazepine receptor. By contrast, Werry (1982), suggests that the selectivity is minor. He feels that the pharmacological effect is similar to the general sedatives, relating the advantages of the benzodiazepines to the flatness of the dose response curve that allows finer tuning and therefore anxiolysis without marked sedation and relatively low toxicity. Side effects include drowsiness, disinhibition, and incoordination. Psychological and physical dependence may develop, with seizures on withdrawal. Other side effects that are very uncommon and rarely serious include nausea, ataxia, constipation, skin sensitivity, and rarely syncopy. Greenblatt and Shader (1974) state that although this class of drugs appears to be relatively innocuous as far as serious side effects, a final conclusion cannot be made and more monitoring needs to be done. In reference to paradoxical reactions, Gittelman (1980) reviews a number of studies. In one of these in 130 children on levels above 30 mg/day of chlordiazepoxide, 13 had reactions of loss of control and going "wild." Five other studies reviewed include 185 cases and find no behavioral deterioration with the benzodiazepines. Based on these data Gittelman-Klein (1978) concludes that "paradoxical behavioral effects of anti-anxiety agents appear to be rare, occurring only with sustained treatment at relatively high doses."

Gittelman (1980) also reviewed three placebo controlled studies of children with behavior disorders in which diazepam had no significant effect over placebo. In a recent placebo controlled study (Petti et al., 1982) chlordiazepoxide in dosages between 15 to 120 mg/day is used in 9 hospitalized boys between ages 7–11. Preliminary results in this heterogeneous hospitalized population suggests that the drug has a positive effect on withdrawn, mildly depressed, and anxious children, and a worsening effect on the behavior of severely impulsive-aggressive or schizophrenic children.

In summary, antihistamines are widely used for developmental anxieties on the basis of clinical anecdotal reports. Studies of effectiveness in children with psychiatric disorders has been mainly in hospitalized children and with inconclusive results. Benzodiazepines similarly are not well studied, but clinical studies and relative safety indicate that further studies should be a high priority. Because of the risk of tardive dyskinesia with neuroleptics, antihistamines and benzodiazepines may play an increasingly important psychopharmacological role.

SUMMARY

Anxiety varies from a mild emotion of everyday life, to moderately intense states accompanying normal developmental stages (developmental anxieties), to a prominent symptom of psychiatric disorders. Evaluating anxiety within this conceptual range will help distinguish anxiety as a normal phenomena from anxiety of pathological significance. There are few methodologically good studies of psychopharmacological treatment of the DSM III Anxiety Disorder Group, except for the demonstration that imipramine has a significant positive effect on return to school in the school phobia variant of Separation Anxiety Disorder. Of major significance is Rapoport's recent finding that climipramine has significant therapeutic benefits for children with Obsessive-Compulsive Disorder. Antihistamines and benzodiazepines are frequently used for developmental and other anxiety states. The relative safety of these agents and the lack of clinical studies on children with primarily anxiety symptoms make studies of these agents on various anxiety conditions a high priority.

REFERENCES

Adams, P. (1979). Psychoneurosis. In J. Noshpitz (Ed.), *Basic handbook of child psychiatry* (Vol. 2, p. 231). New York: Basic Books.

Anthony, E. J. (1975). Neurosis in children. In A. M. Freedman, H. I. Kaplan, & B. J. Sadock (Eds.) *Comprehensive Textbook of Psychiatry* (Vol. 2, pp. 2155–2157). Baltimore: Williams & Wilkins.

Berney, T., Kolvin, I., Bhate, S. R., Garside, R. F., Jeans, J., Kay, S., & Scarth, L. (1981). School phobia: A therapeutic trial with clomipramine and short-term outcome. *British Journal of Psychiatry, 138,* 110–118.

Campbell, M., Anderson, L. T., & Green, W. H. (1983). Behavior-disordered and aggressive children: New advances in pharmacotherapy. *Journal of Developmental and Behavioral Pediatrics, 4*(4), 256–271.

Chess, S., Thomas, A., & Birch, H. C. (1967). Behavior problems revisited: Findings of an anterospective study. *Journal of the American Academy of Child Psychiatry, 6,* 321–331.

Coffey, B., Shader, R. I., & Greenblatt, D. J. (1983). Pharmacokinetics of benzodiazepines and psychostimulants in children. *Journal of Clinical Psychopharmacology, 3*(4), 217–225.

D'Amato, G. (1962). Chlordiazepoxide in management of school phobia. *Diseases of the Nervous System, 23,* 292–295.

American Psychiatric Association. (1980). *Diagnostic and statistical manual of mental disorders* (3rd ed.). American Psychiatric Association: Washington, DC.

Effron, A. S., & Freedman, A. M. (1953). The treatment of behavior disorders in children with Benadryl. *Journal of Pediatrics, 42,* 261–266.

Eisenberg, L. (1958). School phobia: A study in the communication of anxiety. *American Journal of Psychiatry, 114.* 712–718.

Eisenberg, L. (1959). The pediatric management of school phobia. *Journal of Pediatrics, 55,* 758–766.

Elkins, R., Rapoport, J. L., & Lipsky, A. (1980). Obsessive-Compulsive Disorder of childhood and adolescence. *Journal of the American Academy of Psychiatry, 19,* 511–524.

Fish, B. (1968). Drug use in psychiatric disorders of children. *American Journal of Psychiatry, 124,* 8 Fall.

Freedman, A. N., Effron, A. S., & Bender, L. (1955). Pharmacotherapy in children with psychiatric illness. *Transactions of the Society of Biological Psychiatry, 10,* 31.

Freud, A. (1966). Obsessional neurosis. *International Journal Psychoanalysis, 47,* 116–122.

Freud, S. (1913). The disposition to obsessional neurosis. *Standard Edition, 12,* 311–326. London: Hogarth Press, 1955.

Gittelman-Klein, R., & Klein, D. F. (1971). Controlled imipramine treatment of school phobia. *Archives of General Psychiatry, 25,* 204–207.

Gittelman-Klein, R., & Klein, D. F. (1973). School phobia: Diagnostic considerations in the light of imipramine effects. *Journal of Nervous and Mental Diseases, 156,* 199–215.

Gittelman, R. (1980). Diagnosis and drug treatment of childhood disorders. In D. F. Klein, R. Gittelman, F. Quitkin & A. Rifkin, (Eds.), *Diagnosis and drug treatment of psychiatric disorders: Adults and children* (2nd ed.) (pp. 590–776). Baltimore: Williams & Wilkins.

Gittelman-Klein, R. (1975). Pharmacotherapy and management of pathological separation anxiety. In R. Gittelman-Klein (Ed.), *Recent advances in child psychopharmacology* (pp. 255–272). New York: Human Science Press.

Gittelman-Klein, R. (1978). Psychopharmacological treatment of Anxiety Disorders, Mood Disorders and Tourette's Disorder in children. In M. A. Lipton, A. DiMascio & K. F. Killam, *Psychopharmacology: a generation of progress* pp. (1471–1480), New York: Raven Press.

Greenblatt, D. J., & Shader, R. I. (1978). Pharmacotherapy of anxiety with benzodiazepines and B-adrenergic blockers. In M. A. Lipton, A. DiMascio, & K. F. Killam, (Eds.), *Psychopharmacology: A generation of progress.* New York: Raven Press.

Greenblatt, D. J., & Shader, R. I. (1974) *Benzodiazepines in clinical practice.* New York: Raven Press.

Hayes, T. A., Panitch, M. L., & Barker, E. (1975). Imipramine dosage in children: A comment on "Imipramine and electrocardiographic abnormalities in hyperactive children." *American Journal Psychiatry, 132,* 546–547.

Hershberg, S. G., Carlson, G. A., Cantwell, D. P., & Strober, M. (1982). Anxiety and depressive disorders in psychiatrically disturbed children. *Journal of Clinical Psychiatry, 43*(9), 358–361.

Hollingsworth, C. E., Tanguay, P. E., Grossman, L., & Pabst, P. (1980). Long-term outcome of Obsessive-Compulsive Disorder in childhood. *Journal of the American Academy of Child Psychiatry, 19,* 134–144.

Judd, L. L. (1965). Obsessive-compulsive neurosis in children. *Archives of General Psychiatry, 12,* 136–143.

Kandel, E. R. (1983). From metapsychology to molecular biology: Explorations into the nature of anxiety. *American Journal of Psychiatry, 140*(10), 1277–1293.

Klein, D. F., (1964), Delineation of two drug-responsive anxiety syndromes. *Psychopharmacologia, 5,* 397–408.

Klein, D. F., Gittelman, R., Quitkin, F. & Rifkin, A. (1980). *Diagnosis and drug treatment of psychiatric disorder: Adults and children* (3rd ed.). Baltimore: Williams, & Wilkins.

Korein, J., Fish, B., Shapiro, T., Gehner, E. W., & Levidon, L. (1971). EEG and behavioral effects of drug therapy in children: Chlorpromazine and diphenhydramine. *Archives of General Psychiatry, 24,* 552–563.

Lewis, A. (1935). Problems of obsessional illness. *Proceedings of the Royal Society of Medicine,* *29,* 325–336.

Martin, G. I., & Zang, P. J. (1975). Electrocardiographic monitoring of enuretic children receiving therapeutic doses of imipramine. *American Journal of Psychiatry, 132,* 540–547.

Petti, T. A., Fish, B., Shapiro T., Cohen, I. L., & Campbell, M. (1982). Effects of chlordiazepoxide in disturbed children: A pilot study. *Journal of Clinical Psychopharmacology,* *2,* 270–273.

Rapoport, J. I., Mikkelsen, E. J., & Werry, J. S. (1978). Anti-manic, anti-anxiety, hallucinogenic and miscellaneous drugs. In J. S. Werry (Ed.), *Pediatric psychopharmacology* (pp. 316–346). New York: Brunner/Mazel.

Rapoport, J., Elkins, R., Mikkelson, E., Sceerg, W., Buchsbaum, M. S., Gillin, J. C., Murphy, D. L., Zahn, T. P., Lake, R., Ludlow, G., Mendelson, W. (1980). Clinical controlled trial of chlorimipramine in adolescents with Obsessive-Compulsive Disorder. *Psychopharmacological Bulletin,* No. 3, 16–63.

Rapoport, J., Elkins, R., Langer, D. H., Sceerg, W., Buchsbaum, M. S., Gillin, J. C., Murphy, D. L., Zahn, T. P., Lake, R., Ludlow, G., Mendelson, W. (1981). Childhood Obsessive-Compulsive Disorder. *American Journal of Psychiatry, 138,* 1545–1554.

Russo, R., Gururaj, V., & Allen, J. (1976). The effectiveness of dipheny-hydramine HCL in pediatric sleep disorders. *Journal of Clinical Pharmacology, 16,* 284–288.

Salzman, L., & Thaler, F. H. (1981). Obsessive-Compulsive Disorders: A review of the literature. *American Journal of Psychiatry, 138,* 286–296.

Shapiro, A., Shapiro, E., Brunn, R., & Sweet, R. (1978). *Gilles de la Tourette Syndrome.* New York: Raven Press.

Smith, R. E., & Domino, E. F. (1980). Dystonic and dyskinetic reactions induced by H, antihistaminic medication. In W. E. Fann et al. (Eds.), *Tardive dyskinesia* (pp. 325–332). New York: Spectrum Publications.

Thorén, P., Asberg, M., Cronholm, B., Jörnestedt, L., & Präskman, L. (1980a), Clomipramine treatment of Obsessive-Compulsive Disorder. I. A controlled clinical trial. *Archives of General Psychiatry, 37,* 1281–1285.

Thorén, P., Asberg, M., Bertilsson, Mellström, B., Sjöquist, F., & Präskman, L. (1980b). Clomipramine treatment of Obsessive-Compulsive Disorder II. Biochemical aspects. *Archives of General Psychiatry. 37,* 1289–1294.

Tyrer, P. J. (1982). Anti-anxiety drugs. In P. J. Tyrer (Ed.), *Drugs in psychiatric practice.* Cambridge: Butterworth.

Werry, J. S. (1982). An overview of pediatric psychopharmacology. *Journal of the American Academy of Child Psychiatry, 21,* 3–9.

White, J. H. (1977). *Pediatric psychopharmacology.* Baltimore: Williams & Wilkins.

Winsberg, B. G., Goldstein, A., Yepes, L. E. & Perel, J. M. (1975). Imipramine and electrocardiographic abnormalities in hyperactive children. *American Journal of Psychiatry, 132,* 542–545.

Tourette's Syndrome and Tic Disorders

**J. GERALD YOUNG, M.D., LEONARD I. LEVEN, M.D.,
PETER J. KNOTT, PhD, JAMES F. LECKMAN, M.D., and
DONALD J. COHEN, M.D.**

We are grateful to M. Easton for preparation of the manuscript. Research described in this chapter was supported by The Rosenstiel Foundation, The Gateposts Foundation, MHCRC Grant MH 30929, NICHD Grant HD 03008, CCRC Grant RR 00125, The John Merck Fund.

The grunts, grimaces, curses, and unusual movements of Tourette's Syndrome endow it with a uniquely vivid clinical presentation among neuropsychiatric disorders. This lifelong illness may be so debilitating as to require hospitalization or so minor that it is barely noticeable. Tourette gave an extensive description of the disorder one century ago that is accurate today, but clinical observations continue to generate new questions about diagnostic elements that are important determinants of treatment.

Tourette's Disorder may go unrecognized, in part because the diverse symptoms may mimic other disorders; on the other hand the typical features may be immediately recognizable in a passerby on the street. Motor and phonic tics are the most common components of the disease and create the predominant impression upon meeting a patient. A range of other symptomatic behaviors is also characteristic of individuals with Tourette's Syndrome (TS), including compulsions, attentional dysfunction, and impulsivity. The relation of these behaviors to other features of TS is an intriguing puzzle. Symptomatic behaviors are frequent in some individuals, occasional occurrences in others, or are entirely absent in others. Criteria for the diagnosis of TS can be easily applied in most cases, but in a minority of cases the intensity of associated symptomatic behaviors may obscure the diagnosis.

Treatment questions are also complex and physicians may face difficult therapeutic decisions. A business executive's tics are mild but a burden to him. Should they be treated with medication that carries the risk of side effects? Should two medications be administered, and dosages increased, for the homebound teenage boy because of his disabling symptoms and their effects on his family? What treatment can be suggested for the young boy with beginning TS? Should a medication be considered at this early age?

These questions converge on hypotheses concerning the neurobiological basis for TS, the important effects of the environment, and the developmental course of the disorder. Each component must be understood when considering strategies to stabilize the irregular activity of a child's motor and behavioral systems.

CLINICAL PRESENTATION OF TOURETTE'S SYNDROME

Tics are rapid involuntary movements of individual muscle groups. A convenient grouping of disorders involving tics is based upon categorization according to duration of symptoms, the presence of vocal or phonic tics in addition to motor tics, and the complexity of the tics.

Types of Tic Disorders

Transient tic disorders often occur during the early school years and can be observed in up to 15 percent of all children; they include eye blinking, nose wiggling, grimacing, and squinting.

Transient vocalizations are less common and include coughing, throat clearing, humming, or other distracting noises. Childhood tics may be unusual, such as licking the palm, smelling fingers, poking and pinching the genitals, or pointing a finger at another person. Transient tics last from weeks to a few months and usually are not associated with specific behavioral or school problems, although they may be common among children with compulsive personalities or attentional problems. They are especially noticeable during excitement or fatigue. As with all tic syndromes, boys are afflicted three to four times more frequently. Familial aggregation of transient tics is observed. While transient tics by definition do not persist for more than a year, a child may have a series of transient tics over the course of several years.

Chronic tic disorders have a relatively unaltered pattern over many years. While transient tics come and go, with sniffing replaced by forehead furrowing or finger snapping, chronic tics such as neck stretching or blinking may persist unchanged for years. *Chronic multiple tics* (CMT) refer to an individual with several chronic motor tics. The boundaries among transient tics, chronic tics, and chronic multiple tics are often obscure. The disorder of *Gilles de la Tourette* (TS) is characterized by multiform, frequently changing motor and phonic tics and a range of behavioral symptoms. The current diagnostic criteria include an age of onset between 2 and 15 years; recurrent, involuntary, rapid, purposeless motor movements affecting multiple muscle groups; multiple vocal tics; the ability to suppress movements voluntarily for minutes to hours; variations in the intensity of the symptoms over weeks to months (waxing and waning); and a duration of more than one year (American Psychiatric Association, 1980; Shapiro et al., 1978; Friedhoff & Chase, 1982). While these criteria are fundamentally valid, they are not immutable. First, rare cases of TS may emerge after age 15. Second, the concept of "involuntary" is difficult to define operationally, since some patients feel their tics have a volitional component—a capitulation to an internal urge for motor discharge accompanied by psychological tension and anxiety (Bliss et al., 1980). Finally, these criteria do not portray other behavioral symptoms often observed in TS patients, such as attentional problems, compulsions, and obsessions.

Tourette's Syndrome (TS): Description and Classification of Symptoms

Motor and Phonic Tics.   Motor and phonic tics of TS can be characterized by their frequency, complexity, and the degree to which they cause distress and disrupt the patient's daily life (Cohen et al., 1982). Frequent tics, occurring 20–30 times a minute, such as mouth puckering, nodding, or grimacing, may be less disruptive than an infrequent tic, occurring several times an hour, such as slamming to the ground, punching out or screaming.

Simple motor tics are rapid, meaningless involuntary movements that can be painful (e.g., jaw snapping) and embarassing. They are easily distinguished from simple muscular twitches or rapid fasciculations.

Complex motor tics may be slower, more purposeful in appearance, and more easily described by terms used for deliberate actions. Complex motor tics can be any type of movement that the body can produce—for example, gyrating, hopping, clapping, thrusting, tensing arm or neck muscles, fist clenching, and kicking. A patient may hyperextend his thumb or wrist until becoming double-jointed, suddenly thrust his head forward, control his diaphragm, kiss people, punch at the wall, or rub his fingers together next to his ear. At some point on the continuum of complex motor tics, the term "compulsion" seems an appropriate description for the organized, repetitive character of the actions. The need to arrange objects neatly, to do and then undo the same action and to carefully "finish" something a certain number of times are compulsive in quality and accompanied by considerable internal pressure as well as internal resistance. These complex motor tics may greatly impair school work, for example, when a child must tear pages out of textbooks or write over the same letter so many times that the paper is worn thin. Self-destructive behaviors occur—such as head banging, eye poking, picking at scabs, or sticking oneself with sharp objects; more rarely, aggression toward others, such as poking or pinching a loved one, may be a symptom.

Simple phonic tics are linguistically meaningless sounds or noises, such as hissing, coughing, spitting, sucking, snorting, and sniffing. *Complex phonic tics* are recognizable words, phrases, or sentences, for example, "Oh, no!" "Oh, boy, now you've said it," "Yup, that's it," "But, but. . . ." Phonic symptoms may interfere with the smooth flow of speech and resemble a stammer, stutter, or speech clutter. These symptoms often occur at points of linguistic transition of speech. Patients may abruptly alter speech volume, slur a phrase, emphasize a word, or assume an accent.

Coprolalia, the explosive utterance of foul or dirty words or more elaborate sexual and aggressive comments, causes marked social distress. Corpolalia occurs in up to 40 percent of TS patients, depending on the clinical series. It is the most well-known symptom of TS and was described as "pathognomonic" by Tourette (Goetz & Klawans, 1982). Early in the course of coprolalia, a child may mumble the beginnings of words ("fff," "sh, sh") in order to camouflage the obscenity. Finally, the curses can be restrained no longer and he will shout the full expletive. While watching television, playing, or sitting at his desk, curse words will pop into his mind and just as quickly be expressed. A child also may be bothered by mental coprolalia, incessant obscene thoughts or images (Shapiro et al., 1973b).

Some patients progress to more elaborate forms of coprolalia in which swearing is embedded in longer statements or takes the form of sexual, hostile, and insulting comments. These comments may be considered to be simple rudeness until their compulsive quality becomes apparent. Insulting remarks include socially unacceptable descriptions of another person's appearance, social status, or behavior—"You're the fattest fucking son-of-a-bitch I've ever seen," "What tits," "Cubans eat it!", "You're bald. . . oops, I shouldn't say that." Needless to say, the response of the described person may be socially disastrous or dangerous for the patient.

From the time of the onset, a patient with TS becomes remarkably inventive in disguising motor or phonic tics. Blending them into actions with an apparent purpose, such as adjusting his pants or mumbling assent to what a companion is saying, the patient succeeds in leaving the impression of mere behavioral oddities. The repetitive, forced nature of the behaviors is recognizable to a careful observer, and may be a significant contribution to an accurate family history when mildly afflicted relatives are interviewed.

Associated Disorders. TS patients often have sufficient symptoms to meet the criteria for another psychiatric diagnosis. There is controversy about whether these symptoms are an inherent component of TS, secondary to the disorder, or coincidental. Emerging genetic and developmental evidence suggests that attentional and compulsive disorders are manifestations of an underlying, genetic diathesis for TS and a range of related behavioral dimensions (Cohen et al., 1979, 1980).

The most common behavioral problems associated with TS in childhood involve the regulation of attention and activity. Approximately 50 percent of children with TS satisfy the diagnostic criteria for attention deficit disorder (ADD: poor attention, difficulty concentrating, distractibility, impulsivity, and hyperactivity). The ADD and hyperactivity of these patients often originates in the preschool years and precedes the onset of tics, or occurs when tics are so mild they are noticed only in retrospect (Cohen et al., 1980; Rapoport et al., 1982; Comings & Comings, 1984). ADD and hyperactivity tend to parallel tics in severity later in the development of the disorder. Deteriorating attentional capacity appears to reflect underlying psychobiological dysfunctions involving inhibitions in TS, and may be aggravated by the effort required to attend to the outer world, while working hard to remain quiet and still. Attentional problems persist during periods of relative tic remission. Most TS patients do not have primary learning disabilities; while their intelligence is normal, attentional problems and hyperactivity may profoundly effect school achievement. At least 30–40 percent of TS children have serious school performance handicaps that require special intervention. While it is difficult to distinguish specific causes in these multiple handicapped children, 5–20 percent may have a primary learning disability.

A large number of TS patients are burdened with obsessions and compulsions. The actual percentage of patients affected is uncertain because the distinction between a complex motor tic and a compulsion is a clinical judgment. While this remains an open question, our experience suggests that 40 percent of TS patients have obsessions and compulsions (Cohen et al., 1980). The family members of TS patients also have a markedly increased frequency of obsessive-compulsive disorder, suggesting a genetic association between these disorders.

It is often difficult to select the optimal medication in the face of this panoply of symptoms. Two considerations serve as aids to treatment planning. First, a knowledge of the natural history of Tourette's Syndrome provides a broad, practical guide when gauging treatment requirements. Second, the determination of a few target symptoms for treatment (according to the judgment of the child, parents, and physician) lends clarity to later treatment planning.

With these considerations in mind, the physician can estimate what the various drugs might realistically be anticipated to accomplish. Which symptoms are likely to improve and which may be untouched with a treatment? Will there be a substantial cost in side effects? Are the less intrusive therapies capable of comparable results? What treatment can be initiated for those symptoms unresponsive to the medication? These questions are critical guides to the selection of treatment, but any treatment must ultimately be judged in relation to the child's development and the natural history of TS. In this situation the physician can act as an advocate for the child. The family is typically riveted on the current disturbing symptoms and the psychological and social distress they cause the child and themselves; the family's anxiety and their lack of appreciation of the natural history of TS may lead them to neglect a broad appraisal of their child's illness and treatment, which includes his future development.

Natural History: A Hypothetical Case

A common pattern for the development of TS is initiated when behavioral difficulties, such as irritability, poor frustration tolerance, and attentional problems occur during the preschool years; a few transient tics will accompany or follow these problems. Sustained tics are recognizable by seven or eight years of age and are followed by other motor and phonic symptoms. A rostro-caudal progression of motor tics occurs in most individuals; eye blinking and other facial tics are followed by shoulder shrugging, arm movements, truncal symptoms, and leg movements in that general sequence. Simple tics are followed by complex motor tics, while phonic symptoms usually follow the simple motor tics by months or a year; complex phonic symptoms then evolve. Highly organized motor symptoms (compulsions, rituals, and self-destructive acts) and the most complex phonic symptoms (provocatively aggressive comments, graphic descriptions of sexual acts, rude descriptions) usually emerge several years or more after the onset of the simple tics. The most severely afflicted patients tend to have prominent early behavioral difficulties and relatively early onset of motor tics. Of course, there are numerous exceptions to this hypothetical pattern (Leckman & Cohen, 1983).

Ultimate social adaptation may be determined more by behavioral and attentional difficulties than by simple motor or phonic tics. Patients with severe tics can achieve adequate social and vocational adjustment in adult life, although not without considerable emotional pain. The interaction of symptoms and environmental factors mold eventual social adaptation: the severity of attentional problems; the degree of interference by compulsions; the level of school achievement, general intelligence and adaptive capacities; the quality of family support; the understanding of friends at school or work; and the severity and form of complex motor and phonic symptoms.

Long-term use of medication often obscures the natural history of TS and the physician's understanding of emerging social and personality difficulties. Haloperidol is so commonly prescribed that assessment of a very large percentage of TS patients includes the often difficult differentiation of preexisting symptoms and medication side effects. These side effects may diminish the child's emerging sense of self-control, autonomy, self-esteem, and cognitive and social competence. Psychoactive medication may alter a child's experience of his body and the working of his mind, as well as single a child out in school, alter his daily schedule, focus parental and other adult concern on small changes in symptoms and side effects, and tie the child down to the care and attention of many adults.

A generation of adults with TS has developed under the influence of changing doses of haloperidol and other medications. They have been preoccupied with symptoms, medications, side effects, and being "victims" of a disease and its treatments. The developmental tasks of middle childhood and adolescence—individuation, industriousness, autonomy, appreciation of bodily pleasures, coping with confusing motivations—may be neglected while patients grow up feeling uncertain about which feelings are really "their own," which feelings are "the Tourette Syndrome," and which feelings are the result of medication. Patients who are aggressive toward themselves or others are especially subject to confusion about social skills, adaptive channeling of impulses into work habits, and conventional expectations concerning self-control because of their illness. The impossibility of learning about healthy aggression and its flexible application to other pursuits may leave them outside the usual pursuits of their age-mates. Some severely afflicted individuals become profoundly maladapted, dependent, isolated, and "chronic" patients in response to these overwhelming problems. They are burdened by debilitating personality disorders, phobias, and anxiety. The deteriorating course of the illness makes it difficult to distinguish etiological factors related to the severity of the disorder and its natural history on the one hand, and factors related to social and academic consequences, medication, and medical management, on the other. It is not surprising that patients have recurrent minor depressions and occasional major depressions. During adolescence and adulthood, the social isolation, academic failure, and disfiguring symptoms sometimes become intolerable, leading to suicidal thoughts or attempts.

Epidemiology

An estimated 15 percent of school children have transient tics; the prevalence may be somewhat lower for adults. Epidemiological figures tend to be unreliable because of their dependence upon observational methods; the more carefully one looks, the more tics one finds. The peak incidence of transient tics coincides with the mean age of onset of TS (7 years), and probably reflects biological and psychological maturation. There are no adequate incidence and prevalence data for TS. While the disorder had been thought to be rare, with increasing medical recognition and the excellent publicity provided by the national Tourette Syndrome Association, more cases are now being identified. We have estimated the prevalence to be at least 1 in 2000 for the full syndrome, based on known cases in Connecticut. Genetic evidence suggests that TS and multiple tics are related, and this would increase the prevalence of the TS diathesis several fold, perhaps to as common as 1 in 200 or 1 in 300 (Jagger et al., 1982; Schoenberg, 1982; Lucas et al., 1982; Kondo & Nomura, 1982; Nomura & Segawa, 1982; Mak et al., 1982).

Genetics

Familial aggregation of TS was first described in the original nineteenth century reports. There is a strong genetic contribution to TS, with clear familial aggregation of TS and multiple tics. Boys are more often afflicted than girls, who require a stronger genetic predisposition, that is, more afflicted individuals in their family, for expression of the disorder (Kidd et al., 1980; Pauls et al., 1981). The sons of mothers with TS have the highest risk for developing symptoms, possibly as high as 30–50 percent. A mode of genetic transmission has not been established for TS. Some pedigrees suggest a dominant autosomal gene; however, more data fit polygenic models with sex thresholds of expression affecting the trait (Comings & Comings, 1984; Kidd et al., 1980; Pauls et al., 1981; Eldridge et al., 1977). Several mathematical models of genetic transmission are being explored. Environmental factors are important and there are many sporadic cases of TS that lack a family history of TS. Further clinical research hopefully will clarify the mode of genetic transmission; the use of direct interview methods for relatives, rather than family history data, will be essential to the generation of an accurate genetic model (Pauls et al., 1984).

There is increasing evidence of a genetic association between TS and other neuropsychiatric disorders, especially ADD and obsessive-compulsive disorder.

ADD is a common prodromal component of TS, persisting after full expression of the disorder in most children. There are children and adults with ADD and no tics, ADD and motor tics only, or ADD and phonic symptoms, who may be suffering from a milder variant of TS. These individuals may have a variant of TS that has not progressed to full expression, because of biological or environmental protective factors. This hypothesis is especially compelling in relation to children with serious ADD who have siblings or other close relatives with TS or multiple tics. However, the TS variant of ADD may not be rare even in nonfamilial cases, in which the critical factor may be impairment in a regulatory system. Similarly, obsessive-compulsive disorder, without tics or with few tic symptoms, is overrepresented in families of patients with TS. Further biological and genetic studies will clarify the precise nature of the relationship among TS and other disorders. If other disorders are found to be linked genetically with the biological diathesis of TS, these disorders may be genotypically distinctive variants from other forms of ADD, obsessive-compulsive, or anxiety disorders that are not associated with TS. Genetic heterogeneity is more the rule than the exception in biology (Cohen et al., 1979; and 1980; Comings & Comings, 1984).

A BEHAVIORAL AND BIOLOGICAL MODEL TO GUIDE TREATMENT

The heterogeneity of symptoms in TS can be the source of treatment failure in two ways. First, individual behaviors may not be recognized as components of the disorder because they lack a resemblance to more common features. Second, the obvious influence of psychosocial factors on symptomatic expression, together with the child's ability to momentarily suppress overt symptoms, makes it difficult for parents to differentiate TS symptoms from provocative behavior on the part of the child. During periods of severe symptomatology this discrimination may not be possible.

One model that provides a conceptual structure for these symptoms emphasizes the disinhibition characteristic of the disorder. Assessment of individual symptoms suggests that the regulation of behaviors and thoughts is altered by the disease. Behaviors and thoughts that ordinarily remain under control are expresssed publicly. A psychological and behavioral boundary ordinarily taken for granted is absent or permeable, much as the skin of a burn victim no longer functions as a protective and regulatory barrier. Actions are repeated over and over in purposeless sequence long after they have achieved their aims. Sudden emotions are voiced in spite of their provocative sexual or aggressive content, just as the rapid, involuntary movements appear in spite of the embarassment or regret experienced by the patient. This behavioral dysregulation is amplified by stress, even the minor aggravations of daily life.

This view of TS as a disease characterized by an impairment of normal processes of inhibition suggests involvement of the regulatory components of neuronal systems. Impaired regulatory control could occur at a tissue level (e.g., an imbalance among interacting neuronal systems, such as dopaminergic and serotonergic) or at molecular level (e.g., altered receptor sensitivity).

Assigning a fundamental role to disinhibition in the conceptualization of TS illuminates disagreements among clinicians about the definition of TS. The clinical questions ask how broad the definition of TS should be. Should attentional impairments and compulsive behaviors be designated as variably present components of TS (as might be suggested by the disinhibition hypothesis), or is it more useful to consider these problems as co-occuring and treat each separately? Clinical research has not moved sufficiently far to reach a decision on this point. Nevertheless, a broad model has pragmatic value until we have a fuller understanding of underlying disease processes. By extending our attention from pharmacological control of motor tics to the range of treatments that will aid the patient in his or her attempts to achieve better control over his behavior, we gain a perspective that is better attuned to the multiple problems encountered by a child with TS.

In order to clarify how this view might affect treatment, we will consider how assessment procedures determine the course of treatment.

ASSESSMENT

The foundation of a medical and psychiatric evaluation for a child with tics is meticulous attention to history and a thorough examination. Certain components of the evaluation require special consideration if treatment is to be carried out successfully in the face of multiple symptoms following a waxing and waning course.

1. Physicians may have a tendency to emphasize the tics and lose sight of the child. The clinician must assess other areas of functioning and difficulties, particularly school performance, presence of attentional and learning difficulties, and relations with family and peers. Before a family has received a diagnosis, the child and family may think the child is "going crazy." The child may be extremely distressed by his own experiences and by the criticism he has received from parents who have scolded, cajoled, bribed, threatened, or perhaps beaten him in order to stop his strange behavior. During evaluation, therefore, family issues, including parental confusion and guilt, need to be addressed.

2. Thorough assessment of a child with TS requires several hours. The clinician will learn about the fluctuation of symptoms; as the child

becomes more comfortable, he will show his symptoms with less suppression or inhibition. The identification of symptoms and their fluctuation will be essential for establishing a baseline against which treatment can be assessed. The patient must have confidence in the doctor if he is to acknowledge his most frightening and bizarre symptoms.

3.   The description, severity, frequency, and disruptive effects of the motor and phonic tics need to be specified from the time of their appearance until the present. Important features include onset, progression, waxing and waning, and aggravating or ameliorating factors. It is of great practical importance to examine the degree to which they have interfered with the child's social, familial, and school experiences. It is very useful to monitor symptoms over a few months in order to assess their severity and fluctuation, impact on the family, and the nature of the child and family's adaptation (Shapiro et al., 1972). This will be facilitated if the family uses standard rating forms (e.g., a list of tic symptoms and a behavioral checklist, such as the Conners Parent-Teacher Questionnaire).

4.   Neurological examination should include documentation of classical and neuromaturational abnormalities, as well as any stigmata present. About half of TS patients have nonlocalizing, so-called "soft" neurological findings, suggesting disturbances in the body schema and integration of motor control. These findings have no specific implications, but may eventually contribute to the definition of a clinical subgroup. Neurological findings also are important as "baseline" data in order to distinguish them from medication side effects (Shapiro et al., 1973).

While the EEG is often abnormal in TS, the findings are nonspecific. Children with paroxysmally abnormally tracings are occasionally treated as epileptic, but anticonvulsants are of no consistent value in TS (Bergen et al., 1982). Computed tomography of the brain generally fails to indicate any abnormality (Caparulo et al., 1981). While the EEG and computed tomography are not necessary for the diagnosis or treatment of TS, clinicians request these tests because of the seriousness of the illness, the concern of the family and the physician, and the importance of considering other disorders affecting movement (such as a seizure disorder or Wilson's disease). Additional chemical studies may also be included in the medical workup because of their relation to movement disorders: electrolytes, calcium, phsophorus, ceruloplasmin, and liver function tests. In practice, TS is rarely confused with these disorders today, because the history and findings in TS are distinctive.

5. A detailed behavioral pedigree of extended family is required, including tics, compulsions, attentional problems, and learning disorders. A grandfather's TS may have been diagnosed Sydenham's chorea, an uncle may have been thought to be odd or weird. A parent may be embarrassed about acknowledging his or her own symptoms, and deny that he or she has ever had tics.

6. A detailed review of previous medications is required. When a child has received stimulant medications, it is important to determine whether there were preexisting tics or compulsions, and the temporal relation between the stimulants and any new symptoms. There is now substantial evidence that stimulants may facilitate the emergence of tics in a vulnerable individual (Golden, 1974; Lowe et al., 1982). Catecholaminergic agonists are contained in other drugs, such as in antihistamine combinations used to treat allergies or in medications used for asthma. If a patient with TS is on a stimulant or a drug containing a sympathomimetic, it should be discontinued unless there is a compelling therapeutic indication. If such drugs were used in the past, it is important to determine their effects. Children who developed tics while on stimulants may also have had beneficial effects, such as improved attention and learning.

Any medication previously prescribed for TS needs to be assessed, especially dosage, initial positive and negative response to the drug, and reasons for discontinuing. A family may report that haloperidol was not useful for a child or that he had unacceptable side effects. A careful history may reveal that he improved on haloperidol but then developed akathisia that was not recognized, or that the side effects were dose-related and probably controllable. Was the medication used at the correct dosage, with close monitoring, for a long enough time? Patients may not recognize important side effects of a drug. For example, families may not appreciate that their child's fearfulness or school phobia may be related to haloperidol and not primarily to psychological issues.

A child who comes for evaluation while on an ineffective medication requires a judicious clinical approach. The clinician must decide whether to increase the dosage and see if the child improves or discontinue the medication and observe the child's response. Discontinuation from haloperidol may lead to severe withdrawal-emergent exacerbation of symptoms—sometimes far beyond their original severity—for up to two to three months. Thus, if haloperidol is withdrawn, it cannot be expected that the child's "real" status will be visible for quite a while. Some children may improve for a few weeks after haloperidol discontinuation, then experience a short period of exacerbation, and finally gradually improve. With discontinuation of haloperidol, cognitive blunting, feeling dull, poor motivation, school and social phobias, excessive appetite, and sedation may lift quickly, over days to several weeks, while tic symptoms remain or become worse. New dyskinesias, secondary to neuroleptic withdrawal, may appear and remain for 4–12 weeks. Thus, the decision to discontinue haloperidol may be more difficult than the one to initiate it. Families and children may have great difficulty tolerating the accelerating symptoms and disorganization and require support from the physician; hospitalization may be necessary.

If clonidine is not beneficial, tapering withdrawal over one or two weeks may be followed by symptom exacerbation lasting several days to a few weeks. This exacerbation typically is milder than after haloperidol, and children rarely become worse during withdrawal than prior to treatment. Less is known about withdrawal from phenothiazines in TS patients, but withdrawal-emergent dyskinesias occur.

7.   Careful assessment of intellectual ability and school achievement is required for children having school problems. TS children often do not have clearly delineated learning disorders, and the average IQ of TS patients is normal; rather their problems tend to lie in the area of attentional deployment, perseverance, and ability to organize themselves and their work. Many have difficulties with penmanship (graphomotor skills) and compulsions that interfere with writing. Specification of problem areas will aid in the recommendation of alternatives (e.g., use of typewriter or more emphasis on oral reports) (Joshko & Rourke, 1982; Inagnoli & Kane, 1982; Sutherland et al., 1982; Hagin et al., 1982).

8.   Families often ask if TS is a "medical" or "emotional" disorder. A well-conducted assessment, in which all sectors of the child's development are discussed, is an important step in undoing the mischieveous separation of body and mind. This orientation to TS and its treatment can be conveyed implicitly during the assessment—as the clinician analyzes medical, psychosocial, and psychological issues—and usually requires explicit discussion at the end of the evaluation (Cohen et al., 1982).

Parents may themselves have TS or disorders associated with it. There are several implications of this multigenerational sharing of symptoms. A clinician may be reluctant to fully state his impressions of the child's social and personality problems because he may observe similar difficulties in the parents. The relationship between the clinician and family may be strained because of attentional problems, impulsivity, or obsessional features in the parents. Parents may feel additional guilt when they understand the genetic contribution to their child's disorder. On the other side, parents with tics or TS are likely to be more sympathetic with their child's dilemmas.

TREATMENT

Decisions concerning treatment depend upon the diagnosis and the degree to which the symptoms interfere with the child's development. The primary goal should be to help the child navigate the normal developmental tasks—for the school-age child, to feel competent in school, develop friendships, experience trust in his parents, and enjoy life's adventures. Many children with multiple tics and TS continue to move onward with development; for them, pharmacological treatment generally is not indicated. Natural parental upset about the symptoms requires calm discussion and education about available treatments. If treatment is agreed upon by the child, family, and physician, developmental issues must be continually reassessed (Cohen & Leckman, 1984; Bruun, 1984; Van Woert et al., 1982).

There are several approaches to treatment.

Monitoring

Optimally, the clinician can follow a patient for several months before a specific treatment plan is organized. The goals of this first stage of treatment are to establish a baseline of symptoms; define associated difficulties in school, family, and peer relations; obtain necessary medical tests; monitor, through checklists and interviews, the range and fluctuation of symptoms; establish aggravating and alleviating factors; and establish a relationship.

Reassurance

Sometimes the child's tics are of minimal functional significance. A child may satisfy the criteria for TS, yet have good peer relations, school achievement, and sense of self, and no treatment may be needed. Parents may be worried about the child's future. In general, the severity of TS is apparent within a short period after its appearance; by the time a child has had TS for two or three years, one can estimate with reasonable accuracy how severe the disorder ultimately will be. For transient single tics, reassurance is fully appropriate. Families should also be informed about emerging knowledge concerning genetic factors.

Pharmacological Treatment

The only effective treatment for simple and complex motor and phonic tics is pharmacological. Psychotherapy may help children with TS understand the effects of the illness on themselves and on the response of peers, and the usual conflicts accompanying development. While psychotherapy may reduce the severity of tics slightly in individual children as a result of relief of general stress and anxiety, as a rule tics are not responsive to psychotherapy. Behavior modification, hypnotherapy, and relaxation methods have been tried with TS with little success; they may act synergistically with pharmacotherapy, but no firm evidence supports this. Some patients are able to learn methods of self-control, particularly as they grow older. Three types of medication have broad use in the treatment of TS today

Haloperidol. Haloperidol has been the most common treatment for TS since the 1960s. During the first years of its use, dosage was rapidly increased to very high levels (up to 300 mg/day), followed by gradual reduction. However, it is now accepted that haloperidol is most effective at quite low doses. Patients generally are given an initial dose of .5 mg/day, which is slowly increased up to 3–4 mg/day, usually in twice daily dosage. Impressive benefits are seen at these low doses, and patients may have almost complete remission with few side effects (Shapiro et al., 1973, 1978; Shapiro & Shapiro, 1982). Patients for whom low doses of haloperidol are ineffective may benefit from higher doses (10–15 mg), but improvement is often limited and side effects troubling.

Up to 80 percent patients with TS initially benefit from haloperidol, sometimes dramatically. However, long-term follow-up suggests that only a smaller number, perhaps 20–30 percent, continue haloperidol for an extended period of time. Haloperidol is discontinued because of the emergence of side effects, including lethargy, weight gain, dysphoria, pseudoparkinsonian symptoms, intellectual dulling, personality changes, feeling like a "zombie," and akathisia (Cohen et al., 1980; Shapiro et al., 1978; Bruun, 1982; Bogomolny, 1982). Pseudoparkinsonian and acute dystonic reactions can be controlled with antiparkinsonian agents (1–2 mg/day of benztropine). Akathisia is less responsive to anticholinergic agents. A school phobia occasionally appears during the first weeks of treatment with low doses of haloperidol, while tics are improving. Social phobias in adults involve acute anxiety about going to work or performing at work; like school phobia, they can be extremely disabling. When these phobias are not recognized as drug side effects, they can continue for months; they remit within weeks of stopping haloperidol. Intellectual dulling can lead to a marked deterioration of school and work performance. Children who are excellent students and enjoy many friendships may become poor students, unhappy, and isolated after begining haloperidol for tics. Some clinicians prescribe methylphenidate in combination with haloperidol in order to counter the attentional impairment caused by haloperidol. The association between stimulant medications and tics suggests that adding a stimulant to haloperidol should be considered experimental and performed only with informed consent and careful monitoring until long term effects can be assessed.

Haloperidol has been incriminated in the onset of tardive dyskinesia (TD). The appearance of new facial or hand movements may be difficult to assess in a patient with a preexisting movement disorder. Are these tics? Is TD appearing? Orofacial movements suspected to be TD sometimes disappear several weeks after discontinuation of haloperidol (Shapiro & Shapiro, 1982; Klawans et al., 1982; Fog et al., 1982). Some animal studies suggest TD may be more likely to appear after multiple discontinuation and reintroductions of neuroleptics, so it is probably wise not to attempt frequent drug holidays with haloperidol. Withdrawal exacerbations seldom make this feasible in any case.

Antiparkinsonian agents need not be prescribed until required to combat specific side effects (parkinsonian tremor or rigidity, dystonia, oculogyric crisis, or akathisia). However, some clinicians prefer to begin low doses of these agents once the haloperidol is above a certain threshold, perhaps 2 mg/day, because of fear of the occurrence of these frightening side effects in school. Antiparkinsonian agents have their own side effects, so prophylactic use may be unwise. Patients should be instructed about haloperidol's potential side effects and have an antiparkinsonian drug at home and with them on trips in the event that they develop extrapyramidal symptoms. They should also be informed that, in an emergency, acute dystonic reactions can be treated with other drugs, such as Valium, Librium, or Benadryl. Patients and families should be alerted to unusual new symptoms that may be mistaken for TS instead of side effects of haloperidol. For example, a teenager began to have repeated episodes of thrusting his tongue and deviating his jaw. These episodes eventually lengthened, and he would hold his tongue and jaw in a rigid position for hours. He became afraid to go to school or out with friends. This dystonic reaction was not diagnosed until haloperidol was discontinued for other side effects.

Clonidine. The first description of the value of clonidine for treatment of TS appeared in 1979 (Cohen et al., 1979) and was followed by other open and controlled trials indicating that from 40–70 percent of TS patients benefit from its use (Cohen et al., 1979a, 1980; Shapiro & Shapiro, 1982; Bruun, 1982; Leckman et al., 1982). Clonidine has been approved by the Federal Drug Administration (FDA) only for use in hypertension, but clinicians can prescribe it for TS without special government approval as long as they understand its indications and share the basis for their decision with the family and child. Formal FDA approval for the use of clonidine in TS is anticipated. Clonidine primarily inhibits nonadrenergic functions, while haloperidol alters dopaminergic functioning. Interactions between central dopaminergic and noradrenergic systems may be involved in the pathophysiology of TS, and there is evidence that clonidine indirectly affects central dopaminergic systems (Leckman et al., 1983; Antelman & Caggiula, 1977). Clonidine reduces simple motor and phonic tics, and is particularly useful in improving attentional problems and ameliorating complex motor and phonic symptoms. Clonidine treatment should be initiated at low doses of .05mg/day and slowly titrated over several weeks to .15–.30 mg/day (or approximately 3 mg/kg/day). Doses of .4 mg/day are not infrequent, but doses above .5 mg/day are more likely to lead to side effects. When medication is working effectively, patients may experience the need for their next dose by sensing increasing anxiety, frequency of symptoms, or irritability. Haloperidol may bring a clear improvement within a few days, but clonidine has a slower onset of action. This can make the evaluation of its therapeutic effects difficult with an expectant and anxious family. When larger doses are used earlier, improvement may occur sooner, but there may be more sedation. Using a slower titration to therapeutic levels, clonidine may take three weeks or longer to show a beneficial effect. The patient may experience a reduction in tension, a sense of being calm, or having a "longer fuse" before tics are reduced. A gradual decrease in complex motor tics and compulsions also may precede clear improvement in simple tics. Evaluation of the medication's effectiveness may not be possible before three to four months. When there is a positive reponse, improvement may progress for up to a year or more. Patients gain confidence in themselves, adjust better to school, feel less irritable, and have fewer tic symptoms. These therapeutic benefits reinforce each other. Clonidine has only recently been used in TS, so the longest individual period of treatment is five years. Children with extremely severe TS have benefitted after several years of treatment with clonidine, and only slight increases in medication have been required.

The major side effect of clonidine is sedation; it appears early in the course of treatment, especially if the dose is increased quickly, but abates after several weeks. A few patients have dry mouth, but children less often than adults. Clonidine continues to decrease salivary flow even after years of treatment (Selinger et al., in press). Rarely, patients complain that things are "too bright," perhaps due to impairment of pupillary constriction. At higher doses, there may be hypotension and dizziness; this is more likely if clonidine is given at high doses quite early or if it is increased to over .4–.5 mg/day. At lower doses, blood pressure is not clinically affected, although a fall of several millimeters of mercury in diastolic and systolic pressure can be detected. Slight prolongation of the PR interval on the electrocardiogram has been noted, but has not been considered significant. No other medical or clinical side effects have emerged, but careful observation continues.

Before clonidine is prescribed, it is wise to obtain an EKG and routine blood studies. No alterations in standard blood chemistry measures or hemogram have been identified.

The combined use of haloperidol and clonidine has not yet been examined in controlled studies and only anecdotal information is available. The combination has been used in two clinical situations: (1) for patients whose symptoms are not fully controlled on haloperidol, or who are having serious side effects when medication is increased, yet who cannot discontinue haloperidol because of the severity of symptoms; and (2) for patients on clonidine who have inadequate control of motor and phonic symptoms. It appears that patients can be managed with smaller doses of haloperidol when clonidine is added; on the other hand, haloperidol may improve tic control for some patients on clonidine. Small doses of both medications are used when the drugs are combined, and no serious side effects have been reported on other than those seen with the drugs used individually.

Pimozide. This is a potent neuroleptic widely used in Europe for the treatment of psychosis. Several clinical studies have suggested pimozide to be as effective as haloperidol in the treatment of TS and possibly less sedating; controlled comparisons are required (Shapiro & Shapiro, 1982; Ross & Moldofsky, 1977; Shapiro et al., 1983; Moldofsky & Brown, 1982). Clinical experience with children is limited because the drug is not yet available in the United States. Pimozide is a diphenylbutylpiperidine derivative, chemically distinct from haloperidol, clonidine, or the phenothiazines. Its mode of action appears to be preferential blocking of postsynaptic dopamine receptors (Seeman & Lee, 1975; Nose & Takemoto, 1975). Pimozide is an effective therapeutic agent in a double-blind, crossover design comparing it with placebo

(Shapiro & Shapiro, 1984). Side effects are similar to those encountered with haloperidol, but may be less severe and appear to be tolerated by many patients. Individual patients who have not had a favorable result with haloperidol or clonidine occasionally report dramatic improvement with pimozide. Treatment is initiated at 1 mg/day, and dosage may be gradually increased to a maximum of 6–10 mg/day (.2 mg/kg) for children and 20 mg/day for adults. Pimozide has a long half-life (55 hours) and once daily dosage may be feasible. Major side effects include sedation, pseudoparkinsonism, akathisia, insomnia, and dizziness, as well as depression, nervousness, and other adverse behavioral effects. Antiparkinson agents are useful. Tardive dyskinesia should be considered a likely long term risk until proved otherwise (Shapiro & Shapiro, 1984).

Pimozide causes EKG changes in up to 25 percent of patients, including T wave inversion, U waves, QT prolongation, and bradycardia. Electrocardiogram changes are observable within one week and at doses as low as 3 mg/day. The manufacturer recommends discontinuation of pimozide with the occurrence of T wave inversion or U waves, seen in up to 20 percent of patients; dosage should not be increased if there is prolongation of the QT interval (corrected). Discontinuation of pimozide appears to bring normalization of the EKG within one week. A number of cardiac deaths have occurred in physically healthy patients receiving pimozide. In addition to usual clinical and laboratory monitoring, patients receiving pimozide should receive an EKG before treatment, monthly during dosage increases, and at three month intervals thereafter (Shapiro & Shapiro, 1984).

Phenothiazines and Other Medications.   Haloperidol was thought to have a specific therapeutic effect in TS. Increasing experience suggests that some patients have a comparable response to phenothiazines (Borison et al., 1982).

When equivalent doses are used and side effects are also similar, haloperidol may be no more useful than phenothiazines. On the other hand, phenothiazines have no greater value than haloperidol. When a patient cannot tolerate haloperidol, a trial with a phenothiazines may be indicated; dosages are similar to those used in the treatment of schizophrenia and cause the same side effects.

Substituted benzylamines (e.g., metapropramide) have been used in Europe with some success, but pseudoparkinsonian side effects and altered kidney function limit their broad use. Agents that affect cholinergic function are not commonly used in the treatment of TS. Intravenous physostigmine has been used to study cholinergic mechanisms; even those investigators observing a reduction in TS symptoms have been unable to apply agents like physostigmine clinically (Stahl & Berger, 1980, 1981). Lecithin has no benefit in controlled trials or anecdotal reports (Rosenberg & Davis, 1982). Agents affecting serotonergic function have not been useful, but there are few rigorous studies (Van Woert et al., 1982, 1977a and b). It is likely that medications with increasingly specific modes of action will become available during the next several years and be applied to the treatment of TS.

Choice of Medication. The clinician's choice of initial drug is a difficult decision. The greatest cumulative experience is with haloperidol, so that its therapeutic benefits and side effects are well defined. Clonidine may be preferred as a first drug because of its limited side effects and positive effect on attention; however, where a rapid response is needed, haloperidol is more effective. Clonidine has less immediate and dramatic therapeutic effects, and they are less extensively defined. Until more evidence accumulates, or other drugs become available, individual clinical experience will determine which drug should be given an initial several-month course. If a patient is started on haloperidol, discontinuation may be difficult because of withdrawal symptoms that are not attentuated by clonidine at usual doses. Some clinicians have added low dose clonidine to low dose haloperidol with good results, but no controlled studies have been reported. Whether pimozide will become an alternative to haloperidol will depend on the seriousness and frequency of side effects when it is more widely used; the association with cardiac death and the extremely limited study with children suggest caution.

When used alone, antidepressant medications either aggravate or fail to improve TS symptoms. However, if a TS patient develops a serious depression, the use of antidepressant medication should be considered. In this situation, an antidepressant can be added to ongoing TS treatment (haloperidol, clonidine) with good results. Both haloperidol and clonidine may cause lowered spirits or dysphoria, and assessment of depression may be difficult. A period of no medication might be considered before the addition of an antidepressant, especially if depression appears soon after the use of medication and with no apparent psychosocial precipitant. Minor tranquilizers have no apparent benefit on tic symptomatology; however, individual patients have benefited when they are used to alleviate anxiety or improve sleep.

Academic Intervention

Attentional and learning problems necessitate educational intervention for children with TS. They may require special tutoring, a learning laboratory, a self-contained classroom, or special day or residential school settings, depending on the severity of academic and associated behavioral problems. It may be difficult to convince a school district of the need for special school provisions when a bright TS patient does not have specific learning disabilities but has attentional problems limiting his optimal functioning. Tourette's Syndrome is an uncommon disorder, and schools need to be informed about the nature of TS and its effects on attention and learning; at times the physician must be active as a child's advocate.

Children with TS sometimes remain as homebound students because their symptoms are judged to be too disruptive for the classroom. Phonic tics are especially problematic for teachers. When a child is homebound, he is being deprived of his legal right to the least restrictive educational environment and an adequate education. This is an urgent situation, requiring intensive medical and legal intervention. Children who stay at home are likely to experience an exacerbation of symptoms as they exert less control and are exposed to the tedium of no outside diversions and the intense, often negative or ambivalent interactions with parents. A chain reaction is set up in which symptoms lead to worse symptoms and increasing isolation from the modulating effects of socialization. School difficulties and appropriate school placement require prompt clinical intervention, before attention to tics, and should be the initial focus of treatment.

Genetic Counseling

Parents and older TS patients increasingly inquire about the genetic risk for siblings and offspring. The precise mode of inheritance is still not known, so only general advice is possible. Birth into a family with a first degree relative (parent or sibling) with TS increases the risk of disorder for the child from 1 in many hundreds or thousands to 1 in 4 or 5. The risk is much higher for male offspring. Genetic counseling requires tact and sensitivity about the meaning of the information to a young adult with TS. The children of a mother with TS have an especially high risk, and judicious concern is required when counseling the TS mother who desires a child. At present, there is no method for prenatal diagnosis. It is important to emphasize the uncertainties of genetic counseling, as well as the increasing knowledge about treatment.

Multiple-Handicapped TS Patients

The adolescent or adult with longstanding, severe TS and multiple associated social and academic difficulties present complex treatment challenges. It is not uncommon for these most severely afflicted individuals to have few personal or social resources and to have intensely ambivalent relations with their exhausted families. Disentangling what is "Tourette's" and what are the manifold consequences of chronicity, disorganization, and various medications may be a major, long term therapeutic task. Patients may no longer know what is under their control, in any sense of this term, and what is primarily a manifestation of their TS. Reconstructing their experience and trying to understand what they are doing is a goal of the therapeutic work. Medication side effects and withdrawal-emergent effects confuse matters and make it difficult to assess any intervention. Most pathetic are the young adults who exhibit self-mutilation, such as poking their eyes or biting their cheeks or banging their heads, during TS crises; other patients become chronically dependent and unable to function on their own, yet have nobody to turn to. For the young adult who has had serious interference with school achievement, socialization, and personality development, a thorough rehabilitation program is required. The patient may need vocational guidance, a halfway house program, psychotherapy, family counseling, and advocacy, in addition to judicious use of medication. Even in desperate situations, therapeutic commitment combined with the patient's determination and courage may lead to satisfying therapeutic results. The treatment is facilitated if there is a therapeutic team that can be mutually supportive and can work together to find social and financial resources during the many months when the patient may be dependent and demanding.

Episodes of exacerbation are to be expected. Months of hard-won progress may seem to dissipate in days without a trace. It is natural for the physician to become disappointed and angry during these exacerbations, as symptoms return and a patient seems to crumble. The patient may sense the physician's attitude; when he becomes enraged and utterly discouraged, the treatment relationship may end. Clinicians, like parents, may cajole, bribe, and threaten. The physician may not know how to set "limits" that can be used by the patient to regain a sense of inner control, because he recognizes that such behavioral approaches are sometimes an expression of anger. However, if a therapeutic alliance can be maintained, it is possible to weather the storm and for this shared experience to strengthen the treatment relationship as the patient restabilizes. Short term hospitalization may be useful during crisis. However, TS patients may be unwelcome on an inpatient neurology or psychiatry service because of their disruptive and often bizarre behavior. Phonic symptoms are as disturbing in a hospital as in a school. When patients are hospitalized, there is a tendency to use medication for sedation, not only because of the patient's needs but because of the anxiety of the clinical staff and other patients. The availability of an inpatient service willing to accept a TS patient, and knowledgeable about its treatment, can be reassuring and critical to both the patient and the physician.

ETIOLOGY AND NEUROBIOLOGICAL RESEARCH

While genetic factors appear to be a powerful influence in the etiology of TS, they are not found in all cases nor are the underlying mechanisms of transmission and expression known. Intensive research on etiological factors has focused on neurochemical alterations in the brain (Cohen et al., 1979a and b; Butler et al., 1979; Hanin et al., 1979; Young et al., 1981a and b).

Pharmacological and metabolic research suggest alterations in several neurochemical systems. Dopaminergic involvement is supported by the most compelling evidence: the dramatic response to haloperidol and other dopamine receptor blockers, exacerbations produced by stimulant medications, and findings of reduced levels of the principal dopamine metabolite (homovanillic acid, HVA) in the cerebrospinal fluid (CSF) of TS patients (Cohen et al., 1978; Butler et al., 1978; Singer et al., 1982; Koslow & Cross, 1982; Iversen & Alpert, 1982; Bunney & DeRemier, 1982; Stahl & Berger, 1982). Serotonergic mechanisms have been suggested by reduced CSF 5-hydroxyindoleacetic acid (5-HIAA), the principal serotonin metabolite (Cohen et al., 1978; Butler et al., 1978; Singer et al., 1982; Koslow & Cross, 1982; Jacobs et al., 1982). The role of cholinergic systems is obscured by contradictory reports; enhanced cholinergic activity (through use of physostigmine) has been associated with both improvement and worsening of TS (Stahl & Berger, 1980, 1981; Rosenberg & Davis, 1982). Elevated levels of red blood cell choline have been found in TS patients and their relatives, but the relation of this to brain cholinergic function is unclear (Hanin et al., 1979; Comings et al., 1982). Norandrenergic mechanisms have been most persuasively implicated by the observation that clonidine, which inhibits noradrenergic activity through stimulation of an inhibitory autoreceptor, may improve motor and phonic symptoms (Cohen et al., 1979b; Leckman et al., 1983; Young et al., 1981b). Noradrenergic involvement has also been suggested by the increased symptomatology during stress and anxiety. Elevated levels of the chief norepinephrine metabolite (3-methoxy-4-hydroxyphenethylene glycol, MHPG) in the CSF of some severe patients, has been observed, but metabolic studies of CSF and plasma MHPG have not yet clarified the noradrenergic role in TS (Leckman et al., 1983; Young et al., 1981a and b; Ang et al., 1982).

It is possible that the expression of TS involves several neurotransmitter systems, operating in a cascading or reinforcing fashion. Various components of the disorder may involve different neurotransmitters and the balance among them; for example, motor tics may express dopaminergic overactivity while impaired inhibitory mechanisms (e.g., attentional problems) may represent noradrenergic dysregulation. There is evidence for interactions among neurochemical systems (Leckman et al., 1983; Antelman & Caggiula, 1977; Bunney & DeRemier, 1982). For example, both the dopaminergic and serotonergic systems show a pronounced response to D-amphetamine (Cohen et al., 1978). Clonidine directly reduces noradrenergic functioning, but may also influence dopaminergic activity (Leckman et al., 1983). This noradrenergic-dopaminergic interaction appears to require the mediation of the serotonergic system in the raphe nuclei (Bunney & DeRemier, 1982). Other neurotransmitters may also be implicated in TS as well. A role for opioid receptors, for example, is suggested by the amelioration of symptoms reported by patients who have used heroin (Buck & Yamamura, 1982). It is important to recognize that none of these findings assert that a specific neuronal system is the site of the primary pathology. Most or all may only be secondarily affected. New animal research methods may clarify these interactions and suggest mechanisms mediating clinical phenomena, such as stress-induced exacerbation of symptoms (Knott & Hutson, 1982; Shaywitz et al., 1982).

The use of stimulant medication is a particularly important risk factor for tics and TS. In some cohorts over 25 percent of TS patients have had a course of stimulant medication early in the emergence of their behavioral or tic symptoms; they had received an initial diagnosis of ADD and hyperactivity. Several series of cases have been reported in which the use of stimulants (methylphenidate, dextroamphetamine, and pemoline) has been associated with the onset of motor and phonic tics; pemoline may be especially likely to be involved (Golden, 1974; Lowe et al., 1982). Stimulant medications produce complex stereotypies in animals that disappear when the stimulants are terminated (Knott & Hutson, 1982); similarly, several percent of all children treated with stimulant medication develop simple motor tics (such as eye blinking or nose puckering) that disappear with reduction or discontinuation of the medication. It is more controversial to say that stimulants actually trigger or produce prolonged chronic multiple tics or TS that persist following the termination of medication (Comings & Comings, 1984; Shapiro & Shapiro, 1981; Caine et al., 1984). However, many cases have been reported in which this seems to have occurred (Golden, 1974; Lowe et al., 1982). Compelling clinical evidence comes from tic-free children who have had two courses of stimulant medication. During the first course, tics have emerged after months of treatment, but disappeared after discontinuation of the stimulant. After initiation of a second course of stimulants, tics have appeared within days and have persisted for months or permanently after stimulants have been withdrawn. These children seem to have had TS kindled by repeated exposure to stimulants. An important feature of this association is that some children—but, importantly, not all—who have had TS emerge during the course of stimulant treatment, have a family history of TS or tics and might have been genetically vulnerable. Furthermore, it is not possible to know whether a subgroup of ADD children who have developed TS with stimulants were already progressing to TS in any case. Detailed neurochemical, genetic, and clinical studies are needed to specify the interacting factors contributing to stimulant induction and exacerbation of tic symptoms. For example, we do not know if genetically less vulnerable children require longer treatment or larger amounts of stimulants to precipitate TS or are "invulnerable" to TS. It is unclear how stimulants affect receptor function in children carrying a genetic loading for TS. However, it is beyond dispute that stimulants cause transient tics, often (but not always) worsen preexisting tic symptoms, and elicit stereotypes and prolonged alterations in CNS dopaminergic and other systems in animals. Similarly, stimulants occasionally cause transient psychotic symptoms in vulnerable children (Young, 1981). It seems likely that stimulants precipitate the full expression of TS earlier than it might have appeared in some vulnerable children; of course, it also might not have developed at all. There is sufficient information to state that stimulants should be used cautiously with ADD children who have a close relative with tics, should not be used with ADD children with a first-degree relative with TS, and should be discontinued with the onset of tics in children who were previously tic-free.

Several lines of evidence suggest that TS may be heterogeneous biologically: there is variability in the nature and severity of symptoms, in family history, in natural history, and in response to medication. Extremely severe cases of TS with multiform, ceaseless, and devastating symptoms may be etiologically different from milder forms. While TS cases can be subgrouped on the basis of clinical findings, such as the presence of compulsions or ADD, further research is necessary to determine if these groups are distinctive or represent a spectrum of severity.

CONCLUSION

Tourette's Syndrome is a chronic and usually lifelong disorder in which simple motor and phonic tics may interfere less with development than complex tics (compulsions), complex phonic symptoms, and associated attentional and behavioral problems. Evaluation should include careful attention to personality development and school achievement; intervention includes reassurance and support, medication if needed, and guidance and advocacy in relation to appropriate school placement. Target symptoms include not only motor and phonic symptoms but an individual's full range of functioning. The major goal of treatment is to help the child successfully move along the various lines of development. The use of medication that interferes with these achievements runs the risk of creating patients who are socially more disadvantaged than had they been left undiagnosed. Maintenance on psychoactive medications for many years poses medical and behavioral toxicological risks that require careful scrutiny. Family therapy, psychotherapy, and behavior modification approaches have limited value in relation to motor and phonic tics, but they should be considered for the behavioral and psychological problems that may compound TS or occur in a family because of the stress of a chronic neuropsychiatric disorder. Periods of exacerbation are likely to lead to anxiety and stress that may further aggravate the condition. The clinician's availability and a long-standing relationship are especially important at such times.

One reassuring fact for families and patients is that TS has become an area of active clinical research interest and more has been learned in the past few years than in the preceding century. The reliance of TS patients on research progress was dramatized by a 16-year-old young man with incapacitating complex motor tics and compulsions. A bright and successful student of science, he examined the TS treatment literature after medications were frustratingly unsuccessful. These researches led him to urge his parents to allow him to have a neurosurgical treatment for his brain impairment. They eventually decided that the possible side effects were unacceptable. Fortunately, he later had a good response to a trial of pimozide, and has sustained his improvement. Continuing intensive research efforts hold the promise of additional treatment advances and clarification of causes of this debilitating syndrome.

REFERENCES

American Psychiatric Association. (1980). *Diagnostic and Statistical Manual of Mental Disorders (DSM-III)* (3rd ed.). Washington, D.C.: American Psychiatric Association.

Ang, L., Borison, R., Dysken, M., & Davis, J. M. (1982). Reduced excretion of MHPG in Tourette Syndrome. In A. J. Friedhoff & T. N. Chase (Eds.), *Advances in neurology* (Vol. 35). Raven Press: New York.

Antelman, S. M., & Caggiula, A. R. (1977). Norepinephrine-dopamine interactions and behavior. *Science, 195*, 646–653.

Bergen, D., Tanner, C. M., & Wilson, R. (1982). The electroencephalogram in Tourette Syndrome. *Annals of Neurology, 11*, 382–385.

Bliss, J., Cohen, D. J., & Freedman, D. X. (1980). Sensory experiences of Gilles de la Tourette Syndrome. *Archives of General Psychiatry, 37*, 1343–1347.

Bogomolny, A., Erenberg, G., & Rothner, D. (1982). Behavioral effects of haloperidol in young Tourette Syndrome patients. In A. J. Friedhoff & T. N. Chase (Eds.), *Advances in neurology* (Vol. 35). Raven Press: New York.

Borison, R. L., Ang, L. Chang, S., et al. (1982). New pharmacological approaches in the treatment of Tourette Syndrome. In A. J. Friedhoff & T. N. Chase (Eds.), *Advances in neurology* (Vol. 35). Raven Press: New York.

Brunn, R. D. (1982). Clonidine treatment of Tourette Syndrome. In A. J. Friedhoff & T. N. Chase (Eds.), *Advances in neurology* (Vol. 35). Raven Press: New York.

Brunn, R. D. (1982). Dysphoric phenomena associated with haloperidol treatment of Tourette Syndrome. In A. J. Friedhoff & T. N. Chase (Eds.), *Advances in neurology* (Vol. 35). Raven Press: New York.

Brunn, R. D. (1984). Gilles de la Tourette's Syndrome: An overview of clinical experience. *Journal of the American Academy of Child Psychiatry, 23*(2), 123–125.

Buck, S. H., & Yamamura, H. I. (1982). Neuropeptides in normal and pathological basal ganglia. In A. J. Friedhoff & T. N. Chase (Eds.), *Advances in neurology,* (Vol. 35). Raven Press: New York.

Bunney, B. S., & DeRemier, S. (1982). Effect of clonidine on dopaminergic neuron activity in the substantia nigra: Possible indirect mediation by noradrenergic regulation of the serotonergic Raphe System. In A. J. Friedhoff & T. N. Chase (Eds.), *Advances in neurology* (Vol. 35). Raven Press: New York.

Butler, I. J., Koslow, S., Seifert, W., et al. (1979). Biogenic amine metabolism in Tourette Syndrome. *Annals of Neurology, 6*, 37–39.

Caine, E. D., Ludlow, C. L., Polinsky, R. J., & Ebert, M. H. (1984). Provocative drug testing in Tourette's Syndrome: D- and L- amephetamine and haloperidol. *Journal of the American Academy of Child Psychiatry, 23*(2), 147–152.

Caparulo, B. K., Cohen, D. J., Rothman, S. L., et al. (1981). Computed tomographic brain scanning in children with development neuropsychiatric disorders. *Journal of the American Academy of Child Psychiatry, 20*, 338–357.

Cohen, D. J., Detlor, J., Shaywitz, B. A., & Leckman, J. F. (1982). Interaction of biological and psychological factors in the natural history of Tourette Syndrome: A paradigm for childhood neuropsychiatric disorders. In A. J. Friedhoff & T. N. Chase (Eds.), *Advances in neurology* (Vol. 35). Raven Press: New York.

Cohen, D. J., Detlor, J., Young, J. G., & Shaywitz, B. A. (1980). Clonidine ameliorates Gilles de la Tourette Syndrome. *Archives of General Psychiatry, 37*, 1350–1357.

Cohen, D. J. et al. (1978). CSF acid monoamine metabolites after probenecid administration. *Archives of General Psychiatry, 35*, 245–250.

Cohen, D. J., & Leckman, F. J. (1984). Tourette's Syndrome: Advances in treatment and research. Introduction. *Journal of the American Academy of Child Psychiatry, 2*, 123–125.

Cohen, D. J., Shaywitz, B. A., Young, J. G., et al. (1979b). Central biogenic amine metabolism in children with the syndrome of chronic multiple tics of Gilles de la Tourette: Norepinephrine, serotonin, and dopamine. *Journal of the American Academy of Child Psychiatry, 18*, 320–341.

Cohen, D. J., Young, J. G., Nathanson, J. A., & Shaywitz, B. A. (1979a). Clonidine in Tourette's Syndrome. *Lancet 1979, ii*, 551–553.

Comings, D. E., & Comings, G. G. (1984). Tourette's syndrome and attention deficit disorder with hyperactivity: Are they genetically related? *Journal of the American Academy of Child Psychiatry, 23*(2), 138–146.

Comings, D. E., Gursey, B. T., Avelino, E., et al. (1982). Red blood cell choline in Tourette Syndrome. In A. J. Friedhoff & T. N. Chase (Eds.), *Advances in neurology* (Vol 35). Raven Press: New York.

Comings, D. E., Gursey, B. T., Hecht, T., & Blume, K. (1982). HLA typing in Tourette Syndrome. In A. J. Friedhoff & T. N. Chase (Eds.) *Advances in neurology* (Vol. 35). Raven Press: New York.

Eldridge, R., Sweet, R., Lake, C. R., et al. (1977). Gilles de la Tourette's Syndrome: Clinical, genetic, psychologic, and biochemical aspects in 21 selected families. *Neurology, 27*, 115–124.

Fog, R., Pakkenberg, H., Regeur, L., & Pakkenberg, B. (1982). "Tardive" Tourette Syndrome in relation to long-term neuroleptic treatment of multiple tics. In A. J. Friedhoff and T. N. Chase (Eds.), *Advances in neurology* (Vol. 5). Raven Press: New York.

Friedhoff, A. J., & Chase, T. N. (Eds.). (1982). Gilles de la Tourette Syndrome. *Advances in neurology* (Vol. 35). Raven Press: New York.

Goetz, C. G., and Klawans, H. L. (1982). Gilles de la Tourette on Tourette Syndrome. In A. J. Friedhoff & T. N. Chase (Eds.), *Advances in neurology* (Vol. 35). Raven Press: New York.

Golden, G. S. (1974). Gilles de la Tourette's Syndrome following methylphenidate administration. *Developmental Medicine and Child Neurology, 16*, 76–78.

Golden, G. S. (1982). Tourette Syndrome in children: Ethnic and genetic factors and response to stimulant drugs. In A. J. Friedhoff & T. N. Chase (Eds.), *Advances in neurology* (Vol. 35). Raven Press: New York.

Hagin, R. A., Beecher, R., Pagano, G., & Kreeger, H. (1982). Effects of Tourette Syndrome on learning. In A. J. Friedhoff and T. N. Chase (Eds.), *Advances in neurology* (Vol. 35). Raven Press: New York.

Hanin, I., Merikangas, M. R., Merikangas, K. R., et al. (1979). Red-cell choline and Gilles de la Tourette Syndrome. *New England Journal of Medicine, 301*, 661–662.

Harcherik, D. F., Leckman, J. F., Detlor, J., & Cohen, D. J. (1984). A new instrument for clinical studies of Tourette's Syndrome. *Journal of the American Academy of Child Psychiatry, 23*(2), 153–160.

Incagnoli, T., & Kane, R. (1982). Neuropsychological functioning in Tourette Syndrome.

In A. J. Friedhoff & T. N. Chase (Eds.), *Advances in neurology* (Vol. 35). Raven Press: New York.

Iversen, S. D., & Alpert, J. E. (1982). Functional organization of the dopamine system in normal and abnormal behavior. In A. J. Friedhoff and T. N. Chase (Eds.), *Advances in neurology* (Vol. 35). Raven Press: New York.

Jacobs, B. L., Trulson, M. E., Heym, J., & Steinfels, G. F. (1982). On the role of CNS serotonin in the motor abnormalities of Tourette Syndrome: behavioral and single-unit studies. In A. J. Friedhoff & T. N. Chase (Eds.), *Advances in neurology* (Vol. 35). Raven Press: New York.

Jagger, J., Prusoff, B. A., Cohen, D. J. et al. (1982). The epidemiology of Tourette's Syndrome: A pilot study. *Schizophrenia Bulletin, 8,* 267–278.

Joschko, M., & Rourke, B. P. (1982). Neuropsychological dimensions of Tourette Syndrome: Test-retest stability and implications for intervention. In A. J. Friedhoff & T. N. Chase (Eds.), *Advances in neurology* (Vol. 35). Raven Press: New York.

Kidd, K. K. & Pauls, D. L. (1982). Genetic hypothesis for Tourette Syndrome. In A. J. Friedhoff & T. N. Chase (Eds.), *Advances in neurology* (Vol. 35). Raven Press: New York.

Kidd, K. K., Prusoff, B. A., & Cohen, D. J. (1980). Familial pattern of Gilles de la Tourette Syndrome. *Archives of General Psychiatry, 37,* 1336–1339.

Klawans, H. L., Nausieda, P. A., Goetz, C. G., et al. (1982). Tourette-like symptoms following chronic neuroleptic therapy. In A. J. Friedhoff & T. N. Chase (Eds.), *Advances in neurology* (Vol. 35). Raven Press: New York.

Knott, P. J., & Hutson, P. H. (1982). Stress-induced stereotypy in the rat: Neuropharmacological similarities to Tourette Syndrome. In A. J. Friedhoff & T. N. Chase, (Eds.), *Advances in neurology* (Vol. 35). Raven Press: New York.

Kondo, K., & Nomura, Y. (1982). Tourette Syndrome in Japan: Etiologic considerations based on associated factors and familial clustering. In A. J. Friedhoff & T. N. Chase (Eds.), *Advances in neurology* (Vol. 35). Raven Press: New York.

Koslow, S. H., & Cross, C. K. (1982). Cerebrospinal fluid monoamine metabolites in Tourette Syndrome and their neuroendocrine implications. In A. J. Friedhoff and T. N. Chase (Eds.), *Advances in neurology* (Vol. 35). Raven Press: New York.

Leckman, J. F., Cohen, D. J., Detlor, J., et al. (1982). Clonidine in the treatment of Tourette Syndrome: A review of data. In A. J. Friedhoff and T. N. Chase (Eds.), *Advances in neurology* (Vol. 35). Raven Press: New York.

Leckman, J. F., & Cohen, D. J. (1983). Recent advances in Gilles de la Tourette Syndrome: Implications for clinical practice and future research. *Psychiatric Development, 3,* 301–316.

Leckman, J. F., Detlor, J., Harcherik, D. F., et al. (1983). Acute and chronic clonidine treatment in Tourette's Syndrome: A preliminary report on clinical response and effect on plasma and urinary catecholamine metabolites, growth hormone, and blood pressure. *Journal of the American Academy of Child Psychiatry, 22,* 433–440.

Leckman, J. F., Detlor, J., Harcherik, D. F., et al. (1984). Short and long-term treatment of Tourette's disorder with clonidine: A clinical perspective. Submitted for publication.

Lowe, T. L., Cohen, D. J., Detlor, J., et al. (1982). Stimulant medications precipitate Tourette's Syndrome. *Journal of the American Medical Association, 247,* 1729–1731

Lucas, A. R., Beard, C. M., Rajput, A. H., & Kurland, L. T. (1982). Tourette Syndrome in

Rochester, Minnesota, 1968–1979. In A. J. Friedhoff & T. N. Chase (Eds.), *Advances in neurology* (Vol. 35). Raven Press: New York.

Mak, F. L., Chung, S. Y., Lee, P., & Chen, S. (1982). Tourette Syndrome in the Chinese: A follow-up of 15 cases. In A. J. Friedhoff & T. N. Chase (Eds.), *Advances in neurology* (Vol. 35). Raven Press: New York.

Moldofsky, H., & Brown, G. M. (1982). Tics and serum prolactin response to pimozide in Tourette Syndrome. In A. J. Friedhoff & T. N. Chase (Eds.), *Advances in neurology* (Vol. 35). Raven Press: New York.

Nee, L. E., Caine, E. D., Polinsky, R. J., et al. (1980). Gilles de la Tourette syndrome: Clinical and family study of 50 cases. *Annals of Neurology, 7,* 41–49.

Nee, L. E., Polinsky, R. J., & Ebert, M. H. (1982). Tourette Syndrome: Clinical and family studies. In A. J. Friedhoff & T. N. Chase (Eds.), *Advances in neurology* (Vol. 35). Raven Press: New York.

Nomura, Y., & Segawa, M. (1982). Tourette Syndrome in oriental children: Clinical and pathophysiological considerations. In A. J. Friedhoff & T. N. Chase, *Advances in neurology* (Vol. 35). Raven Press: New York.

Nose, T., & Takemoto (1975). The effect of penfluridol and some psychotropic drugs on monoamine metabolism in central nervous system. *European Journal of Pharmacology, 31,* 351–359.

Pauls, D. L., Cohen, D. J., Heimbuch, R., et al. (1981). Familial pattern of transmission of Gilles de la Tourette syndrome and multiple tics. *Archives of General Psychiatry, 38,* 1085–1090.

Pauls, D. l., Kurger, S. D., Leckman, J. F., et al. (1984). The risk of Tourette's syndrome and chronic multiple tics among relatives of Tourette's syndrome patients obtained by direct interview. *Journal of the American Academy of Child Psychiatry, 23*(2), 134–137.

Price, R. A., Kidd, K. K., Cohen, D. J., & Pauls, D. L. (1984). A twin study of Tourette Syndrome. *Behavioral Genetics* (in press).

Rapoport, J., Nee, L., Mitchell, S., et al. (1982). Hyperkinetic Syndrome and Tourette Syndrome. In A. J. Friedhoff & T. N. Chase (Eds.), *Advances in neurology* (Vol. 35). Raven Press: New York.

Rosenberg, G. S., & Davis, K. L. (1982). Precursors of acetylcholine: Considerations underlying their use in Tourette Syndrome. In A. J. Friedhoff & T. N. Chase (Eds.), *Advances in neurology* (Vol. 35). Raven Press: New York.

Ross, M. S., & Moldofsky, N. (1977). Comparison of pimozide with haloperidol in Gilles de la Tourette Syndrome. *Lancet, 1,* 103.

Schoenberg, B. S. (1982). Neuroepidemiologic approach to Tourette Syndrome. In A. J. Friedhoff & T. N. Chase, (Eds.), *Advances in neurology* (Vol. 35). Raven Press: New York.

Seeman, P., & Lee, T. (1975). Antipsychotic drugs: Direct correlation between clinical potency and presynaptic action on dopamine neurons. *Science, 188,* 1217–1219.

Selinger, D., Cohen, D. J., Ort, S., et al. (1984). Parotid salivary response to clonidine in Tourette's Syndrome: Indicator of adrenergic responsivity. *Journal of the American Academy of Child Psychiatry* 23 (4), 392–398.

Shapiro, A. K., & Shapiro, E. (1981). Do stimulants provoke, cause or exacerbate tics or Tourette Syndrome? *Comprehensive Psychiatry, 22*(3), 265–273.

Shapiro, A. K., & Shapiro, E. (1982). Clinical efficacy of haloperidol, pimozide, penfluridol, and clonidine in the treatment of Tourette syndrome. In A. J. Friedhoff & T. N. Chase (Eds.), *Advances in neurology* (Vol. 35). Raven Press: New York.

Shapiro, A. K., & Shapiro, E. (1984). Controlled study of pimozide vs. placebo in Tourette's Syndrome. *Journal of the American Academy of Child Psychiatry, 23*(2), 161–173.

Shapiro, A. K., Shapiro, E., Bruun, R. D., & Sweet, R. D. (1978). *Gilles de la Tourette's Syndrome.* Raven Press: New York.

Shapiro, A. K., Shapiro, E., & Eisenkraft, G. J. (1983). Treatment of Gilles de la Tourette Syndrome with pimozide. *American Journal of Psychiatry, 140,* 1183–1186.

Shapiro, A. K., Shapiro, E., & Wayne, H. (1972). Birth, developmental and family histories and demographic information in Tourette's syndrome. *Journal of Nervous and Mental Diseases, 155,* 335–344.

Shapiro, A. K., Shapiro, E., & Wayne, H. L. (1972). The symptomatology and diagnosis of Gilles de la Tourette's syndrome. *Journal of the American Academy of Child Psychiatry, 12,* 702–273.

Shapiro, A. K., Shapiro, E., & Wayne, H. L. (1973). Treatment of Gilles de la Tourette's Syndrome with haloperidol: Review of 34 cases. *Archives of General Psychiatry, 28,* 92–96.

Shapiro, A. K., Shapiro, E., Wayne, H. L., & Clarkin, J. (1973). Organic factors in Gilles de la Tourette's Syndrome. *British Journal of Psychiatry, 122,* 659–664.

Shapiro, E., & Shapiro, A. K. (1982). Tardive dyskinesia and chronic neuroleptic treatment of Tourette patients. In A. J. Friedhoff & T. N. Chase (Eds.), *Advances in neurology* (Vol. 35). Raven Press: New York.

Shaywitz, B. A., Wolf, A., Shaywitz, S., et al. (1982). Animals models of neuropsychiatric disorders and their relevance for Tourette Syndrome. In A. J. Friedhoff & T. N. Chase (Eds.), *Advances in neurology* (Vol. 35). Raven Press: New York.

Singer, H. S., Tune, L. F., Butler, I. J., et al. (1982). Clinical symptomatology, CSF neurotransmitter metabolites, and serum haloperidol levels in Tourette Syndrome. In A. J. Friedhoff & T. N. Chase (Eds.), *Advances in neurology* (Vol. 35). Raven Press: New York.

Stahl, S. M. & Berger, P. A. (1980). Cholinergic treatment in the Tourette Syndrome. *New England Journal of Medicine, 302,* 1311.

Stahl, S. M., & Berger, P. A. (1981). Physostigmine in Tourette Syndrome: Evidence for cholinergic underactivity. *American Journal of Psychiatry, 138,* 240–242.

Stahl, S. M., & Berger, P. A. (1982). Cholinergic and dopaminergic mechanisms in Tourette Syndrome. In A. J. Friedhoff & T. N. Chase (Eds.), *Advances in neurology,* (Vol. 35). Raven Press: New York.

Sutherland, R. J., Kolb, B., Schoel, W. M., et al. (1982). Neuropsychological assessment of children and adults with Tourette Syndrome: A comparison with learning disabilities and schizophrenia. In A. J. Friedhoff & T. N. Chase (Eds.), *Advances in neurology* (Vol. 35). Raven Press: New York.

Van Woert, M. H., Rosenbaum, D., & Enna, S. J. (1982). Overview of pharmacological approaches to therapy for Tourette Syndrome. In A. J. Friedhoff & T. N. Chase (Eds.), *Advances in neurology* (Vol. 35). Raven Press: New York.

Van Woert, M. H., Rosenbaum, S., Howieson, J., & Bowers, M. B., Jr. (1977b). Long-term therapy of myoclonus and other neurologic disorders with L-5-hydroxytryptophan and carbidopa. *New England Journal of Medicine, 296,* 70–75.

Van Woert, M. H., Yip, L. C., & Balis, M. D. (1977a). Purine phosphoribosyltransferase in Gilles de la Tourette Syndrome. *New England Journal of Medicine, 296,* 210–212.

Volkmar, F. R., Leckman, J. F., Detlor, J., et al. (1984). EEG abnormalities in Tourette's Syndrome. *Journal of the American Academy of Child Psychiatry, 23,* 352–353.

Young, J. G. (1981). Methylphenidate-induced hallucinosis. *Journal of Developmental and Behavioral Pediatrics, 2,* 35–38.

Young, J. G., et al. (1981a). Cerebrospinal fluid, plasma, and urinary MHPG in children. *Life Sciences, 28,* 2837–2845.

Young, J. G., et al. (1981b). Plasma free MHPG and neuro-endocrine responses to challenge doses of clonidine in Tourette's syndrome: Preliminary report. *Life Sciences, 29,* 1467–1475.

Conduct Disorders

DANIEL J. O'DONNELL, M.D.

INTRODUCTION

Conduct disorders are complex conditions for which as yet there are no adequate explanations or predictably reliable treatments. Children included in this diagnostic category represent a very diverse heterogenous group reflecting differences in age of onset, clinical characteristics, family background, socioeconomic features, associated symptoms and conditions, and response to treatment. Our current state of knowledge does not yet permit sufficient explanations or predictably reliable recommendations for treatment of conduct disorders.

Conduct disorders are the most common reason for referral of children for psychiatric evaluation and treatment. In one study, one-third to three-quarters of children brought to treatment centers were referred because of aggressive behavior (Wells & Forehand, in press). The incidence of aggressive conduct disorders in the general population, derived from data-oriented approaches to diagnosis and the use of clear diagnostic criteria appears to be 3–4 percent (Trites et al., 1979; Rutter et al., 1976). American reports on overall prevalence are uncertain because of differences in diagnostic criteria and, until recently, the absence of specific diagnostic criteria and categories. Nevertheless, reports are generally consistent in pointing out that aggressive conduct disorders are among the leading pediatric public health problems in the country. Two-thirds to three-quarters of children with all types of conduct disorders are boys, and boys represent an even higher percentage of children with aggressive conduct disorders.

The seriousness of the public health problem is further underscored by the poor outcome of children with conduct disorders. Approximately one-third go on to have antisocial behavior as adults (see Table 9.1). In addition to those who have persistent sociopathic behavior, another third to half have other personality disorder diagnoses, psychiatric diagnoses, or poor social outcome. Traditional psychological treatments have not been proved effective in improving the outcome in conduct disordered-delinquent children. In a recent review of psychological therapies in child psychiatry, Rutter (1982) asserts that psychodynamically oriented residential institutions and "long-term unfocused individual counselling" are "ineffective." The combination of the serious effects of conduct disorders together with generally poor results from psychosocial treatments and/or environmental manipulations has spurred widespread clinical use of pharmacological agents in these children, despite the absence of data supporting their efficacy. The clinical attitude, understandably, toward both psychosocial and pharmacological treatments has been one of attempting any acceptable approach rather than

250

Study	Method	Subject Sample	Beginning Age	Study Period	Beginning Diagnosis	Terminal Diagnosis
Annesley, 1961	Follow-up	Inpatient psychiatry unit	12–18 years	2–5 years	"Behavior disorder" (violence, stealing, truancy)	40% behavior disorder 1% schizophrenia
Morris et al., 1956	Follow-up	Inpatient unit	4–15 years X = 10	To adulthood	Aggressive behavior disorder (unsocialized aggressive)	59% "poor social adjustment" (18% committed crimes) 20% schizophrenia 21% normal
O'Neal & Robins, 1958	Follow-up	Psychiatry clinic	13 years	30 years	Delinquent Aggressive antisocial (not court contact)	37% sociopathic personality 14% neuroses 6% psychoses 11% ill; no diagnosis 14% normal 9% alcoholism 6% sociopathic personality 30% neuroses 30% psychosis 4% ill; no diagnosis 14% normal

Table 9.1. (Continued)

Study	Method	Subject Sample	Beginning Age	Study Period	Beginning Diagnosis	Terminal Diagnosis
Pritchard & Graham, 1966	Child and adult psychiatry clinic attenders	Psychiatry clinic	5–16 years $X = 11.6$	4–28 years $X = 10.8$ years	Delinquency	37% antisocial personality 19% inadequate personality 19% neuroses 15% immature and schizoid personality 11% psychotic disorders
					Conduct disorder	30% antisocial personality 30% neuroses 30% inadequate personality 10% immature and schizoid personality 0% psychotic disorders

Source: From Wells & Forehand (in press).

let these children drift out of society. Firm data supporting psychosocial, environmental (including familial and societal), physiological, and genetic theories of etiology are inconclusive. In large measure research into cause, outcome, and treatment effects has been hampered by diagnostic variability and heterogeneity, and difficulty controlling multiple variables.

DIAGNOSTIC SYSTEMS

DSM-III describes four subcategories based on social skills and aggressivity (see Table 9.2) Each category requires a "repetitive and persistent pattern" of deviant behavior for the diagnosis to be made, and it would be improper to make a diagnosis on the basis of one or few incidents of aggression, stealing, lying, and the like. In this chapter all treatments are discussed in reference to those children with "repetitive and persistent" behaviors.

While inclusion criteria are specified, there are no exclusion criteria. Few of the inclusion criteria are specific for "conduct disorder." A child may be diagnosed by current criteria as having a conduct disorder and satisfy criteria for other disorders, some of which may indicate established or promising pharmacological treatments. Disorders that can contribute to difficulties in acquiring social skills and/or in controlling impulsivity and aggressivity include: (1) Attention Deficit Disorder (ADD), with and without hyperactivity; (2) schizophrenic, schizophreniform, and paranoid disorders; (3) affective disorders, including unipolar and bipolar types; (4) psychomotor/complex partial seizure disorders; and (5) "episodic dyscontrol" disorders.

Many nonviolent behaviors (such as truancy, running away, stealing, substance abuse, and lying) are included under conduct disorders. However, the major focus of this chapter is on aggressive behavior. The reasons for this are, first, aggressivity is the most frequent and immediately distressing referral problem; and, second, nearly all reports of use and research into the pharmacology of conduct disorders focus on children with aggressive behaviors.

Clinic-referred children with conduct disorders have symptoms or characteristics that covary with aggression in at least two distinct patterns. Symptoms of aggressive behavior that were derived from empirically based factor-analytic studies have been reviewed by Quay (1979) and Achenbach and Edelbrock (1978), compared and summarized by Wells and Forehand (in press). Table 9.3, from Wells and Forehand, outlines the two syndromes.

Table 9.2. DSM-III Subtypes of Conduct Disorder

312.00   Conduct Disorder, Undersocialized, Aggressive

Diagnostic Criteria

A. A repetitive and persistent pattern of aggressive conduct in which the basic rights of others are violated, as manifested by either of the following:

    (1) phyical violence against persons or property (not to defend someone else or oneself), e.g., vandalism, rape, breaking and entering, fire-setting, mugging, assault

    (2) thefts outside the home involving confrontation with the victim (e.g., extortion, purse-snatching, armed robbery)

B. Failure to establish a normal degree of affection, empathy, or bond with others as evidenced by no more than one of the following indications of social attachment:

    (1) has one or more peer-group friendships that have lasted over six months

    (2) extends himself or herself for others even when no immediate advantage is likely

    (3) apparently feels guilt or remorse when such a reaction is appropriate (not just when caught or in difficulty)

    (4) avoids blaming or informing on companions

    (5) shares concerns for the welfare of friends or companions

C. Duration of pattern of aggressive conduct of at least six months.

D. If 18 or older, does not meet the criteria for Antisocial Personality Disorder.

312.10 Conduct Disorder, Undersocialized, Nonaggressive

Diagnostic Criteria

A. A repetitive and persistent pattern of nonaggressive conduct in which either the basic rights of others or major age-appropriate societal norms or rules are violated, as manifested by any of the following:

    (1) chronic violations of a variety of important rules (that are reasonable and age-appropriate for the child) at home or at school (e.g., persistent truancy, substance abuse)

    (2) repeated running away from home overnight

    (3) persistent serious lying in and out of the home

    (4) stealing not involving confrontation with a victim

B. Failure to establish a normal degree of affection, empathy, or bond with others as evidenced by no more than one of the following indications of social attachment:

    (1) has one or more peer-group friendships that have lasted over six months

254

Table 9.2.   *(Continued)*

(2)   extends himself or herself for others even when no immediate advantage is likely

(3)   apparently feels guilt or remorse when such a reaction is appropriate (not just when caught or in difficulty)

(4)   avoids blaming or informing on companions

(5)   shares concerns for the welfare of friends or companions

C.   Duration of pattern of nonaggressive conduct of at least six months.

D.   If 18 or older, does not meet the criteria for Antisocial Personality Disorder.

312.23 Conduct Disorder, Socialized, Aggressive

Disgnostic Criteria

A.   A repetitive and persistent pattern of aggressive conduct in which the basic rights of others are violated, as manifested by either of the following:

(1)   physical violence against persons or property (not to defend someone else or oneself), e.g., vandalism rape, breaking and entering, firesetting, mugging, assault

(2)   thefts outside the home involving confrontation with a victim (e.g., extortion, purse-snatching, armed robbery)

B.   Evidence of social attachment to others as indicated by at least two of the following behavior patterns:

(1)   has one or more peer-group friendships that have lasted over six months

(2)   extends himself or herself for others even when no immediate advantage is likely

(3)   apparently feels guilt or remorse when such a reaction is appropriate (not just when caught or in difficulty)

(4)   avoids blaming or informing on companions

(5)   shares concerns for the welfare of friends or companions

C.   Duration of pattern of aggressive conduct of at least six months.

D.   If 18 or older, does not meet the criteria for Antisocial Personality Disorder.

312.21 Conduct Disorder, Socialized, Nonaggressive

Diagnostic Criteria

A.   A repetitive and persistent pattern of nonaggressive conduct in which either the basic rights of others or major age-appropriate societal norms or rules are violated, as manifested by any of the following:

(1)   chronic violations of a variety of important rules (that are reasonable and age-appropriate for the child) at home or at school (e.g., persistent truancy, substance abuse)

Table 9.2. (*Continued*)

---

(2)   repeated running away from home overnight

(3)   persistent serious lying in and out of the home

(4)   stealing not involving confrontation with a victim

B.   Evidence of social attachment to others as indicated by at least two of the following behavior patterns:

   (1)   has one or more peer-group friendships that have lasted over six months

   (2)   extends himself or herself for others even when no immediate advantage is likely

   (3)   apparently feels guilt or remorse when such a reaction is appropriate (not just when caught or in difficulty)

   (4)   avoids blaming or informing on companions

   (5)   shows concern for the welfare of friends or companions

C.   Duration of pattern of nonaggressive conduct of at least six months.

D.   If 18 or older, does not meet the criteria for Antisocial Personality Disorder.

Source. American Psychiatric Association (1980). *Diagnostic and Statistical Manual of Mental Disorders* (3rd ed.). Washington, DC: American Psychiatric Association.

It can be seen that the first, labeled "conduct disorder" corresponds best with the DSM-III category of "Conduct Disorder, Undersocialized, Aggressive Type." The second empirically based syndrome corresponds to the DSM-III category of "Conduct Disorder, Socialized, Aggressive Type." No empirically based evidence exists for the DSM-III category of conduct disorder, undersocialized, nonaggressive type. In addition, there is no support for the category of socialized, nonaggressive conduct disorder, except for delinquent girls (Achenbach, 1980).

ETIOLOGY AND PREDICTIVE FACTORS

Wells and Forehand (in press) review the outcome literature, and find promise in approaches based on behavioral–social learning theory. These methods have been demonstrated to have at least short term

**Table 9.3. Behavior Characteristics of Conduct Disorder
and Socialized Aggressive Disorder**

Conduct Disorder	Socialized Aggressive Disorder
1. Fighting, hitting, and assaultive behavior	1. Has "bad" companions
2. Temper tantrums	2. Steals in company with others
3. Disobedient and defiant	3. Loyal to delinquent friends
4. Destructiveness	4. Belongs to a gang
5. Impertinent	5. Truant from school
6. Uncooperative	6. Stays out late at night
7. Disruptive, interrupts	
8. Negative; refuses direction	
9. Restless	
10. Boisterous and noisy	
11. Irritable	
12. Attention seeking	

Note. Adapted from Quay (1979), p. 17 and 21 by Wells and Forehand (in press).

efficacy and may have promise for longer range improvement. In addition, Griest and Wells (1983), Forehand and McMahon (1981), Forehand et al. (1975), Loeber and Patterson (1981), Patterson (1976, 1982), Patterson et al. (1975), and Reid and Patterson (1976) have identified family behavior and parenting patterns that promote aggressive behavior in children and are responsive to specific intervention techniques such as parenting skills training. Treatment effects in the child have also been shown to follow changed parental behavior that breaks the coercive cycle by increasing parental use of clear, nonhostile commands, effective time-out procedures for noncompliance and rewards (primarily social) for compliance and prosocial behavior.

Constitutional–tempermental factors may make it more likely that a child will be "difficult" (Thomas, Chess, & Birch, 1968; Thomas & Chess, 1984) and thereby less likely to be socially rewarding to the parent and less able to amiably tolerate or respond to less-than-perfect parenting skills. Rutter et al. (1964) find that these "difficult" children are more likely to have severe temper tantrums and aggressive behavior problems than children with less problematic temperaments. Children with ADD have a much higher rate of multiple legal offenses and delinquency as adolescents than normal controls (Satterfield et al., 1982). Other contributing factors that could seriously affect a child's ability to acquire adequate prosocial behavior or maintain sufficient self-control include depression (Puig-Antich, 1982); neurological impairment and abuse (Lewis et al., 1979); and psychomotor epilepsy (Lewis et al., 1982).

In a similar way, there are many medical, psychological, and environmental factors that can affect a parent's ability to tolerate frustration, control irritability, and be energetic and resourceful enough to nurture and teach a child. Parental psychopathology (Griest & Wells, 1983; Patterson, 1980) has been shown to strongly influence parents' perceptions of the child, interactions, and ability to make adequate progress in therapy.

Genetics

There is evidence for a genetic factor in the development of conduct disorders. In the early 1970s a few reports appeared citing an increased frequency of XYY chromosome patterns in prison populations compared to the population at large (Owen, 1972; Hook, 1973). However, a later controlled study of XYY men found no evidence that XYY men in the general population were more violent or aggressive than XY men (Schiavi et al., 1984).

Studies conducted in Scandinavian countries, where detailed adoption records are kept, show that monozygotic twins, have approximately three times the concordance rate for criminality as dizygotic twins. (Christiansen, 1975). In a Danish study, Hutchings and Mednick (1974) found that for adopted children a history of criminality in an adoptive parent did not elevate a child's risk for developing criminality. However, if a biological parent (genetic factor) but not an adoptive parent was criminal, the child's risk was doubled (to 21%). Furthermore, if both a biological and adoptive parent were criminal the offspring risk was more than tripled (to 36.2%). The above data suggest that family environment alone, without genetic predisposition, is not sufficient to increase the risk of developing criminal behavior, but that genetic predisposition alone increases risk and also increases susceptibility towards criminality by a criminal family environment. However, Wells and Forehand (in press) point out other conditions (alcoholism and depression, characterized by irritability and affective dyscontrol, factors probably relevant to poor parenting and difficulty in acquiring social skills and self-control) are familial and probably genetically influenced and may bias genetic studies by contributing to the apparent heritability of criminal behavior. Nearly all studies are also flawed by a lack of uniform criteria for criminality and delinquency and for not distinguishing between violent crimes, property offenses, and petty criminality.

An extensive study of 862 Swedish adopted men and 913 adopted women was reported in a series of articles by Bohman et al. (1982). Cloniger et al. (1982) and Sigvardsson et al. (1982). The advantage of these studies, in addition to their thoroughness, is that Sweden, unlike Denmark, has a registry of alcohol abusers as well as of adoptees and criminals. They were able to show that biological parents with either alcohol abuse or with criminality alone tend to produce children with the same problem. Also, parents and offspring with criminal behavior alone strongly tended to commit only petty, nonviolent crimes whereas most of the violent and repetitive criminals were alcohol abusers. In addition, the number of crimes committed correlated positively with the severity of the alcoholism. For petty criminals, social status and environment did not contribute to the development of criminal behavior unless there was a genetic predisposition. There were also gender differences; while the genetic antecedents were similar, the predisposition had to be more severe for a female to become criminal. The investigators in these studies strongly emphasize that although congenital predisposition was the largest identified contributor to variability, most (76%) of the variability was not explained. In other words, although it seems to be clear that criminality is genetically influenced, the factors influencing the development of criminal behavior are heterogeneous and their interactions are very complicated.

Predictors of Delinquency

Loeber and Dishion (1983) reviewed studies that intended to establish reliable predictors for the development of delinquency in adolescents. In addition to genetic factors they attempted to elucidate the contribution of the other factors that account for that three-fourths of the variability not "explained" by genes. They concluded that the major factor predicting adolescent aggressive delinquent behavior was the parenting technique applied when the child was younger. In addition, they underscored that deviant child behavior per se predicts later delinquent behavior. Tantrums, aggressive behavior, and noncompliance in a child are not passing "phases," and parents and clinicians should not expect children to "grow out" of their deviant behavior. Criminality or antisocial behavior of family members as well as poor educational achievement in the child also predicted delinquent behavior. Stealing, lying, or truancy not only were strong predictors of subsequent delinquency but also led the list of factors predicting recidivism. Separation from parents or socioeconomic status had little predictive value.

Olweus (1980), using a statistical method that clarifies the casual relationships among multiple covarying factors, showed that four variables were most important in determining adolescent delinquent behavior:

1. Mother's permissiveness for aggression.

2. Mother's negativism toward the child: This provides evidence for the theorized relationship between a rejecting, negative, or indifferent primary caretaker and the development of social deviance (as contrasted to only poor self-image or mood or cognitive difficulties). In addition, it was found that a poor relationship between the parents contributed to the mother's negativism toward the child. Helping the parents improve their marriage may indirectly decrease the probability of aggressive–delinquent behavior in the child.

3. Temperament. The child's constitutional, inherent predisposition to being irritable, short-tempered, negative, for example, correlated with delinquency. This too might contribute both to early identification of problem children and to more effective treatment, in so far as it assists clinicians and parents in understanding and accepting that some children are more difficult to raise than others.

4. Mother's and father's use of power-assertive methods contributed to aggressivity. That is, violent parental outbursts, physical punishment, and threats appeared to promote aggressive behavior in the child.

Summary

Simple, unitary explanations (genetic, temperamental, psychological or environmental) are not adequate. Used alone, traditional treatment approaches have not been proved effective.

What follows is a review, class by class, of pharmacological agents used in aggressive behavioral disorders. It must be emphasized that regardless of the pharmacological treatment attempted, it should only be a part of the overall management. Social skills training, parenting skills training, individual and/or group therapy, identification and proper treatment of parental psychiatric illness, decreasing parental and marital stress, control of parental alcoholism, direct behavioral management of aggressive behavior and proper management of learning disabilities are among the many other tasks in trying to help a family and child with a conduct disorder.

MEDICATION

Even though the purpose of this chapter is a review of pharmacotherapy, this author takes the position that the primary treatment of aggressive conduct disorders must be a combination of behavioral and psychosocial approaches. There are conditions in childhood, which are at least partially responsive to drugs, that tend to make it very difficult, if not impossible, for a child to control his or her behavior. A trial of pharmacotherapy may well help such a child to be more amenable to psychological treatments and environmental changes. But we have no expectation, from research data or clinical experience, that any medication alone will sufficiently change "repetitive and persistent" patterns of aggressive behavior even when psychiatric–physiological contributions (e.g., depression, irritability, cortical dysregulation, short attention span, and low frustration tolerance) to aggressive dyscontrol are pharmacologically well treated.

Neuroleptics

Thioridazine (Alderton & Haddinott, 1969), haloperidol (Rogers, 1965; Cunningham et al., 1968; Werry et al., 1975) and perphenazine (Molling et al., 1962) are reported effective in reducing aggressive behavior in psychotically disturbed children. It is uncertain how much of the apparent antiaggressive effect is due to general sedation. Campbell et al. (1982), in a placebo controlled pilot study compared chlorpromazine, haloperidol, and lithium carbonate in conduct disorder children with aggression, hyperactivity, and explosive affect. They reported beneficial effects from all three medications, but excessive sedation with chlorpromazine (mean dose 150 mg/day, range 100–200 mg/day). Lithium (mean dose 1800 mg/day, range 1250–2000 mg/day; blood levels .76–1.24 mEg/L), and haloperidol (mean dose 9.2 mg/day, range 4–16 mg/day) were as effective as chlorpromazine in reducing aggression but with fewer side effects. Haloperidol has been reported to impair cognitive functioning at higher doses (.05 mg/kg/day) compared to lower doses (.025 mg/kg/day) (Werry et al., 1975). However, haloperidol also has been reported to have only minor effects on cognition at a dose that has beneficial effects on aggressive behavior (ranging from .05–.21 mg/kg/day) (Platt et al., 1981). In a later report, Platt et al. (1984) found haloperidol to have mildly negative effects on cognition, apparently not severe enough to impair classroom performance. Lithium has no adverse effect on cognition.

The same group (Campbell et al., 1984) recently reported a large, placebo controlled, double-blind study of the effects of haloperidol and lithium carbonate in the treatment of carefully diagnosed undersocialized, aggressive type conduct disorder children. These hospitalized children had been refractory to all previous treatment attempts. Both medications were significantly superior to placebo in reducing aggressive behavior. Lithium was preferred over haloperidol because it has less effect on cognition and is safer in light of the incidence of extrapyramidal reactions and dyskinesis associated with haloperidol use. These serious adverse affects are reviewed in Chapters 1 and 4, as well as in separate reviews by Campbell et al. (1983) and Gualtieri et al. (1982, 1984).

In addition to sedation, cognitive effects, extrapyramidal symptoms, and tardive dyskinesias, neuroleptics are known to worsen abnormal electroencephalograms (EEGs) (Bennett et al., 1983). The clinical significance of this is not clear.

In our experience, many children referred for inpatient treatment of severe behavior disorders have been inadequately or inappropriately medicated, often, for example, with low (or homeopathic) doses of neuroleptics. Subtle neuroleptic side effects often go unnoticed in children, who may not report subjective changes. For example, akathisia can worsen overactivity, anxiety, and irritability, sometimes leading to an increase in the medication. On the other hand, we have seen cases of neuroleptic-induced akinetic effects being mistaken for a positive clinical response. Another concern is that neuroleptics may cause enough sedation in large doses to suppress aberrant behaviors regardless of the cause, thereby making it more likely that another form of treatment or a less dangerous pharmacological approach will be overlooked. We recommend deferring the use of neuroleptics in the treatment of conduct disorders until diagnostic possibilities and other pharmacological treatments have been examined.

In summary, neuroleptics are commonly used in the treatment of aggressive children. The one well-controlled study of children with strictly diagnosed undersocialized aggressive conduct disorders shows clear clinical improvement with haloperidol when compared to placebo. However, in the same study haloperidol had no advantage over lithium and had more side effects. Neuroleptics have serious, short and long term effects and should not be used unless necessary, when other medications have failed, and, if needed, should be periodically withdrawn to assess continued need. Monitoring for dyskinesias, both directly induced and withdrawal induced, should be frequent and careful.

LITHIUM

There is increasing evidence that lithium carbonate might be useful in the treatment of children with severe aggressive behavior disorders. In general, there are two types of clinical situations where lithium might be considered. The first is in a child with a conduct disturbance who may have an underlying bipolar disorder. The second is in the treatment of unsocialized aggressive conduct disordered children per se, as reported by Campbell et al. (1984).

Lithium is used relatively little in child psychiatry. However there have been a number of reports of use in mixed behavior disorders and suspected juvenile manic-depressive disorder. Many of these reports describe lithium-responsive children as having explosive anger and marked aggressivity. The most recent reviews (Jefferson, 1982; Lena, 1979; Campbell et al., 1984) raise cautious optimism that lithium may prove useful in the treatment of serious childhood disorders with aggressivity as a major feature, particularly in the presence of affective disturbance.

In two reports (Weinberg & Brumback, 1976; Brumback & Weinberg, 1977) six children were described who appeared to have manic-depressive illness. Four had a parent with an unspecified affective illness, one had a second degree relative with affective illness, and one had an affected adoptive parent. Temper tantrums, destructive behavior, anger, irritability, and aggressivity were prominent among their symptoms, which also included hyperactivity, pressured speech, intrusiveness, and moodiness. Trials of lithium resulted in remission in two children, worsening of depressive symptoms in three (requiring discontinuation of lithium), and development of EEG abnormalities in the sixth.

DeLong (1978) reported 12 patients, all with family histories of affective illnesses, who had severe behavior disorders characterized by extreme hostility and aggressivity with explosive anger; poor attention span and distractibility; extreme, recurrent, short mood swings (in nine); and lying, stealing, and fire-setting (in ten). All the children improved on lithium in open treatment trials and four of the children improved on lithium in a blind, placebo cross over study with results measured by parent reports.

There are recent case reports of young children with more classic hypomania (Sylvester et al., 1984) and mania (Poznanski et al., 1984). Each of the cases had a family history of affective disorders. Controlled studies of seven offspring of adults with bipolar illness (Cytryn et al.,

1980; Zahn-Waxler et al., 1984) identify behavior deviance in children as young as two years of age, compared with controls.

Although, frank bipolar disorder is rare in prepubertal children, we have been impressed that these children are often referred to treatment for conduct disorders. Another striking feature of these children is the different impressions they give to parents, teachers, and clinicians at different times. As underscored by Delong (1978), the aggressivity of these children is often extreme and dramatic.

The literature is unclear on the prominence of aggression in the clinical presentation of adolescents with possible lithium-responsive conditions. However, the age of onset of at least one-fifth of manic-depressives is during adolescence (Pope & Lipinski, 1978). Adolescent mania also may appear more schizophreniform than later onset mania (Ballenger et al., 1982). In our experience, nearly all adolescents with manic-depressive illness have significant clashes with authority, at least with parents and teachers if not with the legal authorities. Adolescents with bipolar disorder may be misdiagnosed as conduct disordered. Their irritability, self-doubt, disordered thinking, grandiosity, poor concentration, variable self-abnegation, low frustration tolerance, and tendency to abuse drugs and alcohol all make it difficult if not impossible for many of them to function acceptably in school, community, or neighborhood. Long-standing mood swings can have serious deleterious effects on personality development, affecting sense of confidence, object relations, sense of internal cohesiveness and development of the ability to predict self and other's affective responses to events. The serious effects of early onset bipolar disorder on the developmental tasks of adolescence has been pointed out by Waters and Calleia (1983).

It is our clinical sense that a significant subset of conduct-disordered adolescents might benefit from a trial of lithium. The socially ostracized adolescent in legal trouble who responds to lithium is an excellent example of the need for combined pharmacotherapy and psychotherapy. After the control of mood swings these adolescents require extensive help to acquire a sense of themselves as stable members of society. They are often discouraged by the reputations they carry and tend to revert to previous behaviors because of the difficulty of the tasks required to catch up in school, to make new friends, to reorder family relationships, to regain the lost trust of parents, teachers, peers, and judges. We have many examples of adolescents who have done well on lithium only to be refused permission to return to school.

Lithium responsivity in a patient does not prove a bipolar diagnosis. Schou (1979) reviewed the use of lithium in the treatment of other disorders, including nonpsychiatric disorders, such as hyperthyroidism;

granulocytopenia (including leukemia and cancer chemotherapy induced); Felty's syndrome; headaches, particularly cluster types; cyclical vomiting; and the off-and-on phenomena in Parkinson's disease.

Of importance in the discussion of conduct disorders is the antiaggression effects of lithium. Campbell et al. (1982, 1984) and Campbell, Perry, and Green (1984) reviewed the efficacy of lithium in reducing both animal and human aggression. Campbell et al. (1972), in a comparison of lithium and chlorpromazine in the treatment of 10 severely disturbed hyperactive young children with mixed diagnoses, noted the dramatic reduction in self-mutilating behavior and explosive aggressivity in one six-year-old autistic child. They suggested that lithium might prove to be useful in the treatment of severely aggressive children with explosive affect.

Uncontrolled studies of the antiaggression effects in man were promising (Tupin et al., 1973; Sheard & Marini, 1976). Following animal studies and open studies in man, a large well-designed, double-blind, controlled study was undertaken on severely aggressive prisoners, many of whom were adolescents (Sheard et al., 1976). This study demonstrated a highly significant antiaggression effect of lithium in men not thought to have affective disorders (see Figure 9.1) although that diagnosis may be difficult to make (Cutler & Heiser, 1978; Klein et al., 1980). However, as pointed out by Tupin (1978), it seems likely that explosive violence and "hair trigger" sensitivity to stimuli may be lithium-responsive regardless of the presence or absence of affective disorder.

Campbell et al. (1982, 1984) report the outcome of the only double-blind, placebo controlled study of the effects of lithium in 61 carefully diagnosed undersocialized aggressive conduct disorder children. The results were statistically significant and clinically meaningful; both haloperidol and lithium were clearly superior to placebo in reducing aggressive behavior (see Figure 9.2).

Children in all conditions had untoward effects (haloperidol 100%, lithium 85%, placebo 50%). The number of untoward effects did not differ significantly among conditions, but the daily functioning of children receiving haloperidol was interfered with more than those receiving lithium or placebo. As mentioned above under the section on neuroleptics, lithium is equally efficacious as haloperidol in improving aggressive outbursts and appears to be generally safer, with fewer short and long term problems.

Of course, lithium is not free of serious side effects or clinical management problems. The toxicity and numerous side effects have been reviewed by Reisberg and Gershon (1979). They include: central nervous system, neuromuscular, and renal effects.

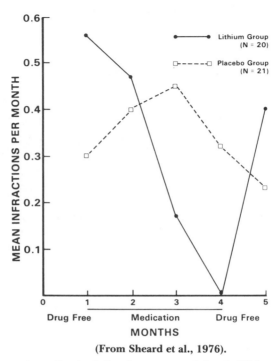

(From Sheard et al., 1976).

Fig. 9.1. Comparison of major infractions per month for the lithium and placebo groups.

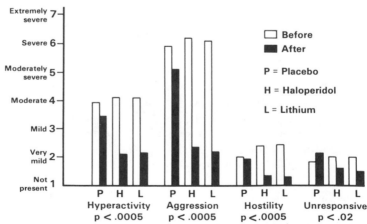

Fig. 9.2. Ratings of two child psychiatrists on the Children's Psychiatric Rating Scale, before and after treatment.

266

Central Nervous System Effects. Bennett et al. (1983) demonstrated characteristic lithium-induced EEG changes in children with conduct disorder (58% of whom had abnormalities at baseline). At therapeutic doses the changes do not seem to be related to any clinical problems. Although neurologic toxic effects (confusion, rigidity, convulsions, coma) are extremely rare at therapeutic blood levels, they have been reported at levels below 1.5 mEq/L (Reisberg & Gershon, 1979). Lithium poisoning causes severe neurotoxicity.

Neuromuscular Effects. Hand tremor is present to some degree in nearly half of patients taking lithium. This is generally a very fine tremor of the fingers, often unnoticeable except when specifically looked for. The B-adrenergic blocking agent propanalol may be useful in treating bothersome cases that cannot be managed by the reduction of the lithium dose (Reisberg & Gershon, 1979).

Renal Effects. The most frequent is lithium-induced diabetes insipidus. Complaints of transient polyurea and polydipsisa are frequent, and a smaller number of patients will go on to have frank diabetes insipidus. One of our patients, a five-and-a-half-year-old boy with severe cyclic mood swings and a strongly positive family history of manic-depressive illness was followed with weekly urine concentrating tests and antidiuretic hormone levels because of polydipsia and polyuria (unpublished observations). His lithium levels dropped, and his dose was increased to maintain a therapeutic level. His urinary function stabilized over a period of about three weeks. His severe behavior disturbance had dramatically improved on lithium, worsened on withdrawal, and he could not be adequately treated without lithium. In cases of frank diabetes insipidus the concentrating defect can be overcome by the use of hydrochlorothiazide diuretic in such a way that the lithium can be continued (Levy et al., 1973). We have done this with good results in adolescents but have not needed to attempt combined thiazide and lithium treatment in children. As a rule, in adult-sized adolescents, after establishing the diagnosis of lithium-induced diabetes insipidus, hydrochlorothiazide can be started at a dose of 25–50 mg b.i.d. and the lithium dose reduced by half to prevent lithium toxicity as the renal concentrating ability returns. The diuretic dose is adjusted to normalize urine output, and the lithium dose is readjusted by following blood levels as frequently as if it were being started for the first time. Electrolyte levels, particularly potassium, must also be closely followed. Lithium-induced diabetes insipidus is completely reversible following lithium withdrawal (Reisberg & Gershon, 1979).

The issue of chronic, morphological renal damage has been summarized by Jenner (1979). Renal biopsies of chronic lithium patients have revealed distal convuluted tubule and collecting duct lesions and chronic interstitial atrophy in a small percentage (12–15%) of patients. There was little correlation between kidney abnormalities and duration of lithium treatment. More important, none of the reported lesions are lithium specific and few other factors such as age, drug use, and other medical conditions, have been controlled. Lithium has not been related to any case of actual renal failure. Baseline and follow-up kidney function tests have been reported for four children who were chronically maintained on lithium for three to five years and showed no impairment of renal function (Khandelwal et al., 1984).

There are other less common or less bothersome effects at therapeutic levels (Reisberg & Gershon, 1979). Cardiac effects are common with T wave flattening or inversion, but with little evidence of clinical significance except in patients with preexisting cardiac pathology. Gastrointestinal effects are frequent but usually mild and tend to decrease over time. Endocrine effects include subtle weight gain and increased carbohydrate craving. Lithium is known to be related to decreased thyroid functioning, but is also reported to be associated with hyperthyroidism. Lithium can cause a characteristic maculopapular rash that is annoying, often disappears, is benign, and should not be considered as an allergic reaction. The management of lithium should be undertaken only by physicians familiar with its use. It requires detailed medical baseline studies, including electrocardiogram, electroencephalogram, liver function tests, electrolytes, renal function tests (including BUN, creatinine, creatinine clearance, 24-hour collection, and ideally antidiuretic hormone levels and concentrating tests), thyroid function tests, general physical examinations, neurological examinations, and a detailed medical history. Children are not as capable as adults of identifying and reporting medication-related problems and the prescribing physician must be sufficiently familiar with lithium and its problems to identify and manage its adverse effects. When properly managed, lithium is a generally safe medication. A responsible adult should always maintain control over medication administration and monitoring compliance.

In summary, lithium may be useful in the management of aggressive conduct disorders. Many of the children reported to have mixed behavior disorders that responded to lithium were characterized by explosive anger, hostility, and irritability, and many of them would satisfy DSM-III criteria for undersocialized, aggressive conduct disorder. Lithium has been shown to have antiaggressive effects in men even in the absence of affective disorders, and has been shown in one well-designed study to be significantly beneficial in the treatment of undersocialized, aggressive conduct-disordered children who were free of affective disorder. In experienced hands, lithium is a relatively safe and well-tolerated medication although the clinical management is complicatd. Clearly, more research must be done before lithium can claim a secure place in the treatment of childhood conduct disorders. A carefully monitored trial of lithium is warranted in many children with otherwise uncontrolled aggression and severe conduct disorders.

Anticonvulsants

There are few subjects in medicine about which there is more unresolved controversy and confusion than the relationship between epileptic disorders and aggressive behavior. Epilepsy itself is difficult to define precisely. As to the question "Are anticonvulsants useful in the treatment of aggression?" the literature supports a simple "no" answer (Lefkowitz, 1969; Looker & Conners, 1970; Conners et al., 1971). Yet there is evidence that many children diagnosed as conduct disordered and many violent "sociopathic" adults suffer from epileptic or epileptoid conditions that contribute to their violence (Mark & Ervin, 1970; Monroe, 1973; Maletzky, 1973; Maletzky & Klotter, 1974; Elliott, 1976; Lewis et al., 1979; Lewis et al., 1982; and Rickler, 1982).

That anticonvulsant medications may also have psychotropic properties further confuses the issue. Carbamazepine, in particular, appears to have specific antimanic properties as well as usefulness in treating trigeminal neuralgia, pain syndromes, diabetes insipidus, and dystonic disorders (Ballenger & Post, 1980). Therefore, positive results with carbamazepine do not mean that the condition was necessarily epileptoid in nature.

In general, the question of whether or not a trial of an anticonvulsant should be attempted for a patient with aggressive behavior arises in one of four situations. First, patients may have aggression associated with frank clinical epilepsy, usually with, but at times without, a positive EEG. The violence may be suspected to be ictal or interictal, or connected to psychological or personality factors supposedly related to epilepsy. Second, aggression may occur in patients who have abnormal EEGs but do not have clinical epilepsy. Third, episodic violence may occur without evidence of clinical epilepsy and with a normal EEG. This violence, when out of character or context, may resemble what is referred to as "episodic dyscontrol," often associated with at least vaguely abnormal EEGs (Mark & Ervin, 1970; Maletzky, 1973; Maletzky & Klotter, 1974; Elliott, 1976; Rickler, 1982). Fourth, because of reported positive results in uncontrolled studies with diphenylhydantoin in some patients with aggressivity (Bogoch & Dreyfuss, 1970), clinicians might employ it in patients with "pure" conduct disorders—that is, in patients in whom there is little basis to suspect paroxysmal phenomena.

There is some evidence that in an extremely small number of patients violence and aggression are ictal phenomena. Glasser and Dixon (1956) reported on 25 children from ages 1–16 with known psychomotor seizure disorders; seven of the children were reported as having "aggressive activity" during their seizures, usually associated with an affective component such as fear or anger. Fourteen were described as having "aggressiveness" as interictal behaviors. Most of these children's symptoms (presumably including the aggressivity) improved with treatment with a variety of anticonvulsants. Nuffield (1961) described a group of epileptic children with a temporal lobe focus in whom aggressivity was more common. In a review of ictal manifestations of complex partial seizures, Daly (1975) states that fear occurs frequently but anger is extremely rare. Lewis et al. (1979) and Lewis and Pincus (1982) demonstrated a relationship among violence, paranoia, and psychomotor epilepsy in a study of 97 incarcerated delinquent boys. Approximately one-fifth of the boys had previously undiscovered psychomotor epilepsy and the severity of delinquency was associated with psychomotor symptomatology. Sonis et al. (1981) provides a detailed case report of a nine-year-old boy referred because of chronic severe aggresivity. He was observed to have a focal seizure and the EEG revealed a temporal lobe focus. His irritability, aggressivity, and EEG improved with carbamazepine in a baseline-carbamazepine-placebo-carbamazepine single-case experimental design.

The general question of whether or not directed aggressivity can be an actual seizure phenomena was studied in 13 patients highly selected as likely to have ictal aggressivity (Delgado-Escueta et al., 1981). A panel of experienced neurologists reviewed the videotaped behaviors of 5400 epileptic patients and concluded that seven exhibited ictal aggression. The aggressive behavor was stereotyped, simple, and never a series of purposeful moments, and very unlikely to be mistaken for volitional aggressivity. Pincus (1981) points out that this study does not answer the question of whether or not a violent crime could be attributed to a seizure.

Harris (1978) and Stevens and Hermann (1981) point out the serious methodological flaws in the reports associating personality disorders with epilepsy, particularly psychomotor epilepsy. However, Lewis and Pincus et al. (1982) report that a significant number of delinquent boys might have undiagnosed psychomotor epilepsy related to their aggressivity, either as ictal or interictal phenomena.

Clearly, a patient with a known seizure disorder should be treated with appropriate anticonvulsants. If aggressivity improves, so much the better. In this type of cases there is little clinical dilemma unless clinical seizures abate but aggressivity, marked irritability, and/or impulsivity remain. Then the question is whether or not seizure control is adequate or whether an increase or change in anticonvulsant is indicated. There are no clear clinical guidelines to help with that decision.

The issue of the significance of abnormal EEGs in a group of aggressive patients who do not have clinical seizures is even more complex and unclear. The term often used to describe many of these patients is "syndrome of episodic dyscontrol" (Mark & Ervin, 1970; Bach-Y-Rita, et al., 1971; Maletzky, 1973; Maletzy & Klotter, 1974; Elliott, 1976; Rickler, 1982). Most of the reports of the results of treatment with anticonvulsants with such patients have been uncontrolled and have been with diphenylhydantoin or carbamazepine (Bach-Y-Rita et al., 1971; Maletzky, 1973; and Elliott, 1976). Maletzky (1974), in a controlled study of diphenylhydantoin using a double-blind trial, reported clearly beneficial effects from diphenylhydantoin compared with placebo. The uncontrolled studies also have shown frequent dramatic decreases in aggressive outbursts in patients who had previously failed to respond to a variety of psychotherapeutic and pharmacological treatments. There is the implication that these conditions are variants of psychomotor epilepsy or manifestations or epileptoid dysfunction of the limbic system. Based on clinical experience and superiority of carbamazepine over diphenylhydantoin in the treatment of psychomotor seizures, carbamazepine seems to be the preferred anticonvulsant in the treatment of this condition (Rickler, 1982).

Although the term "syndrome of episodic dyscontrol" is not in official use, the diagnostic criteria for "Intermittent Explosive Disorder" (APA, 1980) are very similar and include:

"A. Several discrete episodes of loss of control of aggressive impulses resulting in serious assault or destruction of property.

B. Behavior that is grossly out of proportion to any precipitating psychosocial property.

C. Absence of signs of generalized impulsivity or aggressions between episodes.

D. Not due to Schizophrenia, Antisocial Personality Disorder, or Conduct Disorder" (p. 297).

EEG abnormalities, history of central nervous system damage, clinical seizures, auras, or other psychomotor phenomena are not required.

There are no reports specifically of children with intermittent explosive disorders or syndromes of "episodic dyscontrol," although there are obvious similarities between the aggressive dyscontrol described in adults and the behavior of many conduct-disordered children. Diphenylhydantoin and carbamazepine are the only anticonvulsants reported in conduct-disordered children.

Diphenylhydantoin. Lefkowitz (1969) treated 50 institutionalized delinquent boys with marked aggressivity and disruptive behavior, failing to show significant benefit over placebo for diphenylhydantoin at doses of 200 mg/day for 26 days. Both active drug and placebo groups had significant improvement over baseline. However, the diphenylhydantoin patients actually had worse outcome measures of distress, unhappiness, negativism, and aggressiveness.

Looker and Conners (1970) conducted a double-blind placebo controlled, crossover study of 17 children with severe temper tantrums. Forty-one percent had abnormal EEGs, 47 percent had abnormal birth histories and 85 percent had pathological family environments. There were no significant differences between drug and placebo. However, the authors pointed out that a small number of children responded dramatically to diphenylhydantoin.

In a subsequent study Conners et al. (1971) reported on 43 incarcerated delinquent boys in a double-blind placebo controlled design using diphenylhydantoin and methylphenidate. No treatment effects were detectable for either drug. However, the authors speculate that the medication might have been more effective in a more disturbed group. They also noted that the study group as a whole appeared to be less behaviorally disturbed than other groups of institutionalized delinquents, and that many of the children may have been placed there more because of lack of social support than because of severity of symptoms.

Certainly the weight of available evidence does not support claims of efficacy for diphenylhydantoin in the treatment of aggressive, conduct-disordered children who do not have clinical seizure disorders. A safe but hedged conclusion is that diphenylhydantoin most likely has no place in the treatment of conduct disorders.

Carbamazepine. This medication has close structural similarities to tricyclic antidepressants as well as to stimulants and some of the major tranquilizers (Rivinus 1982). It blocks norepinephrine reuptake (Post et al., 1982) and has been reported to decrease disruptive behavior, overactivity, and abnormally elevated mood in severely mentally handicapped adults, with or without EEG abnormalities (Reid et al., 1981). Of all the anticonvulsants it has the greatest specificity for limbic system structures (Penry & Newmark, 1979; and Post et al., 1982). Dalby (1975), in a review of the behavioral effects of carbamazepine, summarized reports of mood enhancement. However, Rivinus (1982) points out that in most of the reports of positive psychotropic effects of carbamazepine, the authors failed to take into account the possible negative mood effects of oversedation from previously administered anticonvulsants. Rett (1978) reported on 900 Austrian children treated with carbamazepine and asserted that it appears to lead to mood enhancement only when it follows treatment with other medication. He speculates that the apparent psychotropic effect is due to improved clinical seizure control and fewer negative psychotropic effects than the prior medications.

Remschmidt (1978) reviewed carbamazepine use in children with behavioral disorders in reports of over 800 patients. He concluded that there was evidence of beneficial effects on "psychomotor function, drive and mood." The vast majority of the studies were uncontrolled. Out of seven double-blind studies, five showed superiority of carbamazepine over placebo, with no difference in two studies. Kuhn-Gebhart (1978) summarized the retrospective assessment of open trials in 50 child patients. His general conclusion was that carbamazepine was probably effective. However, it must be emphasized that this impression was based on uncontrolled trials and retrospective clinical impressions.

Groh (1978) conducted a double-blind crossover trial of carbamazepine in 20 nonepileptic children with "various disturbed patterns of behavior" and found the medication to be superior to placebo. In an attempt to assess which symptoms were most likely to respond to carbamazepine he reviewed the open treatment of 62 children. Those with symptoms of emotional ability, moodiness, irritability, and paranoia and who tended to react violently at minimal provocation were the most likely to respond. These patients appear to be similar to the delinquents described by Lewis et al. (1979). Nineteen of the 20 patients in the double-blind study, despite the fact that they were selected entirely on clinical criteria, had positive EEGs, making them even more similar to the patients described subsequently by Lewis et al. (1982).

Puente (1978) reported on open and controlled trials of carbamazepine in the treatment of behaviorally disturbed children who were characterized as having inattentiveness, disobedience, impulsiveness, aggressiveness, low frustration tolerance, destructiveness, hyperkinesia and emotional instability. The author concluded that the active medication led to a considerable reduction in symptoms of the behavioral disorder. Although improvement was reported it was not clear which symptoms improved or to what degree. EEGs were not done and the nature of the cerebral damage was not specified. The implication, however, was that the children did not have seizure disorders. It is not possible from the data presented to know if these children, in either the open or controlled study, would be diagnosed by DSM-III as having aggressive conduct disorders. Nevertheless, destructiveness, disobedience and aggressivity were prominent symptoms, appearing at least similar to children who might be called conduct disordered or delinquent.

Anticonvulsants have potentially serious adverse effects and significant toxicity at doses not much greater than therapeutic doses. Chronic treatment with diphenylhydantoin frequently causes gingival hyperplasia, hypertrichosis, and coarsening of facial features, and has been reported to cause persistent ataxia and mild peripheral neuropathy (Penry & Newmark, 1979). It also has well-known, less common behavioral toxicities and encephalopathic states with aggravation of preexisting behavioral disorders, delirium, confusional states, and mood alteration. Schizophreniform reactions, including delusions, paranoia, and hallucinations have been reported (Rivinus, 1982). Carbamazepine's adverse effects include vertigo, drowsiness, diplopia, water intoxication, and rare blood dyscrasias (Penry & Newmark, 1979). Two cases have been reported of possible carbamazepine-induced mania in two children with strong family histories of bipolar affective disease (Reiss & O'Donnell, 1984). Blood levels must be monitored, with most laboratories reporting therapeutic levels at 10–20 µg/ml for diphenylhydantoin and 8–12 µg/ml for carbamazepine.

Summary and Clinical Recommendations. It is easy to make recommendations for the treatment of children with conduct disorders who have known seizure disorders: Treat with an appropriate anticonvulsant, then take the most reasonable psychotherapeutic and psychosocial steps indicated for patient and family education and support, treatment of residual behavioral symptoms, and adjustment problems. However, there is as yet no clear basis for treating even severely aggressive conduct disorders with anticonvulsants in the absence of clinical seizure disorder, with or without abnormal EEGs.

As Lewis et al. (1982) point out, there may be a significant number of undiagnosed temporal lobe epileptics among populations of severe delinquents. Hermann et al. (1980) and Pritchard et al. (1980) report that psychological dysfunction is more likely to develop with early onset of temporal lobe epilepsy. It is important to specifically question for the presence of psychomotor phenomena, such as sudden, unexplained sensations of fear, anger, hunger, euphoria or sexual drive; sensation of *deja* or *jamais vu;* macro or microscopia; olfactory, visual, or gustatory hallucination; out-of-body experiences; other dissociative phenomena such as sensations of unreality and time distortions; sudden mystical or religious experiences; unusual somatic sensations; and periods of confusion or poor memory. The presence of these symptoms, particularly when the electroencephalogram is positive, raises the odds that the patient suffers from psychomotor seizures and warrants a trial of an anticonvulsant.

Fifty-six percent of our last 126 admissions of children ages 6–13 had the admission diagnosis of conduct disorder. Of these, only 17% had abnormal EEGs. Nine children with abnormal EEGs did well on anticonvulsants, predominantly carbamazepine, and four with normal EEGs did not improve significantly (Reiss & O'Donnell, unpublished data).

For a treatment resistant, severely aggressive conduct disorder, particularly with even a nonspecifically abnormal EEG, a carefully monitored treatment trial can be conducted in only a few weeks, with very little risk to the patient. If the trial appears to be effective, the clinician, patient, and family can then weigh the advantages and disadvantages of continuing medication treatment.

There is an obvious need for large, well-designed studies of clearly diagnosed patients. In light of the effects of lithium reported by Campbell et al. (1984), the large number of such children with EEG abnormalities (Bennett et al., 1983) and the effectiveness of carbamazepine in the treatment of manic-depressive disorder (Ballenger & Post, 1980), it would be interesting to compare the efficacy of placebo, lithium, and carbamazepine. There are as yet no such studies.

Other Medications

Stimulants and tricyclic antidepressants may have a place in the treatment of children diagnosed, at least initially, as conduct disordered. The uses of these medications in attention deficit disorders and depression are reviewed in detail in Chapters 5 and 6, respectively. Only their relationship to conduct disorders and aggressivity will be reviewed here.

Stimulants. It is a common clinical experience that children with Attention Deficit Disorder (ADD) and hyperactivity often have associated conduct disorders that can range from oppositionalism to severe aggressivity and antisocial behavior. It may be that some type of physiological overreactivity makes it difficult to respond to the ordinary rewards in life as well as the ones built into treatment. Clinically we have observed that attention deficit disordered children seem to require much more frequent reward schedules in behavior programs.

There are some data tending to support an association between ADD and aggressive conduct disorder. Children with ADD are reported to have approximately a 20% rate of delinquency when followed into adolescence (Weiss et al., 1971; Mendelson et al., 1971). The persistence of impulsivity and short attention span has been noted into adulthood and adult patients are reported to have employment instability, interpersonal relationship difficulties, and greater than expected legal difficulties (Wood et al., 1976). In a report describing the outcome of a multimodal treatment approach in the 100 hyperactive boys Satterfield et al. (1981) noted an association between hyperactivity and conduct disorders. Better outcome, including less antisocial behavior, was associated with greater length of treatment. However, they had no control group and differences in length of treatment were primarily due to the high dropout rate of approximately 50%; thus it is possible that those who stayed in treatment and had a better outcome were a better prognosis group. The authors noted that medication treatment alone did not appear to be an improvement over no treatment at all. In a prospective study comparing delinquency rates in 110 adolescent boys with ADD with 88 normal adolescent boys, Satterfield et al. (1982) reported a much higher rate of serious offenses and institutionalization for delinquency in the group with ADD. In addition to their findings of strong relationship between childhood ADD and delinquency, they noted that length of pharmacotherapy was not related to outcome. However, in a four-year follow-up study of hyperactive boys with and without conduct disorders August et al. (1983) reported that only those children who had hyperactivity and conduct disorders as young children had conduct disorders at follow-up and that children with only hyperactivity continued to be free of conduct disorder later in life.

There are few studies assessing the use of stimulants in conduct disorders or similar conditions. Werry et al. (1975) compared haloperidol and methylphenidate in hyperactive children and/or conduct-disordered children and tended to show that either drug was superior to placebo. However, the data did not show if conduct disorder-aggressive behavior improves only if it was associated with hyperactivity or if it improved independently. The study by Conners et al. (1971), comparing methylphenidate and diphenylhydantoin in the treatment of young delinquent boys, was summarized above and showed no effect for either medication. However, the active treatment time was very short. Maletsky (1973) reported that dextroamphetamine improved antisocial behavior in 28 outpatient hyperactive boys treated for three months.

At least it can be said that there is no evidence that stimulants are useful in the treatment of conduct-disordered children uncomplicated by ADD. The question of whether or not ADD predisposes to conduct disorders is also not clearly answered. There does seem to be a frequent association between the two conditions. Considering the high rate of hyperactivity in school-age children (Trites et al., 1979) this condition itself is a significant pediatric public health problem and would be expected to effect a large number of conduct-disordered children by chance alone.

Antidepressants. Cytryn and McKnew (1972) noted that many children with "masked depression" present with aggressive behavior and delinquency. Puig-Antich (1978), in a pilot study of 13 children with prepubertal major depressive disorder, reported that all five boys over 10 years of age also had conduct disorders with symptoms that included fire-setting, frequent lying, stealing, and chronic rule violation. In four of the five with conduct disorder the antisocial behavior followed the onset of depression.

Carlson and Cantwell (1980) evaluated 102 outpatient children; of 28 children diagnosed as having an affective disorder, eight also met criteria for ADD or conduct disorder. They concluded that more traditional methods of assessment overlooked the diagnosis of depression in 60% of children who satisfied criteria for affective disorder and that the majority of missed depressions had been initially diagnosed as unsocialized aggressive reactions or adjustment reactions. Sixty-eight percent of a population of serious juvenile offenders was found to have been suicidal in the previous year (Alessi et al., 1984). Most of those suicidal patients were diagnosed as having either major affective disorders or borderline personality disorders. Chiles et al. (1980) identified major affective disorders in 23% of an adolescent delinquent population, ages 13–15, in a correctional facility. The depressed delinquents' antisocial behavior did not differ in severity or type from the behavior of the nondepressed delinquents. However, the depressed group had more drug and alcohol use as well as a higher incidence of depression and alcoholism in their families.

Puig-Antich (1982) reported a 33 percent association between conduct disorders and prepubertal major depressive disorders. Since the study was designed to study depression, not conduct disorders or their association, the data were presented as a pilot report of the incidental findings. The conduct disorder behaviors followed the onset of depressive symptoms in 87 percent of cases and the depressive symptoms had been present for a long time, usually from one to two years. All 13 boys with both depression and conduct disorder who were treated with imipramine had a full antidepressant response and 11 became free of conduct disorder behaviors. Relapses of antisocial behavior occurred only when depressive symptoms recurred and usually abated after the depression was again treated. The author warns that the data are preliminary and that well-designed, placebo controlled, prospective studies of children with both conduct and depressive disorders are needed. There are no studies of tricyclic antidepressants in the treatment of children who have only a conduct disorder diagnosis.

Again, these medications are very toxic and no child should have access to them. A reliable adult must be responsible for their safekeeping and administration.

In summary, it appears that a substantial number of antisocial and delinquent children also have affective disorders. It may be that the depressive illness itself can predispose to conduct disorder and antisocial patterns of behavior. It is also possible, that the development of conduct disorders and perhaps of a significant subgroup of antisocial adults could be prevented with early identification and treatment of depression in children. The incidence of depression, both major and minor, in school-age children is surprisingly high at 4.3% (Kashani et al., 1983) and a large, lengthy, and ethically sensitive study would be required to assess the effects of early treatment of depression on the development of conduct disorders. Also, Conners et al. (1979) report that the children of unipolar depressed parents may have a higher rate of conduct disorder behavior than the children of bipolar depressed parents. It seems to be reasonable at this time to urge that all conduct-disordered children be very carefully evaluated for depression.

Propranolol. Propranolol, a B-adrenergic blocker, has been reported to effectively control sudden rage outbursts and violent behavior in adult patients with acute brain damage from multiple causes (Elliott, 1977; Yudofsky et al., 1981) and in one 12-year-old boy with postencephalitic psychosis (Schreier, 1979). Williams et al. (1982) reported that propranolol appeared to be effective in controlling rage outbursts in children and adolescents with more subtle and chronic brain damage. Of their 30 patients, 25 met criteria for DSM-III conduct disorder, undersocialized, aggressive type. They had all been unresponsive to previous pharmacological and psychotherapeutic treatments. Their "organic" brain dysfunction included: nine patients with "minimal brain dysfunction," (determined by the presence of soft neurological signs); eleven had uncontrolled seizures disorders; and three had a history of seizures. Approximately 70 percent of available EEGs were abnormal. The duration of neurologic dysfunction ranged from six months to 33 years, with a median of 12 years. Of the 30 patients, 11 were children and 15 were adolescents. Seventy-five percent of the patients were reported to have had at least some improvement in their rage outbursts. However, the study has substantial flaws that make its significance difficult to assess. We are not aware of any controlled studies of this medication in aggressive or conduct-disordered children, with or without brain damage.

CONCLUSION

No clear guidelines can be given for the pharmacological treatment of conduct disorders. The literature as a whole is confusing because of the variety of diagnostic schemes, vagueness of terminology, heterogeneity of study groups, varying doses of medication, and study design flaws that make interpretation difficult.

The term "conduct disorder" should not be thought of as a guide to any particular type of treatment. We recommend that each child diagnosed as having a conduct disorder be very thoroughly evaluated for other, more treatable, conditions. Severely aggressive children and adolescents, particularly those severe enough to warrant hospitalization or incarceration, have a much higher likelihood of also suffering from psychosis, affective disorders, epileptic disorders, or ADD. There is evidence that their proper treatment may lead to amelioration of the conduct disorder symptoms. It is particularly important that clinicians not fall into the trap of accepting an apparently adequate explanation for a patient's behavior and fail to investigate alternate or additional explananations. This is equally true for clinicians who are prone to overlook psychological factors as well as for those who are inclined to overlook organic factors. In our experience much time is spent in discussion, among consultants and in diagnostic and treatment conferences, about whether a patient's entire disorder is functional or organic because some incidents of the behavior appear to be purely functional or predominantly organic. Chronic, physiologically based disorders of impulse control, cognitive processing, affect regulation and drive regulation can shape a patient's personality over time such that the aberrant behavior appears to be purely an effect rather than at least partially a cause.

Any attempted therapy of conduct-disordered children must be accompanied by some method of monitoring results. This is true for psychological as well as pharmacological treatments. The state of the art of treatment of conduct disorders with any treatment method warrants neither unchecked confidence or therapeutic nihilism.

The complicated, difficult, and very serious nature of these conditions should be explained as clearly as possible to everyone involved in a given case: parents, patients, judges, attorneys, probation officers, and school authorities. All involved should know that any component of the recommended treatment, whether psychological or pharmacological, will be undertaken only as a part of a general, comprehensive treatment plan and should not be considered adequate treatment alone. For example, a judge should be discouraged from thinking that a parent is adequately complying with treatment if a medication is properly administered, but psychotherapy appointments are missed or adequate school attendance is not enforced.

In summary, it is likely that many children and adolescents diagnosed as having conduct disorders also suffer from undiagnosed neurological or psychiatric disorders that contribute to the development or continuation of the conduct disorder. Medications specific for those conditions such as neuroleptics, lithium carbonate, anticonvulsants, stimulants and tricyclic antidepressants should be used when there is sufficient evidence of the presence of a responsive condition regardless of the apparent sufficiency of the sociological or psychological explanations for the conduct disorder behavior. Also, there is new evidence that lithium carbonate may be an effective and relatively safe treatment for undersocialized, aggressive conduct disorders per se. Pending further, more definitive studies, clinicians must continue to accept and struggle with the many unanswered questions regarding pharmacotherapies and conduct disorders.

REFERENCES

Achenbach, T. M. (1978). The child behavior profile: I. Boys aged 6 through 11. *Journal of Consulting and Clinical Psychology, 46,* 478–488.

Achenbach, T. M. (1980). DSM-III in light of empirical research on the classification of child psychopathology. *Journal of the American Academy of Child Psychiatry, 19,* 395–412.

Achenbach, T. M., & Edelbrock, C. S. (1978). The classification of child psychopathology: A review and analysis of empirical efforts. *Psychological Bulletin, 85,* 1275–1302.

Alderton, H., & Hoddinott, B. (1969). A controlled study of the use of thioridazine in the treatment of hyperactive and aggressive children in a children's psychiatric hospital. *Canadian Psychiatric Association Journal, 9,* 239–247.

Alessi, N. E., McManus, M., Brickman, A., & Grapentine, L. (1984). Suicidal behavior among serious juvenile offenders. *American Journal of Psychiatry, 141,* 286–287.

American Psychiatric Association. (1980). Diagnostic and statistical manual of mental disorders (DSM-III) (3rd ed.). Washington, DC: American Psychiatric Association.

Annesley, P. T. (1961). Psychiatric illness in adolescence: Presentation and prognosis. *Journal of Mental Science, 107,* 268–278.

August, G. J., Stewart, M. A., & Holmes, C. S. (1983). A four-year follow-up of hyperactive boys with and without conduct disorder. *British Journal of Psychiatry, 143,* 192–198.

Bach-Y-Rita, G., Lion, J. R., Climent, C. E., & Ervin, F. R. (1971). Episodic dyscontrol: A study of 130 violent patients. *American Journal of Psychiatry, 127,* 1473–1478.

Ballenger, J. C., & Post, R. M. (1980). Carbamazepine in manic-depressive illness: A new treatment. *American Journal of Psychiatry, 137,* 782–790.

Bennett, W. G., Korein, J., Kalmijn, M., Greaa, D. M., & Campbell, M. (1983). EEG and treatment of hospitalized aggressive children with haloperidol or lithium. *Biological Psychiatry, 18,* 1427–1440.

Bogoch, S., & Dreyfus, J. (1970). *The broad range of use of diphenylhydantoin* (Vol. 1). Dreyfus Medical Foundation, New York.

Bohman, M., Cloninger, C. R., Sigvardsson, S., & von Khorring, A. (1982). Predisposition to petty criminality in Swedish adoptees. I. Genetic and environmental heterogeneity. *Archives of General Psychiatry, 39,* 1233–1241.

Brumback, R. A., & Weinberg, W. A. (1977). Mania in childhood: II Therapeutic trial of lithium carbonate and further description of manic-depressive illness in children. *American Journal of Diseases of Children, 131,* 1122–1126.

Campbell, M., Cohen, I. L., & Small, A. M. (1982). Drugs in aggressive behavior. *Journal of the American Academy of Child Psychiatry, 21,* 107–117.

Campbell, M., Fish, B., Korein, J., Shapiro, T., Collins, P., & Koh, C. (1972). Lithium and chlorpromazine: A controlled crossover study of hyperactive severely disturbed young children. *Journal of Autism and Childhood Schizophrenia, 2,* 234–263.

Campbell, M., Grega, D. M., Green, W. H., & Bennett, W. G. (1983). Neuroleptic-induced dyskinesias in children. *Clinical Neuropharmacology, 6,* 207–222.

Campbell, M., Perry R., & Green, W. H. (1984). The use of lithium in children and adolescents. *Psychosomatics, 25,* 95–106.

Campbell, M., Small, A. M., Green, W. H., Jennings, S. J., Perry, R., Bennett, W. G., Padron-Gayol, M., & Anderson, L. (1982). Lithium and haloperidol in hospitalized aggressive children. *Psychopharmacology Bulletin, 18,* 126–130.

Campbell, M., Small, A. M., Green, W. H., et al. (1984). A comparison of haloperidol and lithium in hospitalized aggressive conduct disordered children. *Archives of General Psychiatry, 41,* 650–656.

Carlson, G. A., & Cantwell, D. P. (1980). Unmasking masked depression in children and adolescents. *American Journal of Psychiatry, 137,* 455–449.

Chiles, J. A., Miller, M. L., & Cox, G. B. (1980). Depression in an adolescent delinquent population. *Archives of General Psychiatry, 37,* 1179–1184.

Christiansen, K. O. (1974). Seriousness of criminality and concordance among Danish twins. In R. Hood (Ed.), *Crime, criminology and public policy.* London: Heidemann.

Clarkin, J. F., Friedman, R. C., Hurt, S. W., Conn, R., & Aronoff, M. (1984). Affective and character pathology of suicidal adolescent and young adult inpatients. *Journal of Clinical Psychiatry, 45,* 19–22.

Cloninger, C. R., Sigvardsson, S., Bohman, M., & von Khorring, A. (1982). Predisposition to petty criminality in Swedish adoptees II. Cross-fostering analysis of gene-environment interactions. *Archives of General Psychiatry, 39,* 1242–1247.

Conners, C. K., Himmelhoch, J., Goyette, C. H., Ulrich, R., & Neil, J. F. (1979). Children of parents with affective illness. *Journal of the American Academy of Child Psychiatry, 18,* 600–607.

Conners, C. K., Kramer, R., Rothschild, G. H., Schwartz, L., & Stone, A. (1971). Treatment of young delinquent boys with diphenylhydantoin sodium and methylphenidate. *Archives of General Psychiatry, 24,* 156–160.

Cunningham, M. A., Pillai, V., & Blachford-Rogers, W. J. (1968). Haloperidol in the treatment of children with severe behavior disorders. *British Journal of Psychiatry, 114,* 845–854.

Cutler, N., & Heiser, J. F. (1978). Retrospective diagnosis of hypomania following successful treatment of episodic violence with lithium: A case report. *American Journal of Psychiatry, 134,* 753–754.

Cytryn, L., McKnew, D. H., & Bunney, W. E. (1980). Diagnosis of depression in children: A reassessment. *American Journal of Psychiatry, 137,* 22–25.

Cytryn, L., & McKnew, D. H. (1972). Proposed classification of childhood depression. *American Journal of Psychiatry, 129,* 149–155.

Dalby, M. A. (1975). Behavioral effects of carbamazepine. In J. K. Penry & D. D. Daly (Eds.), *Advances in neurology* (Vol. II). Raven Press: New York.

Daly, D. D. (1975). Ictal clinical manifestations of complex partial seizures. In J. K. Penry & D. D. Daly (Eds.), *Advances in neurology* (Vol II). Raven Press: New York.

Delgado-Escueta A. V., Mattson, R. H., King, L., Goldenjohn, E. S., Spiegel, H., Madsen, J., Crandall, P., Dreyfuss, F., & Porter, R. J. (1981). The nature of aggression during epileptic seizures. *The New England Journal of Medicine, 305,* 711–716.

DeLong, G. R. (1978). Lithium carbonate treatment of select behavior disorders in children suggesting manic-depressive illness. *The Journal of Pediatrics, 93,* 689–694.

Elliott, F. A. (1976). The neurology of explosive rage: The dyscontrol syndrome. *The Practitioner, 217,* 51–60.

Elliott, F. A. (1977). Propranolol for the control of the belligerent behavior following acute brain damage. *Annals of Neurology, 1,* 489–491.

Forehand, R., King, H. E., Peed, S., & Yoder, P. (1975). Mother-child interactions: Comparisons of a noncompliant clinic group. *Behavior Research and Therapy, 13,* 79–84.

Forehand, R., & McMahon, R. J. (1981). *Helping the noncomplaint child: A clinician's guide to parent training.* New York: Guilford.

Glasser, G. H., & Dixon, M. S. (1956). Psychomotor seizures in childhood: A clinical study. *Pediatric Neurology,* 646–655.

Griest, D. L., & Wells, K. C. (1983). Behavioral family therapy with conduct disorders in children. *Behavior Therapy, 14,* 37–73.

Groh, C. (1978). The psychotropic effect of Tegretol in non-epileptic children, with particular reference to the drug's indications. In W. Birxmayer (Ed.), *Epileptic seizures—Behavior—Pain.* Berne, Switzerland: Hans & Huber.

Gualtieri, C. T., Breuning, S. E., Shroeder, S. R., & Quade, D. (1982). Tardive dyskinesia in mentally retarded children, adolescents and young adults. North Carolina and Michigan Studies. *Psychopharmacology Bulletin, 18*(1), 62–65.

Gualtieri, C. T., Quade, D., Hicks, R. E., Mayo, J. P., & Shroeder, S. R. (1984). Tardive dyskinesia and other clinical consequences of neuroleptic treatment in children and adolescents. *American Journal of Psychiatry, 141,* 20–23.

Harris, R. (1978). Relationship between EEG abnormality and aggressive and anti-social behavior—a critical appraisal. In L. A. Herson & D. Shaffer (Eds.), *Aggression and antisocial behavior in children and adolescence*. Pergamon Press.

Hermann, B. P., Schwartz, M. S., Karnes, W. E., & Vahdat, P. (1980). Psychopathology in epilepsy: Relationship of seizure type to age at onset. *Epilepsia, 21,* 15–23.

Hook, E. B. (1973). Behavioral implication of the human XYY genotype. *Science, 179,* 139–150.

Hutchings, B., & Mednick, S. A. (1974). Registered criminality in the adoptive and biological parents of registered male criminal adoptees. In S. A. Mednick, F. Schulsinger, J. Higgins, & B. Bell (Eds.), *Genetics, environment and psychopathology*. Amsterdam: North Holland/Elsevier.

Jefferson, J. W. (1982). The use of lithium in childhood and adolescence: An overview. *Journal of Clinical Psychiatry, 43,* 174–177.

Jenner, F. A. (1979). Lithium and the question of kidney damage. *Archives of General Psychiatry, 36,* 888–890.

Kashani, J. H., McGee, R. O., Clarkson, S. E., Anderson, J. C., Walton, L. A., Williams, S., Silva, P. A., Robins, A. J., Cytryn, L., & McKnew, D. H. (1983). Depression in a sample of 9-year old children. *Archives of General Psychiatry, 40,* 1217–1223.

Khandelwal, M. D., Varma, V. K., & Murthy, R. S. (1984). Renal function in children receiving long-term lithium prophylaxis. *American Journal of Psychiatry, 141,* 278–279.

Klein, D. F., Gittleman, R., Quitkin, F., & Rifkin. (1980). *Diagnosis and drug treatment of psychiatric disorders: Adults and children* (2nd ed.). Baltimore: William and Wilkins.

Kovacs, M. (1981). Rating scales to assess depression in school aged children. *Acta Paedopsychiatria, 46,* 305–315.

Kuhn-Gebhart, V. (1978). Behavioral disorders in non-epileptic children and their treatment with carbamazepine. In W. Birxmayer (Ed.), *Epileptic seizures—Behavior—Pain*. Berne, Switzerland: Hans and Huber.

Lefkowitz, M. M. (1969). Effects of diphenylhydantoin on disruptive behavior: Study of male delinquents. *Archives of General Psychiatry, 20,* 643–651.

Lena, B. (1979). Lithium in child and adolescent psychiatry. *Archives of General Psychiatry, 36,* 854–855.

Levy, S. T., Forrest, J. M., & Heninger, E. R. (1973). Lithium-induced diabetes insipidus: Manic symptoms, brain and electrolyte correlates and chlorthiazide treatment. *American Journal of Psychiatry, 130,* 1014–1018.

Lewis, D. O. Pincus, J. G., Shanok, S. S., & Glaser, G. H. (1982). Psychomotor epilepsy and violence in a group of incarcerated adolescent boys. *American Journal of Psychiatry, 139,* 882–887.

Lewis, D. O., Shanok, S. S., Pincus, J. H., & Glaser, G. H. (1979). Violent juvenile delinquents: Psychiatric, neurological, psychological and abuse factors. *Journal of the American Academy of Child Psychiatry, 18,* 307–319.

Loeber, R., & Dishion, T. (1983). Early predictors of male delinquency: A review. *Psychological Bulletin, 94*(1) 68–99.

Loeber, R., & Patterson, G. R. (1981). The aggressive child: A concomitant of a coercive system. *Advances in Family Intervention, Assessment and Theory, 2,* 47–87.

Looker, A., & Conners, C. K. (1970). Diphenylhydantoin in children with severe temper tantrums. *Archives of General Psychiatry, 23,* 80–89.

Maletzky, B. M. (1973). The episodic dyscontrol syndrome. *Diseases of the Nervous System, 34,* 178–185.

Maletzky, B. M. (1974). D-amphetamine and delinquency: Hyperkinesis persisting? *Diseases of the Nervous System, 35,* 543–547.

Maletzky, B. M., & Klotter, J. (1974). Episodic dyscontrol: A controlled replication. *Diseases of the Nervous System, 37,* 175–179.

Mark, V. H. & Ervin, F. R. (1970). *Violence and the brain.* New York: Harper & Row.

Mendelson, W., Johnson, N., & Stewart, A. (1971). Hyperactive children as teenagers: A follow-up study. *Journal of Nervous and Mental Diseases, 153,* 273–279.

Molling, P. A., Lockner, A. W., Sauls, R. J., & Eisenberg, L. (1962). Committed delinquent boys. *Archives of General Psychiatry, 7,* 70–76.

Monroe, R. K. (1973). Anticonvulsants in the treatment of aggression. *The Journal of Nervous and Mental Disease, 160,* 119–126.

Morris, H. H., Escoll, P. j., & Wexler, R. (1956). Aggressive behavior disorders of childhood: A follow-up study. *American Journal of Psychiatry, 112,* 991–997.

Nuffield, E. J. A. (1961). Neurophysiology and behavior disorders in epileptic children. *Journal of Mental Science, 107,* 438–458.

Olweus, D. (1980). Familial and temperamental determinants of aggressive behavior in adolescent boys: A causal analysis. *Developmental Psychology, 16,* 644–660.

O'Neal, P., & Robins, L. N.(1958). The relation of childhood behavior problems to adult psychiatric status: A 30-year follow-up study of 156 subjects. *American Journal of Psychiatry, 114,* 961–969.

Owen, D. R. (1972). The 47 XYY male: A review. *Psychological Bulletin, 78,* 209–233.

Patterson, G. R. (1976). The aggressive child: Victim and architect of a coercive system. In E. J. Mash, L. A. Hammerlynck, & L. C. Handy (Eds.), *Behavior modification and families.* New York: Brunner/Mazel.

Patterson, G. R. (1982). *Coercive family process.* Eugene, Oregon: Castalia Press.

Patterson, G. R., Reid, J. B., Jones, R. R., & Conger, R. E. (1975). *A social learning approach to family intervention: Families with aggressive children.* Eugene, Oregon: Castalia Press.

Penry, J. K., & Newmark, M. E. (1979). The use of antiepileptic drugs. *Annals of Internal Medicine, 90,* 207–218.

Pincus, J. H. (1980). Can violence be a manifestation of epilepsy? *Neurology, 30,* 304–307.

Pincus, J. H. (1981). Violence and epilepsy. *The New England Journal of Medicine, 305,* 696–698.

Platt, J. E., Campbell, M., Green, W. H., & Gregs, D. M. (1984). Cognitive effects of lithium carbonate and haloperidol in treatment resistant aggressive children. *Archives of General Psychiatry, 41,* 657–662.

Platt, J. E., Campbell, M., Green, W. H., Perry, R., & Cohen, I. L. (1981). Effects of lithium carbonate and haloperidol on cognition in aggressive hospitalized school-age children. *Journal of Clinical Psychopharmacology, 1,* 8–13.

Pope, H. G., & Lipinski, J. F. (1978). Diagnosis in schizophrenia and manic-depressive illness: A reassessment of the specificity of schizophrenic symptoms in the light of current research. *Archives of General Psychiatry, 35,* 811–828.

Post, R. M., Uhde, T. W., Putnam, F. W., Ballenger, J. C., & Berrettini, W. H. (1982). Kindling and carbamazepine in affective illness. *The Journal of Nervous and Mental Disease, 170,* 717–732.

Poznanski, E. O., Israel, M. C., & Grossman, J. (1984). Hypomania in a four-year-old. *Journal of the American Academy of Child Psychiatry, 23,* 105–110.

Pritchard M., & Graham, P. (1966). An investigation of a group of patients who have attended both the child and adult departments of the same psychiatric hospital. *British Journal of Psychiatry, 112,* 603–612.

Pritchard, P. B., Lombroso, C. T., & McIntyre, M. (1980). Psychological complications of temporal lobe epilepsy. *Neurology, 30,* 227–232.

Puente, R. M. (1978). The use of carbamazepine in the treatment of behavioral disorders in children. In W. Birxmayer (Ed.), *Epileptic seizures—Behavior—Pain.* Berne, Switzerland: Hans & Huber.

Puig-Antich J., Blau, S., Marx, N., Greenhill, L. L., & Chambers, W. (1978). Prepubertal major depressive disorder: A pilot study. *Journal of the American Academy of Child Psychiatry, 17,* 695–708.

Puig-Antich, J. (1982). Major depression and conduct disorder in prepuberty. *Journal of the American Academy of Child Psychiatry, 21,* 118–128.

Quay, H. C. (1979). Classification. In H. C. Quay & J. Werry (Eds.), *Psychopathological disorders of childhood* (2nd ed.). New York: Wiley.

Reid, A. H., Naylor, G. J., and Kay, D. G. (1981). A double-blind placebo controlled crossover trial of carbamazepine in overactive, severely mentally handicapped patients. *Psychological Medicine, 11,* 109–113.

Reid, J. D., & Patterson, G. R. (1976). The modification of aggression and stealing behvior of boys in the home setting. In A. Bandura & E. Ribes-Inesta (Eds.), *Behavior modification: Experimental analyses of aggression and delinquency.* Hillsdale, NJ: Erlbaum.

Reisberg, B., & Gershon, S. (1979). Side effects associated with lithium therapy. *Archives of General Psychiatry, 36,* 879–887.

Reiss, A. L. & O'Donnell, D. J. (1984). Carbamazepine-induced mania in two children. *Journal of Clinical Psychiatry, 45,* 272–274.

Reiss, A. L., & O'Donnell, D. J. (Unpublished data, 1984). Survey of conduct disordered children on an in-patient children's psychiatric unit.

Remschmidt, H. (1978). The psychotropic effect of carbamazepine in non-epileptic patients, with particular reference to problems posed by clinical studies in children with behavioral disorders. In W. Birxmayer (Ed.), *Epileptic seizures—behavior—pain.* Berne, Switzerland: Hans & Huber.

Rett, A. (1978). The so-called psychotropic effect of Tegretol in the treatment of convulsions of cerebral origin in children. In W. Birxmayer (Ed.), *Epileptic Seizures—Behavior—Pain.* Berne, Switzerland: Hans & Huber.

Rickler, K. C. (1982). Episodic dyscontrol. In D. F. Benson and D. Blumer (Eds.) *Psychiatric Aspects of Neurological Disease.* New York: Grune & Stratton.

Riddle, K. D., & Rappaport, J. L. (1976). A two-year follow-up of 72 hyperkinetic boys. *Journal of Nervous and Mental Diseases, 162,* 126–134.

Rivinus, T. M. (1982). Psychiatric effects of the anti-convulsant regimens. *Journal of Clinical Psychopharmacology, 2,* 165–192.

Rogers, W. J. B. (1965). Use of haloperidol in children's psychiatric disorders. *Journal of Clinical Trials, 2,* 162–165.

Rutter, M. (1982). Psychological therapies in child psychiatry: Issues and prospects. *Psychological Medicine, 12,* 723–740.

Rutter, M., Birch, H. G., Thomas, A., & Chess, S. (1964). Temperamental characteristics in infancy and the later development of behavioral disorders. *British Journal of Psychiatry, 110,* 651–660.

Rutter, M., Tizard, J., Yule, W., Graham, P., & Whitmore, K. (1976). Research Report: Isle of Wight Studies, 1964–1974. *Psychological Medicine, 6,* 313–332.

Satterfield, J. H., Hoppe, C. M., & Schell, A. M. (1982). A prospective study of delinquency in 110 adolescent boys with attention deficit disorder and 88 normal adolescent boys. *American Journal of Psychiatry, 139,* 795–798.

Schiavi, R. C., Theilgraard, A., Owen, D. R., & White, D. (1984). Sex chromosome anomalies, hormones and aggressivity. *Archives of General Psychiatry, 41,* 93–99.

Schou, M. (1979). Lithium in the treatment of other psychiatric and non-psychiatric disorders. *Archives of General Psychiatry, 36,* 856–859.

Schreier, H. (1979). Use of propranolol in the treatment of postencephalitic psychosis. *American Journal of Psychiatry, 136,* 840–841.

Sheard, M. H., & Marini, J. L. (1976). Treatment of human aggressive behavior: Four case studies of the effect of lithium. *Comprehensive Psychiatry, 19,* 37–45.

Sheard, M. H., Marini, J. L., & Bridges, C. I. (1976). The effect of lithium on impulsive aggressive behavior in man. *American Journal of Psychiatry, 133,* 1409–1413.

Sigvardsson A., Cloninger, C. R., Bohman, M., & Von Knorring, A. (1982). Predisposition to petty criminality in Swedish adoptees: III. Sex differences and validation of the male typology. *Archives of General Psychiatry, 39,* 1248–1253.

Sonis, W. A., Petti, T. A., & Richey, E. T. (1981). Epilepsy and psychopathology in childhood. *Journal of the American Academy of Child Psychiatry, 20,* 398–408.

Stevens, J. R. & Hermann, B. P. (1981). Temporal lobe epilepsy, psychopathology and violence: The state of the evidence. *Neurology, 31,* 1127–1132.

Strober, M., & Carlson, G. (1982). Bipolar illness in adolescents with major depression. *Archives of General Psychiatry, 39,* 549–555.

Sylvester, C. E., Burke, P. M., McCauley, E. A., & Clark, C. J. (1984). Manic psychosis in childhood: Report of two cases. *The Journal of Nervous and Mental Disease, 172,* 12–15.

Thomas, A., & Chess, S. (1984). Genesis and evolution of behavioral disorders: From infancy to early adult life. *American Journal of Psychiatry, 141,* 1–9.

Thomas, A., Chess, S., & Birch, G. H. (1968). *Temperament and behavior disorders in children.* New York: New York University Press.

Trites, R. L., Dugas, E., Lynch, G., & Ferguson, H. B. (1979). Prevalence of hyperactivity. *Journal of Pediatric Psychology, 4,* 179–188.

Tupin, J. P. (1978). Usefulness of lithium for aggressiveness (letter). *American Journal of Psychiatry, 135,* 9, 1118.

Tupin, J. P., Smith, D. B., & Clanon, I. L. (1973). The long-term use of lithium in aggressive prisoners. *Comprehensive Psychiatry, 14,* 311–317.

Waters, B., & Calleia, S. (1983). The effect of juvenile-onset manic-depressive disorder on the developmental tasks of adolescence. *American Journal of Psychotherapy, 38,* 182–189.

Weinberg, W. A., & Brumback, R. A. (1976). Mania in childhood. Case studies and literature review. *American Journal of Diseases of Children, 130,* 380–385.

Weiss, G., Minde, K., & Werry, J. W. (1971). Studies on the hyperactive child. *Archives of General Psychiatry, 24,* 409–414.

Wells, K. C., & Forehand, R. (in press). Conduct and oppositional disorders. In P. H.

Bornstein & A. E. Kazdin (Eds.), *Handbook and clinical behavior therapy with children.* New York: Dorsey Press.

Werry, J. S., Aman, M. G., & Lampen, E. (1975). Haloperidol and methylphenidate in hyperactive children. *Acta Paedopsychiatrica, 42,* 26–40.

Williams, D. T., Mehl, K., Yudofsky, S., Adams, D., & Roseman, B. (1982). The effect of propranolol on uncontrolled rage outbursts in children and adolescents with organic brain dysfunction. *Journal of the American Academy of Child Psychiatry, 21,* 129–135.

Wood, D. R., Reimherr, F. W., Wender, P. H., & Johnson, G. W. (1976). Diagnosis and treatment of minimal brain dysfunction in adults. *Archives of General Psychiatry, 33,* 1453–1460.

Yudofsky, W., Williams, D., & Gorman, J. (1981). Propranolol in the treatment of rage and violent behavior in patients with chronic brain syndromes. *American Journal of Psychiatry, 138,* 218–220.

Zahn-Waxler, C., McKnew, D. H., Cummings, E. M., Davenport, Y. B., & Radike-Yarrow, M. (1984). Problem behaviors and peer interactions of young children with a manic-depressive parent. *American Journal of Psychiatry, 141,* 236–240.

Eating Disorders: Anorexia Nervosa and Bulimia

ROBERT L. HENDREN, D.O.

The author wishes to acknowledge the support and suggestions of Joan Barber, M.D., Co-Director of the Eating Disorder Program, George Washington University Medical School, in the preparation of this chapter.

Anorexia nervosa, once considered a rare disorder, is now thought to be relatively common, occurring in as many as one in 250 females in the high risk group between 12 and 18 years *(American Psychiatric Association,* 1980). Characterized by a drive for thinness, its incidence appears to be increasing (Jones et al., 1980; Kendal et al., 1973), as are the number of studies of the disorder. More recent reports consider bulimia, in which food consumed is disposed of by vomiting or laxative abuse, as a variant of anorexia nervosa (Russell, 1979). Various treatment modalities are recommended for both disorders.

In this chapter, the diagnostic categories of anorexia nervosa and bulimia are reviewed, as are recent findings suggesting an association between eating disorders and affective disorders. The rationale for medication, different medications proposed for usage, and their adverse effects in eating disordered patients are presented and reviewed.

DIAGNOSIS

Various diagnostic criteria for anorexia nervosa include those by Feighner (1972) and Bruch (1966). Currently the *Diagnostic and Statistical Manual* (1980) criteria for anorexia nervosa are commonly used, including an intense fear of becoming obese, a disturbance of body image, weight loss of at least 25 percent, a refusal to maintain weight over a minimal normal weight, and no known physical illness that would account for the weight loss.

The other principal eating disorder, bulimia, is described in DSM-III as recurrent episodes of binge eating often followed by self-induced vomiting or laxative abuse. Individuals with bulimia usually are aware that their eating pattern is abnormal. Bulimics often experience depression and self-deprecating thoughts after a binge and while binging are afraid they will be unable to stop.

Anorexia nervosa and bulimia may overlap in that individuals with anorexia nervosa may binge and vomit, and bulimics initially may have had anorexia nervosa. This area of overlap is referred to as "bulimia-nervosa" in the British literature (Russell, 1979). There also appears to be an overlap of bulimia and obesity (Garfinkle & Garner, 1983) as represented in Figure 10.1.

Considerable controversy exists about whether anorexia nervosa and bulimia represent distinct entities or simply symptom complexes that may include other psychiatric illnesses. Bruch (1966) makes a distinction between primary and secondary anorexia nervosa and points out that symptoms of anorexia nervosa may exist in individuals with schizophre-

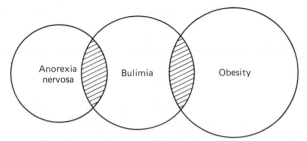

Fig. 10.1. Overlap among anorexia nervosa, bulimia, and obesity.

nia, hysteria, and other psychiatric disorders. These individuals are distinguished from those with "primary" anorexia nervosa by strict adherence to diagnostic criteria. However, this distinction is not always clear, and a mixed picture may exist (Lucas, 1981). In addition, subgroupings of both anorexia nervosa and bulimia is proposed based on personality traits, depressive symptomatology, and other associated psychiatric symptomatology (Garfinkle & Garner, 1983). Diagnostic criteria and the influence of other psychiatric disorders are important considerations when evaluating claims of successful treatment in various populations of eating disordered patients. The diagnosis of anorexia nervosa and/or bulimia does not exclude the possibility of additional psychiatric or physical disorders.

ANOREXIA NERVOSA, BULIMIA, AND AFFECTIVE DISORDER

Recent studies suggest a link between anorexia nervosa, bulimia, and affective disorder. This association arises from four major sources: (1) reports that a high percentage of eating disordered patients demonstrate signs of depression during the illness and at follow-up; (2) family history studies that identify a high incidence of affective disorders in relatives of eating disordered patients; (3) similarities in some neuroendocrine abnormalities between eating-disordered and affective-disordered patients; and (4) reports of response to antidepressant medication.

Dysphoria is commonly reported in patients with anorexia nervosa and is one of the DSM-III criteria for bulimia. Warren's (1968) study of 20 girls with anorexia nervosa reports depression of varying severity in 85 percent of his sample. Depression was noted in 14 of 30 anorexia nervosa patients in Rowland's review (1970). Of 94 patients in Theander's (1970) study, 24 (29 percent) were depressed, 20 had relatives with depressions, and 27 were depressed at follow-up. Hendren (1983) reports on 84 patients with a diagnosis of primary anorexia nervosa; 56 percent met Research Diagnostic Criteria (RDC) for a major depressive disorder.

Cantwell et al. (1977) report follow-up data on 26 patients with a mean length of follow-up of 4.9 years. Twelve of the patient were diagnosed as having affective disorder on the basis of parental interviews. Fifty-six percent had dysphoric mood according to patients' reports and 67 percent according to parents reports. In addition, there was a strong family history of major affective disorders in the patient group. These authors suggest that at least some cases of anorexia nervosa may be a variant of affective disorder. Morgan and Russell (1975) report 42 percent of their 41 patients had depressive symptoms four or more years after discharge, based upon patient and/or relative reports. Hsu et al. (1979) report 38 of their 100 patients deressed at follow-up four to eight years after their presentation for anorexia nervosa. These results were also based upon patient and/or relative reports. Stonehill and Crisp (1977) find anorexia patients to be significantly more depressed than controls, but less depressed than a group of depressed outpatients, based upon follow-up clinical interviews and questionnaires.

Winokur et al. (1980) find a 22 percent incidence of primary affective disorder in relatives of patients with anorexia nervosa compared to 10 percent in the relatives of controls, suggesting a subgroup of anorexia nervosa patients who have a genetic loading for affective disorder.

Several studies demonstrate a strong link between bulimia and depression. Russell (1979) reports depression as a common accompaniment of "bulimia-nervosa," but seldom finds it to be as severe as in endogenous depressive illness. Other studies (Garfinkle, 1980; Casper, 1980; Wold, 1983) find mood swings and depressive symptoms more frequent in bulimic patients than in "restricting" anorexics. Hudson et al. (1983a) report a 27 percent risk for major affective disorder in the relatives of subjects with anorexia nervosa and bulimia in a sample of 89 eating-disordered patients. In one report, relatives of bulimic patients have a higher incidence of affective disorder than do relatives of restricting anorexics (Strober, 1982).

Neuroendocrine studies have furthered the understanding of anorexia nervosa and bulimia and their association with depression. Findings in anorexia nervosa include high cortisol levels, low urinary 3-methoxy-4-hydroxyphenyl glycol (MHPG) levels, and inadequate responses to the Dexamethosone Suppression Test (DST) (Gerner & Gwirtzman, 1981). Enduring central and peripheral decreases in norepinephrine (NE) and NE metabolites are also reported (Kaye, 1983). Delayed thyroid-stimulating-hormone (TSH) release after thyrotropin-releasing-hormone (TRH) administration, is reported in some patients with anorexia nervosa (Casper, 1982; Gold et al. 1980) and increased growth hormone also in reported after TRH stimulation (Gold et al. 1980). Because of the influence of malnutrition and stress in altering hypothalamic-pituitary function in anorexia nervosa, the association of these dysfunctions with those found in affective disorders is not clear (Garfinkle & Garner, 1983). Many researchers conclude that the neuro-endocrine changes seen in primary anorexia nervosa are not the same as the changes seen in the affective disorders (Gerner & Gwirtzman, 1981; Walsh, 1982).

Neuroendocrine abnormalities also are reported in bulimia. Hudson et al. (1983b) report 47 percent of their sample of bulimics have a positive DST. Similarly, Gwirtzman et al. (1983) find 67 percent of their sample fail to suppress on the DST, and 80 percent show blunted TSH after TRH stimulation. These authors are less hesitant in linking bulimia with affective illness, since in bulimia the neuroendocrine abnormalities are not solely an artifact of low weight. However, vomiting and erratic eating patterns may well have some as yet unappreciated influence upon hypothalamic-pituitary function.

Response to antidepressant medication is another finding used to support the association of eating disorders and affective illness and will be covered in the next section on drug treatment of anorexia nervosa and bulimia.

DRUG TREATMENT

Antidepressants

The possibility of an association between anorexia nervosa and bulimia with affective disorder led several investigators to treat these illnesses with antidepressant medication. Initially, tricyclic antidepressants (TCAs) were studied in open trials on a limited number of cases (Mills, 1976; Needleman & Waber, 1977; White & Schnaulty, 1977). Despite claims of success, meaningful conclusions could not be drawn because of insufficient cases or controls. More recent methodologically acceptable studies do not demonstrate appreciable benefits from antidepressant treatment of anorexia nervosa. Lacey and Crisp (1980) report a double-blind placebo controlled study of clomipramine in the treatment of 16 patients with anorexia nervosa. Both placebo and treatment groups reached their goal weights. Clomipramine was significantly associated with increased hunger, appetite, and energy levels. The authors suggest that clomipramine, acting at the level of the hypothalamus, alters hunger and eating behaviors according to the body weight of the patient. Biederman et al. (1982) report on a double-blind placebo controlled study of amitriptyline at a dosage of up to 3 mg/kg/day with a maximum of 150 mg/day, in the treatment of 43 patients with anorexia nervosa. Overall, no statistically significant difference favored the amitriptyline group over either the placebo or the no-medication groups, unrelated to whether or not the patients were depressed.

Reports of the treatment of bulimia with both tricyclic antidepressants and monoamine oxidase inhibitors (MAOIs) are more favorable. Pope et al. (1983) report a placebo controlled double-blind study of imipramine in doses up to 200 mg/day in 22 chronically bulimic women. Eighteen of 20 treated subjects responded to imipramine or a subsequent antidepressant. Improvement was maintained at follow-up one to eight months later. In this study imipramine is significantly superior to placebo in reducing the frequency of binge eating and depressive symptomatology. The authors suggest this response is due to the antidepressant actions of imipramine and lend support to the theory that bulimia is a form of affective disorder.

However, Sabine et al. (1983) treated 50 patients diagnosed as "bulimia-nervosa" with Mianserin (a tetracyclic antidepressant) or with placebo in a double-blind study. They find no significant differences in mood, binging or purging between the treatment and control groups, concluding that bulimia is not a manifestation of underlying affective disorder and that the mood changes are a secondary part of the disorder.

Monoamine oxidase inhibitors (MAOI) are reported effective in the treatment of bulimia, especially when associated with an "atypical" depression with reactive mood and increased appetite, hypersomnia, fatigue, or sensitivity to personal rejection (Walsh, 1982). This initial report by Walsh describes the dramatic response of 6 patients with bulimia and atypical depression to phenelzine (up to 90 mg/day) or tranylcypromine (40 mg/day). This was expanded (Walsh, 1983) to the successful treatment of 7 out of 10 bulimic patients with MAOI. Binge frequency and depressive symptoms were both reduced in the responding group, but these trials were not controlled and a double-blind trial is suggested by the authors.

The treatment of eating disorders with antidepressant medications is as yet an unconfirmed approach. While the association with affective illness is intriguing, it is noted that everything which improves with antidepressants is not depression (Glassman & Walsh, 1983). Further studies are required to determine the efficacy and usefulness of antidepressants in the treatment of eating disorders. At this point, the evidence suggests a therapeutic trial of tricyclic medication may be warranted in chronic bulimic patients with depressive features, and of MAOI in the bulimic patient with atypical depression. It is important to utilize adequate dosages of medications to achieve maximum clinical effect. For most tricyclic antidepressants, use up to 150 mg/day or until side effects occur. Imipramine has been given in doses up to 200 mg/day (Pope et al., 1983). Phenylzine, the most frequently used MAOI usually requires 60–90 mg/day for response. There is so far no convincing evidence that antidepressants are useful in the treatment of anorexia nervosa.

There are risks in using antidepressant medications with eating-disordered patients. Undernourished, low weight patients are more susceptible to hypotension, and other anticholinergic side effects. Biederman et al. (1982) report the following incidence of adverse effects in anorexia nervosa patients treated with amitriptyline: hypotension—18 percent, diaphoresis—18 percents; blurred vision—9 percent, urinary retention—9 percent; leukopenia—9 percent; and drowsiness—55 percent. No important cardiac rhythm or conduction disturbances are reported. Medication absorption and blood levels are affected by induced vomiting. Vomiters and laxative abusers are at even greater risk if placed on antidepressants known to increase cardiac irritability. The bulimic patient's difficulty with impulse control leads to a greater risk of serious complications while taking MAOI. Strict adherence to a tyramine-free diet may be an unrealistic expectation of patients who complain of losing control of their eating (Fairburn & Cooper, 1983). If these risks are of concern the patient should be hospitalized during the medication trial (Walsh et al., 1982).

Lithium Carbonate

Two rationales exist for the use of lithium carbonate in the treatment of anorexia nervosa. One is in the treatment of patients with cyclothymic mood disturbance and family histories of bipolar disorders (Barcai, 1977; Stein et al., 1982). The other is in producing weight gain as a side effect of lithium carbonate treatment (Gross et al. 1981). While the explanation for weight gain with lithium is uncertain, it is believed to be due to its insulinlike effect on the cell membrane (Plenge et al., 1970).

Barcai (1977) administered lithium carbonate to two patients with long-standing anorexia nervosa and labile moods who responded with improvement in mental symptoms and weight gain. Stein et al. (1982)

treated a patient with severe anorexia nervosa and mood swings who also responded to lithium carbonate with weight gain and less emotional lability.

Since lithium carbonate is reported to produce weight gain in depressed patients, Gross et al. (1981) used it to treat eight young women with primary anorexia nervosa in a double-blind controlled study. Patients taking lithium showed greater weight gain at weeks three and four than did those on placebo. Lithium did not affect the patient's perception of hunger.

Lithium toxicity is of special concern in the treatment of anorexia nervosa patients for many of the same reasons that antidepressants require caution. However, the risks are even greater with lithium because of its narrow range of therapeutic levels. The risk of cardiac abnormalities such as ventricular ectopy is reported for those anorextic patients who are malnourished (Gottdiner et al., 1978) and are therefore at greater risk if lithium toxicity occurs (Gross et al., 1981). There is added danger if the patient is vomiting or abusing laxatives. All of the authors cited above recommend close monitoring of patients. When the risks are weighed against the benefits, lithium treatment has demonstrated little usefulness in the treatment of anorexia nervosa except when there is a concomitant cyclic mood disturbance.

Cyproheptadine (Periactin)

Cyproheptadine is a serotonin and histamine antagonist with anticholinergic and sedative effects. Vigersky and Loriaux (1977) performed a double-blind controlled trial of cyproheptadine with 24 anorextic patients for a period of eight weeks. Four patients treated with cyproheptadine responded with weight gain as did two patients in the placebo group. The differences were not statistically significant.

Goldberg, Halmi, Eckert et al. (1979, 1980) have reported studies on the treatment of patients with anorexia nervosa with cyproheptadine or placebo with or without behavior modification. No significant differences in weight gain were found between the placebo or cyproheptadine group. A subsequent report from this group (Goldberg et al., 1980) added patients to their sample size and found differences favoring cyproheptadine on several measures of eating attitudes and two lowered scores on the MMPI scale. In addition, they performed a double-blind trial of amitriptyline versus cyproheptadine versus placebo and found significant drug effect most noticable with the cyproheptadine on measures of weight gain and improved Hamilton depression scores (Halmi et al., 1982). They suggest cyproheptadine may have antidepressant effects because of its serotonin antagonist action.

Dosages range from 2–8 mg four times a day and have exceeded the maximum range recommended in the package insert without significant side effects (Halmi et al., 1982). The few adverse reactions are related to the atropinelike action of medication, the most common of which is sedation. The relative safety of cryproheptadine is one of its advantages. However, claims of its effectiveness so far are not compelling and require further studies.

Anticonvulsants

Anticonvulsant medications are reported successful in the treatment of some eating-disordered patients especially those with an abnormal EEG. Green and Rau (1977) treated 26 patients who had compulsive eating disorders with diphenylhydantoin at a dosage of 400 mg/day. Nine patients responded positiely but 17 failed to respond or had an inadequate trial. Six of the 12 patients with abnormal EEGs responded positively as did three of the 14 with normal EEGs. Seven of the 26 patients described their eating episodes as "irregular, unpredictable and ego dystonic" and reported nonfood related impulsive behaviors. Five of these seven patients had abnormal EEGs and 6 responded to diphenylhydantoin treatment. Patients in this group described their binge eating episodes as seizurelike, followed by a phase of sleepiness and confusion.

In a placebo controlled study of 20 patients, Wermuth et al. (1977) report decreased binge eating in the diphenylhydantoin group. Seven of these patients displayed some abnormality on their EEG. While this study suggests improvement in a distinct group of binge eaters, the two patients with anorexia nervosa did not improve.

Carbamazepine, commonly used as an anticonvulsant, is also reported to be effective in the treatment of bipolar disorder. Its effectiveness is thought to be due to its preferential suppression of electrical transmission in limbic and other subcortical structures. Kaplan et al. (1982) treated six bulimic patients with carbamazepine and report dramatic responses in one patient who also had a history suggestive of bipolar disorder. They postulate a subgroup of bulimic patients with a link to affective illness and a common underlying neurophysiologic limbic system abnormality.

A therapeutic trial of anticonvulsant medication with bulimic patients might be considered when binges are episodic, uncontrollable, ego dystonic, and resemble seizurelike activity (Moore and Rakes, 1982). An abnormal EEG would lend further support to a therapeutic trial. The use of anticonvulsant medication has not been shown to be beneficial in patients with anorexia nervosa or in the routine treatment of patients with bulimia. With further studies, it may prove useful in the treatment of a subgroup of bulimics with abnormal EEGs.

Antipsychotics

Phenothiazines have been widely used in the treatment of eating disorders, particularly in the United Kingdom (Garfinkle & Garner, 1983). Early reports by Dally and Sargent (1960) advocate the use of chlorpromazine and insulin as effective in producing weight gain. Later they suggest chlorpromazine alone is equally successful (Dally & Sargent, 1966).

The rationales for antipsychotic treatment include: (1) unmodulated or increased activity of dopaminergic (and perhaps noradrenergic) pathways in anorexia nervosa (Barry & Klawans, 1976); (2) weight gain associated with antipsychotics; (3) reduction in initial anxiety and resistance to eating; and (4) sedation.

Pimozide (a selective dopaminergic receptor blocker) was studied in a double-blind controlled crossover study of 18 patients with severe anorexia nervosa (Vandereycken & Pierloot, 1982). Weight gain was enhanced initially with pimozide treatment and it appeared to improve motivation and acceptance of weight gain. However, the drug had only a marginal influence on patient attitudes based on the rating scales used.

Recommended dosages of neuroleptic medications vary. Dally and Sargent (1966) start with oral doses of chlorpromazine of 150 mg/day and increase to the patient's tolerance, which may be as high as 1000–1500 mg. Crisp (1965) recommends smaller doses (400–500 mg/day) and uses it only as an adjunct to psychotherapy. Vandereycken and Pierloot (1982) gave 4–5 mg/day of pimozide to the patients in their study.

The adverse effects of antipsychotic medications are particularly worrisome in patients with anorexia nervosa, including a worsening of already existing hypotensive symptoms. In addition, antipsychotics may further reduce body temperature, aggravate leukopenia, and lower the convulsive threshold. An increased frequency of postdischarge bulimia in chlorpromazine-treated anorexia nervosa patients also is reported (Dally & Sargent, 1966).

Neuroleptic medications are not routinely prescribed in the treatment of anorexia nervosa or bulimia. In certain cases, they may be useful initially in the tretment of patients who have marked food-related anxiety and an inability to eat. Careful monitoring is necessary. Even early advocates of antipsychotic treatment for all anorexics now recommend its use only in particular patients with marked anxiety (Dally, 1977).

Minor Tranquilizers

Benzodiazepines have been utilized in the treatment of anorexia nervosa for their anxiolytic effects. Since their use is associated with less slowing of mental processes and fewer unwanted side effects, some recommend their usage over major tranquilizers (Garfinkle & Garner, 1983). This is particularly so for internists treating anorexia nervosa who are more likely to prescribe minor tranquilizers than are psychiatrists who are more likely to prescribe major tranquilizers (Bhanji, 1979).

If minor tranquilizers are to be used, this should be done only for short term relief of anxiety while a working alliance is established. A short acting minor tranquilizer might be given one hour prior to meals for one or two weeks until the patient is more involved in the treatment program. Problems with using minor tranquilizers include sedation and their high potential for dependency, especially among bulimic patients.

Other Medications

Delta-9-tetrahydrocannabinol (THC), the most prominent psychoactive substance in marijuana, is reported to stimulate appetite, promote weight gain, and have an antiemetic effect. However, in a double-blind trial of THC versus diazepam and placebo, it was found not efficacious in the treatment of 11 patients with primary anorexia nervosa (Gross et al., 1983). Three patients experienced severe dysphoria, paranoid ideation, and feelings of loss of control when taking THC. Its usage is not recommended in the treatment of anorexia nervosa.

Naloxone was used in the treatment of eight patients with anorexia nervosa who were concomitantly being treated with behavioral techniques, supportive psychotherapy, and antidepressants (Moore et al., 1981). Naloxone was administered by constant intravenous infusion, and patients demonstrated significantly greater weight gain when receiving the medication than before or after the infusion. Several mechanisms for this weight gain have been proposed and include inhibition of opioids, which may influence the symptoms of anorexia (Gillman & Lichtfeld, 1981). Further studies of Naloxone are needed to elucidate its usefulness in the treatment of eating disorders.

L-dopa has been recommended in the treatment of anorexia nervosa by Johanson and Knorr (1977). They treated nine patients with low doses of L-dopa and report that five experienced a small weight gain (3–

5.5 kg) while in the hospital. One of these relapsed after discharge. The study was not controlled and the results were unimpressive. The rationale proposed for its usage in anorexia nervosa is faulty (Garfinkle & Garner, 1983) and it appears of no value in the treatment of eating disorders.

SUMMARY

No single medication demonstrates clear benefits or advantages in the treatment of patients with anorexia nervosa or bulimia. Tricyclic antidepressants suggest some promise in the treatment of patients with chronic bulimia and usage of MAOI in a subgroup with atypical depression is encouraging. Lithium carbonate, cyproheptadine, and possibly Naloxone, are reported of some benefit in increasing body weight in patients with anorexia nervosa. Anticonvulsants may prove helpful in treating a subgroup of bulimic patients with abnormal EEGs whose binging episodes have a seizurelike quality. Carbamazepine may prove especially useful in this group since it also benefits cyclic mood swings.

Antipsychotic medications have been used to increase weight gain, but the associated risks make its routine usage unwise. Minor tranquilizers are used to decrease anxiety, but one must exercise caution in their usage because of their high potential for dependency.

Other medications such as THC and L-dopa have not proven useful in the treatment of eating disorders.

During the next several years, there is likely to be a greater increase in our understanding of the pathophysiology of anorexia nervosa and bulimia. Medication trials will increase in sophistication and new medications that affect the hypothalamic-pituitary axis will be developed. With this kowledge, the usefulness of medications in the management of eating disorders is likely to be clarified.

REFERENCES

American Psychiatric Association, (1980). *Diagnostic and statistical manual of mental disorders* (3rd ed.). Washington, DC: American Psychiatric Association.

Barcai, A. (1977). Lithium in anorexia nervosa: A pilot study on two patients. *Acta Psychiatrica et Neurologica Scandinavia, 55,* 97–101.

Barry, V. C., & Klawans, H. L. (1976). On the role of dopamine in the pathophysiology of anorexia nervosa. *Journal of Neural Transmission, 38,* 107–122.

Bhanji, S. (1979). Anorexia nervosa: Physicians' and psychiatrists' opinion and practice. *Journal of Psychosomatic Research, 23,* 7–11.

Biederman, J., Herzog, D. B., Rivinus, T., Harper, G., Ferber, R., Rosenbaum, J., Harmatz, J. S., Tandorf, R., Orsulak, P., & Schildkraut, J. (1982). Amitriptyline in the treatment of anorexia nervosa: A double blind placebo controlled study. Presented at the annual meeting of the American Academy of Child Psychiatry, October, 1982, Washington, D. C.

Bruch, H. (1966). Anorexia Nervosa and its differential diagnosis. *Journal of Nervous and Mental Disease, 141,* 555–566.

Cantwell, D. P., Sturzenberger, S., Burroughs, J., & Salkin, B. (1977). Anorexia nervosa: An affective disorder? *Archives of General Psychiatry, 34,* 1087–1093.

Casper, R. C., Eckert, E. D., Halmi, K. A., Goldberg, S. C., & Davis, J. J. (1980). Bulimia: Its incidence and clinical importance in patients with anorexia nervosa. *Archives of General Psychiatry, 37,* 1030–1035.

Casper, R. C., & Frohman, L. A. (1982). Delayed TSH release in anorexia nervosa following injection of thyrotropin-releasing hormone (TRH). *Psychoendocrinology, 7,* 59–68.

Crisp, A. H. (1965). Clinical and therapeutic aspects of anorexia nervosa—a study of 30 cases. *Journal of Psychosomatic Research, 9,* 67–78.

Dally, P. J., (1977). Anorexia Nervosa: Do we need a scapegoat? *Proceedings of the Royal Society of Medicine, 70,* 470–474.

Dally, P. J., & Sargent, W. (1960). A new treatment of anorexia nervosa. *British Medical Journal, 1,* 1770–1773.

Dally, P. J., & Sargent, W. (1966). Treatment and outcome of anorexia nervosa. *British Medical Journal, 2,* 793–795.

Fairburn, C. G., & Cooper, P. J. (1983). MAOIs in the treatment of bulimia. *American Journal of Psychiatry, 140,* 949–950.

Feighner, J. P., Robins, E., Guze, S. G., Woodruff, R. A., Winokur, G., & Munoz, R. (1972). Diagnostic criteria for use in psychiatric research. *Archives of General Psychiatry, 26,* 57–63.

Garfinkle, P. E., & Garner, D. M. (1983). *Anorexia nervosa: A multidimensional perspective.* New York: Brunner/Mazel.

Garfinkle, P. E., Moldotsky, H., & Garner, D. M. (1983). The heterogeneity of anorexia nervosa: Bulimia as a distinct subgroup. *Archives of General Psychiatry, 37,* 1036–1040.

Gerner, R. H., & Gwirtsman, H. E. (1981). Abnormalities of dexamethasone suppression test and urinary MHPG in anorexia nervosa. *American Journal of Psychiatry, 138,* 650–653.

Gillman, M. A., & Lichtfeld, F. J. (1981). Naloxone in anorexia nervosa: Role of the opiate system. *Journal Royal Society of Medicine, 74,* 631.

Glassman, A. H., & Walsh, B. T. (1983). Link between bulimia and depression unclear. Letter to the editor. *Journal of Clinical Psychopharmacology, 3,* 203.

Gold, M. S., Pottash, A. L. C., Sweeney, D. R., Martin, D. M., & Davies, R. K. (1980). Further evidence of hypothalamic-pituitary dysfunction in anorexia nervosa. *American Journal of Psychiatry, 137,* 101–102.

Goldberg, S. C., Halmi, K. A., Eckert, E. D., Casper, R. C., & Davies, J. M. (1979). Cyproheptadine in anorexia nervosa. *British Journal of Psychiatry, 134,* 67–70.

Goldberg, S. C., Halmi, K. A., Eckert, E. D., Casper, R. C., Davies, J. M., & Roper, M.

(1980). Effects of cyrpoheptadine on symptoms and attitudes in anorexia nervosa. (letter). *Archives of General Psychiatry, 37,* 1083.

Gottdiener, J. S., Gross, H. A., Henry, W. L., Borer, J. S., & Ebert, M. H. (1978). Effects of self-induced starvation on cardiac size and function in anorexia nervosa. *Circulation, 58,* 425–433.

Green, R. S., & Rau, J. H. (1977). The use of diphenylhydantoin in compulsive eating disorders: Further studies. In R. A. Vigersky (Ed.), *Anorexia Nervosa* (pp. 377–382). New York: Raven Press.

Gross, H. A., Ebert, M. H., Faden, V. B., Goldberg, S. C., Nee, L. E., & Kaye, W. H. (1981). A double-blind controlled trial of lithium carbonate in primary anorexia nervosa. *Journal of Clinical Psychopharmacology, 1,* 376–381.

Gross, H. A., Ebert, M. H., Faden, V. B., Goldberg, S. C., Kaye, W. H., Caine, E. D., Hawks, R., & Zinberg, N. (1983). A double-blind trial of delta-9-tetrahydrocannabinol in primary anorexia nervosa. *Journal of Clinical Psychopharmacology, 3,* 165–171.

Gwirtsman, H. E., Roy-Byrne, P., Yager, J., & Gerner, R. H. (1983). Neuroendocrine abnormalities in bulimia. *American Journal of Psychiatry, 140,*559–563.

Halmi, K. A., Eckert, E., & Falk, J. R. (1982). Cyproheptadine for anorexia nervosa. (letter) *Lancet, 1*(8285), 1357–1358.

Hendren, R. L. (1983) Depression in anorexia nervosa. *Journal of the Academy of Child Psychiatry, 22,* 59–62.

Hsu, L. K. G., Grisp, A. H., & Hardin, B. (1979). Outcome of anorexia nervosa. *Lancet, 1,* 61–65.

Hudson, J. I., Pope, H. G., Jones, j. M., & Yurgelun-Todd, D. (1983a). Family history study of anorexia nervosa and bulimia. *British Journal of Psychiatry, 142,* 133–138.

Hudson, J. I., Pope, H. G., Jonas, J. M., Laffer, P. S., Hudson, M. S., & Melby, J. C. (1983b). Hypothalamic-pituitary-adrenal axis hyperactivity in bulimia. *Psychiatry Research, 8,* 111–117.

Jones, D. J., Fou, M. M., Babigian, H. M., & Hutton, A. E. (1980). Epidemiology of anorexia nervosa in Monroe County, New York 1960–76. *Psychosomatic Medicine, 42,* 551–558.

Kaplan, A. S., Garfinkle, P. E., Darby, P. L., & Garner, D. M. (1983). Carbamazepine in the treatment of bulimia. *American Journal of Psychiatry, 140,* 1225–1226.

Kaye, W. H., Jimerson, D. C., Lake, R., & Ebert, M. H., (1983). Enduring norepinephrine disturbances in anorexia. Presented at the annual meeting of the American Psychiatric Association, May 2, 1983, New York City.

Kendal, R. E., Hall, D. J., Hailey, A., & Babigian, H. M. (1973). The epidemiology of anorexia nervosa. *Psychosomatic Medicine, 3,* 200–203.

Lacey, J. H., and Crisp, A. H. (1980). Hunger, food intake, and weight: The inpact of clomipramine on a refeeding anorexia nervosa population. *Postgraduate Medical Journal, 56* (suppl. 1.), 79–85.

Lucas, A. R. (1981). Toward the understanding of anorexia nervosa as a disease entity. *Mayo Clinic Proceedings, 56,* 254–264.

Mills, I. H. (1976). Amitriptyline therapy in anorexia nervosa (letter). *Lancet, 2,* 687.

Moore, R., Mills, I. H., & Foster, A. (1981). Naloxone in the treatment of anorexia nervosa: Effect on weight gain and lipolysis. *Journal Royal Society of Medicine, 74,* 129–131.

Moore, S. L., & Rakes, S. M. (1982). Binge eating—therapeutic response to diphenylhydantoin: Case report. *Journal of Clinical Psychiatry, 43,* 385–386.

Morgan, H. G., & Russell, G. F. M. (1975). Value of family background and clinical features as predictors of long-term outcome in anorexia nervosa: four-year follow-up study of 41 patients. *Psychological Medicine, 5,* 355–371.

Needleman, H. L., & Waber, D. (1977). The use of amitriptyline in anorexia nervosa. In R. Vigersky (Ed.), *Anorexia nervosa* (pp. 341–348). New York: Raven Press.

Plenge, P., Mellerup, E. T., & Rafaelsen, O. J. (1970). Lithium action on glycogen synthesis in rat, brain, livers, diaphragm. *Journal of Psychiatric Research, 8,* 29–36.

Pope, H. G., Hudson, J. I., Jonas, J. M., & Yurgelun-Todd, D. (1983). Bulimia treated with imipramine: A placebo-controlled, double-blind study. *American Journal of Psychiatry, 140,* 554–558.

Reilly, P. P. (1977). Anorexia nervosa. *Rhode Island Medical Journal, 60,* 419–422.

Rowland, C. V., Jr. (1970). Anorexia nervosa: a survey of the literature and review of 30 cases. *International Psychiatry Clinics Journal, 7,* 37–137.

Russell, G. (1979). Bulimia nervosa: an ominous variant of anorexia nervosa. *Psychological Medicine, 9,* 429–448.

Sabine, E. J., Yonace, A., Farrington, A. J., Barratt, K. H., & Wakeling, A. (1983). Bulimia nervosa: A placebo controlled, double-blind therapeutic trial of mianserin. *British Journal Pharmacology, 15,* 1955–1025.

Stein, G. S., Hartshorn, S., Jones, J., & Steinberg, D. (1982). Lithium in a case of severe anorexia nervosa. *British Journal of Psychiatry, 140,* 526–528.

Stonehill, E., & Crisp, A. H., (1977). Psychoneurotic characteristics of patients with anorexia nervosa before and after treatment and follow-up 4–7 years later. *Journal Psychosomatic Research, 21,* 187–193.

Strober, M., Salkin, B., Burroughs, J., & Morrell, W. (1982). Validity of the bulimic-restrictor distinction in anorexia nervosa. *Journal Nervous Mental Disorders, 170,* 345–351.

Theander, S. (1970). Anorexia nervosa. *Acta Psychiatrica et Neurologica Scandanavia, 214,* (supplement).

Vandereycken, W., & Pierlot, R. (1982). Pimozide combined with behavior therapy in the short term treatment of anorexia nervosa. *Acta Psychiatrica et Neurologica Scandanavia, 66,* 445–450.

Vigersky, R. A., & Loriaux, D. L. (1977). The effects of cyproheptadine in anorexia nervosa: a double-blind trial. In R. A. Vigersky, (Ed.), *Anorexia nervosa* (pp. 349–356). New York: Raven Press.

Walsh, B. T. (1982). Endocrine disturbances in anorexia nervosa and depression. *Psychosomatic Medicine, 44,* 85–91.

Walsh, B. T., Stewart, J. W., Wright, L., Harrison, W., Roose, S. P., & Glassman, A. H. (1982). Treatment of bulimia with monoamine oxidase inhibitors. *American Journal of Psychiatry, 139,* 1629–1630.

Walsh, B. T., Stewart, J. W., Wright, L., Roose, S. P., & Glassman, A. H. (1983). Treatment of bulimia with monoamine oxidase inhibitors. Presented at the annual meeting of the American Psychiatric Association, May, 1983, New York City.

Warren, W. (1968). A study of anorexia nervosa in young girls. *Journal of Child Psychology and Psychiatry, 9,* 27–40.

Wermuth, B. M., Davis, K. L., Hollister, L. E., & Strunkard, A. J. (1977). Phenytoin treatment of the binge-eating syndrome. *American Journal of Psychiatry, 134,* 1249–1253.

White, J. H., & Schnaulty, N. L. (1977). Successful treatment of anorexia nervosa with imipramine. *Diseases of the Nervous System, 38,* 567–568.

Winokur, A., March, V., & Mendals, J. (1980). Primary affective disorder in relatives of patients with anorexia nervosa. *American Journal of Psychiatry, 137,* 695–698.

Wold, P. N. (1983). Anorexic syndromes and affective disorder. *Psychiatric Journal University of Ottawa, 8,* 116–119.

Enuresis and Sleep Disorders

DAVID SHAFFER, M.D. and PAUL J. AMBROSINI, M.D.

Nocturnal enuresis is usually defined as the involuntary passage of urine during sleep in the absence of any identified physical abnormality, in children aged four or five years. The choice of four or five to define enuresis as a problem behavior is not arbitrary. A number of studies (Kaffman & Elizur, 1977; Miller et al., 1960; Oppel et al., 1968) indicate that children who are still wetting at the age of four are different from those who are wetting at an earlier age in that the former have a sharply reduced probability of becoming dry during the following year. Kaffman and Elizur (1977) also have shown that while four year olds who wet the bed have more behavioral problems than those who are dry, this is not so with three year olds. Taken together this suggests that wetting up until age three is part of the normal spectrum of development, but that children who wet after age four differ qualitatively from those who have aquired continence.

PREVALENCE AND NATURAL HISTORY

The prevalance of enuresis varies with which frequency of wetting (Rutter et al., 1973) is taken to define the problem. Seven percent of seven year old boys wet more than weekly, but 15 percent wet less frequently than that. The prevalence of enuresis in adults is not known although Forsythe and Redmond (1974) found that three percent of enuretic children were still enuretic after the age of 20. Between the age of four and six enuresis is as common in girls as it is in boys; however, after the age of seven, the ratio of boy to girl wetters increases so that by the age of 11 boys are twice as likely to be wet as girls (Essen & Peckham, 1976; Rutter et al., 1973; Oppel et al., 1968; Douglas, 1973; Miller, 1973). In part this is because girls become continent earlier than boys, and in part because boys are more likely to develop secondary enuresis (Essen & Peckham, 1976).

The prognosis for becoming dry (Essen & Peckham, 1976; Miller et al., 1960) is greater for children who wet intermittently than for those who wet nightly; for primary than for secondary enuretics; for girls than for boys (after age 11 years); and for children from middle or upper class families.

ETIOLOGY

The cause of bedwetting cannot usually be identified in an individual child. Nevertheless, a number of associations have been noted in different research studies.

306

Genetics

Enuresis commonly runs in families. Approximately 70 percent of all enuretics have a first degree relative who is, or has been, afflicted with the same condition (Bawkin, 1961). Twin studies (Hallgren, 1960; Bakwin, 1973) show that concordance for enuresis is significantly greater in uniovular than in binovular twins (68% vs. 36% in Bakwin's study).

Family history does not seem to have direct clinical significance. It is unrelated to the prevalence of associated psychiatric disorder (Mikkelson et al., 1980; Shaffer et al., 1985) and it is as common among primary enuretics as among secondary (Fritz & Anders, 1979; Shaffer et al., 1985). However, Shaffer et al. (1985) found that enuretics whose mother was enuretic will more often have a home in which there is significant marital discord and their previously enuretic mothers will have more psychiatric symptoms.

Association with Urinary Infection

Enuresis is five times as common in girls with pyelonephritis than it is in the general population (Dodge et al., 1970; Jones et al., 1972; Meadow et al., 1969). Conversely, urinary infections are five times as common in enuretics as in the general population (Kunin et al., 1962; Shaffer et al., 1968). This association is clinically important and enuretic girls should be viewed as a high risk group in whom a full bacteriologoical examination is mandatory. It is not clear whether enuresis *results* from genitourinary abnormalities of the sort that lead to or *result* from urinary infection or whether enuresis itself facilitates ascending infection, thus *causing* infection. However, abnormalities on an intraveneous pyelogram or on micturating cystography are present in less than 1 percent of enuretic children (Forsythe & Redmond, 1974; McKendry & Stuart, 1974) and, when found there are virtually always other features that would lead the clinician to suspect an organic lesion (Redman & Seibert, 1979). This applies to both diurnal and nocturnal enuretics. Accordingly, it is recommended that all cases of enuresis be investigated by examination and culture of the urine, but that radiographic investigation be reserved for children with documented urinary tract infection (American Academy of Pediatrics, 1980).

Outflow-Tract Obstruction

The notion that enuresis is associated with subtle degrees of urethral or bladder neck obstruction (Mahoney, 1971) has been critically reviewed by Smith (1964) and Shaffer (1985), who conclude that this hypothesis does not explain most cases of enuresis. There is *no* evidence that urethral dilation or bladder neck repair are effective treatments for enuresis, although the presence of a high-pressure bladder may call for ureteric implantation to treat vesico-ureteric reflux. Johnston et al. (1978) have shown that enuretics with reflux will nearly always have concomitant urinary infection.

Bladder Size and Function

Troup and Hodgson (1971) and Starfield (1967) found that on average the maximum volume passed by enuretics after a fluid load is significantly less than that passed by either their nonenuretic siblings or other controls. This does not appear to be related to anatomical size of the bladder.

Shaffer et al. (1985) found that 55 percent of a population of enuretics at school clinics had a functional bladder volume one standard deviation below the expected volume. Low functional bladder volume was found significantly more often in behaviorally disturbed children and in children with current speech or language difficulties but with equal frequency in primary and secondary enuretics and in those without a positive family history of wetting.

An overlap in functional bladder capacity between enuretics and nonenuretics has been noted in all studies so that a small functional bladder capacity is not in itself sufficient basis for enuresis. It may be that a young child with a low functional bladder volume and possibly other developmental delays will have greater difficulty in initially "learning" bladder control and that it is only one of a number of factors that may mitigate against the development of continence at the usual time. The pathophysiology of this reduced "functional bladder capacity" is not known. However, the association with speech and language delay and with behavior problems suggests central rather than peripheral mechanisms.

Enuresis and Sleep

—Mikkelson et al. (1980) found that enuretic events occur on a random basis in any sleep stage; that the frequency of events within any one stage is proportional to the amount of time spent by the individual in that sleep stage and that the overall sleep architecture is no different in enuretics and nonenuretics.—

Neuroleptic-Induced Enuresis

Urinary incontinence during sleep has been reported to occur during administration of the neuroleptics thioridazine (Mellaril) and thiothixene (Navane) among both adult (Nurnberg & Ambrosini, 1979; Shenoy, 1980) and child (Boon, 1981) psychiatric patients with no prior history of enuresis. In all cases the problem has remitted after the neuroleptic drug was discontinued. It is not clear whether the effect was specific for these drugs or is a more general phenomenon with neuroleptics. Incontinence may also occur in phenothiazine-induced catatonic states and stress incontinence may take place in patients receiving chlorpromazine (VanPutten et al., 1972); however, these may be different phenomena. The mechanisms involved are unknown.

Developmental Delays

Enuretics are twice as likely as other children to have a motor or speech delay (Essen & Peckham, 1976). This may account for the high rate of psychiatric disorders in enuretics (see below). Enuretics with a psychiatric disturbance are more likely to have associated speech or language difficulties (Shaffer et al., 1985) and have more neurological soft signs than enuretics without psychiatric symptoms (Mikkelsen et al., 1980).

Toilet Training

In a prospective study, Kaffmann and Elizur (1977) found that persistent wetting is related to training delay. The rate among six to eight-year-old children whose training had started after 20 months was nearly four times greater than among those whose training had started earlier.

Enuresis as a Psychiatric or Psychosocial Disorder

Parents often assume that bedwetting is a sign of "nervousness." The psychoanalytical literature is replete with psychological explanations for enuresis, for example, that it is an exhibitionistic defense against castration anxiety (Angel, 1935) or that a repressed (hostile or sexual) drive is being satisfied through wetting (Michaels, 1961), or that the shame and guilt that accompanies enuresis reflects superego responses to aggressive impulses. Other theories that have been invoked (see Shaffer, 1973, for a review) include regarding enuresis as an immature form of gratification; as a manifestation of anxiety, mediated by a direct autonomic effect on bladder function; or as an expression of hostility in children who have difficulty showing aggression in more direct ways.

Regardless of the reasons, an association between enuresis and emotional–behavioral disturbance has been found in large scale surveys of the general population after taking into account social background differences (Essen & Peckham, 1976; Rutter et al., 1973). The association is stronger in girls and in children who wet by day, as well as by night, but there is no consistent association with age or with the frequency of wetting (Hallgren, 1956; Rutter et al., 1973). However, only a minority of enuretics are disturbed. This means that enuresis cannot invariably be regarded as a sign of psychiatric disorder. The emotional–behavioral difficulties associated with enuresis do not follow any consistent pattern (Lickorish, 1964; Rutter et al, 1973); and, there is no marked tendency for enuresis to be associated with tics, temper tantrums, nailbiting, (Oppel et al., 1968; Rutter et al., 1973), fire-setting, or cruelty to animals (Felthous & Bernard, 1978).

The mechanisms involved in the association between bedwetting and psychiatric disturbance remains obscure (see Shaffer, 1985). There are a number of factors that are common in the histories of both bedwetters and disturbed children, and it is possible that these conditions arise from a similar cause but by separate mechanisms. It should be emphasized that there is no evidence that wetting is either "necessary" or beneficial to the disturbed child, and it should be assumed that treatment of enuresis is helpful. The coexistence of disturbance and enuresis is, therefore, an indication rather than a contraindication to initiate effective symptomatic treatment.

TREATMENT OF BEDWETTING

Comparatively few bedwetters receive treatment. In 1960, Miller et al. found that fewer than 30 percent of 11-year-old enuretics had ever been assessed or treated for their complaint. In view of the generally good response to treatment, it must be assumed that the high prevalence rates reported in more recent studies reflect a similar situation. There has been no research on why parents do not seek treatment for their enuretic children, although clinical experience suggests that many families accept bedwetting as an unavoidable part of growing up.

An unknown number of children stop wetting as soon as a clinic appointment is made for them. Others stop wetting the night after they have seen the doctor for the first time and before any treatment has been started, yet others stop wetting as soon as a bell and pad is fitted to their bed. As the bell never rings to waken them, conditioning cannot have taken place. We know little about these responses to nonspecific intervention, nor do we know if the children who respond in this way are themselves distinctive, or whether the quality or duration of their cure is satisfactory. However, responses of this sort often anger the parents of the newly dry child, confirming a belief that the child could have stopped wetting before, had he or she so wished.

Surgical Treatment

The rationale for the surgical treatment of enuresis is that it relieves outflow-tract obstruction, an unsustained hypothetical cause of enuresis. There is no basis for such treatment. No controlled studies have been reported on surgical procedures, which include urethral dilation, meatotomy, or bladder neck repair or cystoplasty to enlarge the bladder (Kvarstein & Mathison, 1981). These interventions do not appear to alter the urodynamic properties of the bladder. Attempts to modify the neurological control of the bladder by division of the sacral nerves (Torrens & Hald, 1979) or the detrusor by bladder transection have also been disappointing (Janknegt et al., 1979). The hazards of such surgery are well documented (Smith, 1969); they include urinary incontinence, recurrent epidydimitis, and aspermia and it is distressing that relatively few surgical studies report that an adequate trial of behavior therapy has preceded intervention.

Night Lifting and Fluid Restriction

These procedures are often adopted by the parents of younger children who are still wetting the bed. Roberts and Schoellkopf (1951) investigated these practices and concluded that they did little to increase the chances of a dry night. The only controlled study (Hagglund, 1965) found that lifting produced a short-lived reduction in wetting frequency. However, lifting and restriction may be more effective in those bedwetters who are never referred for specialist treatment. A good response to lifting may be one of the reasons why professional advice is not sought.

Retention-Control Training

Paschalis et al. (1972) reported on a procedure in which children were instructed to delay micturition in increments of two to three minutes each day after feeling the urge to void. The treatment continues for 20 days, by which time the child should be deferring micturition for 45 minutes on each occasion. The efficacy of this treatment in a proportion of children was reported by Paschalis et al. (1972) and also by Stedman (1972) and Miller (1973).

However, Harris (1977) reported equivocal results and in the largest and most carefully designed study, Fielding (1980) reported on 75 children randomly assigned to treatment by the bell and pad only or the bell and pad preceded by four weeks of retention-control training. The bell and pad was far superior to retention control in reducing night wetting in the enuretic children, regardless of whether or not their incontinence was confined to sleep or whether they were also daytime wetters. Given that the retention control training is time-consuming and may be stressful for both the parent and the child, it cannot be recommended.

Treatment Involving Night Walking

Pfaundler (1904) devised an alarm system to alert nurses after their patients had wet the bed. He noted that when this was carried out the children soon ceased to wet. Despite this early report of a successful treatment for enuresis, the method was not generally applied for another 30 years, when Mowrer and Mowrer (1938) described a similar device. The Mowrer apparatus, with some technical refinements, has continued to be used and constitutes the most effective form of therapy now available. The device usually consists of an auditory signal linked to two electrodes in the form of perforated metal or foil sheets upon which the child sleeps. The sheets are separated by an ordinary cotton sheet. When the child passes urine, contact is made between the two electrodes and an auditory signal is emitted.

A number of theories have been advanced to explain the efficacy of the alarm system. In the classical conditioning paradigm, bladder distension or the micturition contraction is assumed to be the indifferent stimulus (IS). Treatment introduces an unconditiond stimulus (US) (the auditory signal) in proximity to the IS, which then acquires the properties of a conditioned stimulus leading to a conditioned response (CR) (waking). Support for a conditioning model is provided by the findings that (a) when the introduction of the US is delayed, treatment is ineffective, and (b) extinction of the CR after initial cure can be inhibited by intermittent reinforcement (Finley et al. 1973) and by overlearning (Young & Morgan, 1972) (see below).

However, it seems likely that other learning processes are also involved. The "gadget effect" whereby the child becomes dry when the apparatus is placed on the bed but not switched on (DeLeon & Mandell,

1966) suggests that avoidance learning, a form of operant conditioning, may also be important. The effectiveness of twin-signal apparatus designed by Lovibond (1964) and Hansen (1979) lends support to this. The apparatus emits a moderate volume auditory signal when micturition is first detected and a second much louder aversive noise several seconds later. Hansen has demonstrated its efficacy in enuretic children who did not respond to conventional bell and pad treatment and postulates that avoidance learning (to avoid the second loud, aversive noise) may be being coupled with classic conditioning to result in cure. Turner (1973) has pointed out that the use of the bell and pad focuses the family's attention on the wetting habits of the child and that dry nights are more liable to be noted and rewarded by praise. He suggests that social learning is an important component in the bell's efficacy.

"Cure rates," defined as 14 nights of continuous dryness, vary from 50 to 100 percent. Cure is usually reached during the second month of treatment (Kolvin et al., 1972), or by six months in mentally retarded children (Smith, 1981). Response may be hastened by increasing the intensity of the auditory stimulus (Finley & Wansley, 1977) or by the simultaneous use of a stimulant drug, such as methylamphetamine (Young & Turner 1965). This also increases the likelihood of relapse. Young and Morgan (1973) and Dische et al. (1983) have examined the characteristics associated with a delayed response to treatment. Significant factors are maternal anxiety, disturbed home background, and a failure of the child to waken with the alarm. Age of the child and initial wetting frequency was not significantly related to dalay.

Azrin et al. (1974) reported that the time taken to reach cure criterion with the bell and pad could be shortened if a number of other procedures subsumed under the name of the "dry bed" program were undertaken. These included retention control training (see above), training in rapid awakening, rapid reinforcement for correct micturition, and so on.

The "dry bed" procedure (Azrin & Thienes, 1978) is a complicated one. It starts in the afternoon when the child is encouraged to drink large quantities of their favorite beverage to increase the frequency of micturition. If the child feels the need to urinate they are asked to hold for increasingly longer period of time; when the child has to urinate, they are asked to lie on the bed as if they were asleep, then go to the bathroom, role playing what they will have to do at night. This is then rewarded with praise and another drink.

Just before bedtime, the child is asked to role play a self-correction procedure taking off his or her pajamas, removing sheets and putting them back on, and also to role-play what to do in the middle of the night.

Fluids continue to be given until the child falls asleep. There is a discussion about the rewards for being dry, and once the child has fallen asleep they are awoken hourly until 1 a.m. The child is given additional fluids on each awakening until two hous before the final awakening. If they are dry they are asked to rehearse yet again what they will have to do if they fell the need to pass urine and, if they are able to urinate, they are praised for correct toileting. If an accident occurs the parent awakens the child and reprimands them for wetting, directs the child to the bathroom to finish urination, and gives cleanliness training that involves changing of night clothes. If the child is dry the next morning, he or she is allowed to stay up for an extra hour the next night, which provides social reinforcement. If wet the next morning, the child is once again required to change bed and pajamas and does a large number of positive practices in correct toileting, both in the morning and one-half hour before bed the following night.⁓

However, it seems likely (Nettelbeck & Langeluddecke, 1979) that without the simultaneous use of a urine alarm apparatus, the so-called "dry bed" training produces substantially the same results as no treatment at all. Furthermore, Mattsson and Ollendick (1977) have reported adverse affects from this very intensive approach stating that preschool children may react with temper tantrums or withdrawing behavior and the parents may also become upset and need a good deal of support. Given that the simultaneous use of the bell and pad is essential to achieve cure, it is questionable whether its use can be justified.

Treatment Problems

A high proportion of families discontinue treatment before cure. Turner (1973) has indicated failure to understand or to follow the instructions; failure of the apparatus to wake the child, and irritation at false alarms are all predictive of discontinuation.

Relapse after initial cure also presents a problem. Turner (1973) computed that the average relapse rate within a year is 35 percent. Young and Morgan (1973) found that relapse is more likely in older children. Two techniques have been designed to reduce the relapse rate. (1) *Intermittent reinforcement*—this may involve the use of special apparatus designed to waken the patient after only a proportion of micturitions (Finley et al., 1973). Lovibond (1964) has suggested that by using ordinary apparatus during three or four days each week, similar results may be obtained. It should be noted that when this approach is used initial cure may be delayed. (2) *Overlearning*—Young and Morgan (1972) have found that if children are given a fluid load of two pints after having reached dryness criterion, the relapse rate is reduced from 35 to 11 percent. This approach has the advantage of not delaying the initial "cure.".

As mentioned above, the bell and pad offers the opportunity of a cure to the great majority of bedwetters. However, its successful use requires that the therapist be acquainted with practical problems that are likely to arise during treatment and that he be available for a fairly intensive level of support and guidance during the early stages of the treatment process.

Drug Treatment

The use of modern pharmacotherapeutic agents to treat enuresis began when atropine and belladonna derivatives were used to increase bladder tonicity and vesical capacity. Since then a wide range of drugs have been tested for their clinical efficacy (see Blackwell & Currah, 1973 for a review). Although a variety of agents from stimulants to sedatives, pituitary snuff to neuroleptics have been used to treat enuresis, only the tricyclic antidepressants (TCA) and more recently the vasopeptide, DDAVP, have been shown in methodologically adequate studies to be superior to placebo.

Tricyclic Antidepressants. In 1960, MacLean first reported an anecdotal account of the efficacy of imipramine in childhood enuresis. The drug had been tried following the clinical observation that adult depressives treated with imipramine had difficulty initiating micturition. This clinical finding was subsequently confirmed in a large number of well-designed studies (Poussaint et al., 1967; Shaffer et al., 1968). It is now widely accepted that TCAs can significantly reduce wetting frequency in most enuretics regardless of their behavioral, urological, or intellectual status (Smith & Gonzales, 1967; Milner & Hills, 1968; Shaffer et al., 1968; Kunin et al., 1970; Petersen et al., 1973; Mikkelsen et al., 1980).

Most of the currently available tricyclics have been tried in double-blind studies, and all seem equally efficacious. Tricyclics classified as either primary or seconday amines and those whose predominant pharmacological effects are to inhibit reuptake of either norepinephrine *or* serotonin neurotransmitters are similarly effective although no definitive study has yet compared the efficacy of TCAs with differing pharmacological profiles directly in the same patients.

The response of enuresis to treatment with TCAs has a consistent pattern, characterized by rapidity, degree, duration or persistence, and dose range of response. Tricyclics generally control enuresis within the first week of use if not earlier. When the dose remains constant, there is no cumulative effect. An analysis of response during a four-week double-blind study showed no consistent change in wetting frequency when comparing the first fortnight with the latter, even though the tricyclic dose was increased (Korczyn & Kish, 1979). Rapoport et al. (1980), monitoring tricyclic plasma levels and EEG changes over a 55-day period, in a double-blind crossover design, found all children who sustained a good response showed immediate improvement; there were no good responders with a delayed response.

No study has shown total remission of enuresis in more than 50 percent of subjects and more often only 10 to 20 percent of children completely stop bedwetting (Blackwell & Currah, 1973). Reduction of wetting frequency is the most likely outcome. In several, representative, well-controlled studies of outpatient enuretic children between 51–66 percent will have at least a 50 percent reduction of wetting frequency; the remainder will wet at more than half their previous rate or show no apparent response (Bindelglas et al., 1968; Forsythe & Merrett, 1969; Liederman et al., 1969).

Some children show an initial improvement but then develop tolerance between the second and sixth week of treatment even though plasma tricyclic levels remain stable (Rapoport et al., 1980). Enuresis generally recurs when the tricyclic is discontinued regardless of whether the tricyclic is abruptly withdrawn or tapered off over weeks (Shaffer et al., 1968). Pharmacotherapy with TCAs, therefore, has little influence on the pathophysiology of enuresis. Wetting frequency relapses rapidly and gains may be totally lost within two weeks after discontinuing medication.

Although tricyclic antidepressants are the most common pharmacological agents used to treat enuresis, their mode of action remains obscure. Enuresis that is generally nonepisodic and by no means always associated with psychiatric disorder, cannot be regarded as a "depressive equivalent." Moreover, the antienuretic effect of the TCAs is very rapid in contrast to its delayed antidepressant activity (Rapoport & Mikkelson, 1978); and the drugs are equally effective in enuretics with and without an associated psychiatric disorder (Shaffer et al., 1968; Mikkelson et al., 1980). The TCAs affect sleep architecture, decreasing the number of wakenings, the time spent in rapid eye movement (REM) sleep, and increasing stage four sleep (Baldessarini, 1980). However, enuretic events are not confined to any one sleep stage (see above). Finally, although

TCAs have significant anticholinergic and antiadrenergic properties, tricyclics with no anticholinergic activity (Petersen et al., 1974) are effective in enuresis while primary anticholinergics (Wallace & Forsythe, 1969) and antiadrenergic (Shaffer et al., 1978) agents are not. In summary, none of the known effects of the TCAs, that is, antidepressant activity, their effect on levels of sleep and arousal, or their anticholinergic and adrenolytic effects on bladder function, seem likely to be effective mechanisms.

Other Pharmacological Agents. Other pharmacological agents which have shown some promise in the treatment of enuresis include DDVP, Oxybutynin, chlordiazepoxide and amantadine hydrochloride.

Aladjem et al. (1982) have reported on the results of a double-blind clinical trial of the vasopeptide desamino-D-arginine vasopressin (DDVP). In a double-blind, random assignment study, Aladjem et al. (1982) found 40 percent of treated children ceased wetting completely and a further 40 percent showed a satisfactory response, results that are comparable to those found with the tricyclic antidepressants. However, as with the TCAs, when medication is discounted, most children will wet again at the same rate as before treatment. The treatment did not appear to have been mediated by an antidiuretic effect because urine osmolality was unchanged.

Oxybutynin is an antispasmodic that reduces uninhibited detrusor muscle contraction of the urinary bladder and increases vesical volume at both the first reflex contraction and at the first desire to void (Thompson & Lauvets, 1975; Koff et al., 1978). This antispasmodic activity is not shared by imiprimine (Diokno et al., 1972). In one uncontrolled study of 39 primary enuretics, aged 5–28, who were nightly wetters and not helped by imipramine, weekly wetting decreased to three or less times per week. It may be that oxybutynin is effective in individuals with uninhibited vesical contractions, and a methodologically adequate study is called for.

The minor tranquilizer, chloradiazepoxide, has been reported beneficial in enuresis by Salmon (1973) and Noark (1964). Salmon noted a significant reduction in wetting frequency when administering 10 mg of chlordiazepoxide three times per day in a double-blind placebo controlled study. Werry et al. (1975) found chlorodiazepoxide ineffective in comparison to imipramine.

Amantadine hydrochloride, an antiviral agent and dopamine agonist, has been reported in a four-week pilot study to effectively reduce wetting frequency by 46 percent (Ambrosini & Fried, 1983). This medication was given once or twice daily and the total average dose was approximately 150 mg/day. This response persisted during a two-week follow-up period off medication. Side effects were minimal.

⌐PRACTICAL GUIDE TO ASSESSMENT OF ENURESIS⌐

In assessing the enuretic child the physician should:

1.   Inquire into symptoms suggestive of associated urinary tract infection, such as frequency, urgency and dysuria, unexplained vomiting or fevers. Urine should be examined microscopically and bacteriologically. Simple chemical examination for the presence or absence of albumen is of no value in detecting or excluding urinary infection.

2.   Enquire into other conditions that are often associated with wetting, such as encopresis and educational and behavioral difficulties.

3.   Enquire into factors that might influence the choice of treatment such as:

Sleeping and housing arrangements.

Parental attitudes toward the enuretic child. Where there is a good deal of hostility, resentment, or indifference, it may be difficult to enlist the parents' cooperation and patience without which symptomatic treatment is unlikely to work.

Parental attitudes toward different types of treatment. Some parents view the bell and pad as a punitive device and will be reluctant to use it without explanation and support. Others will have similarly strong feelings about the use of drugs.

4.   Enquire into ways in which the symptom might be self-reinforcing. For example, some children regularly go into their parents' bed at night after they have wet. This may be a source of gratification to either parent or child that they will be reluctant to give up.

5.   Ask the family to collect an objective record of wetting frequency.

Treatment should always be preceded by such a period of observation. During this time the child may wet infrequently, or stop altogether. Observations are recorded on a chart onto which the child places a sticker whenever he has a dry night. If this is displayed for the rest of the family to see, the social rewards for being dry may themselves have a therapeutic effect. During this period of baseline observation—which should last for at last two weeks—various simple interventions, such as lifting or fluid restriction can be assesed. ⁓

PRACTICAL GUIDE TO TREATMENT OF ENURESIS

⁓Alarm Treatment⁓

There is as yet insufficient evidence to advocate the use of daytime training. Every effort, therefore, should be made to treat the child with the bell and pad. This is a safe, relatively brief form of treatment more likely to result in a permanent cure than any other.

Ideally, instruction on how to fit the bell and pad on the patient's bed should be given with both parents and child being present on a clinic bed made up for this purpose. Initial follow-up should take place a few days after the bell and pad have been supplied to deal with any difficulties that the patient or parents might experience. Most families who abandon treatment, do so during this early period.

Many children are not woken by the alarm and parents should be warned of this possibility before treatment is started. Sleeping arrangements may need to be altered so that the parent can hear the bell and waken the child after it has sounded. Booster alarms of differing volumes and tones are available and are often helpful. Some children will turn the bell off before going to bed, and parents should be advised to place it as far from the bed as possible so that it is out of reach. They should also check that the switch is still on before they retire to bed.

Once the bell has rung the child should be taught to get up, turn off the alarm, and empty their bladder. He or she should then be encouraged to assist the parents in removing the wet sheets and replacing them with dry ones. The bell is switched back on, and the child will in almost all cases return to sleep without delay. If a second micturition should occur during sleep, it is reasonable to advise parents not to reset the alarm a third time.

False alarms are a source of irritation to the family and may be due to contact between the clips or metal sheets through movement or else through a worn intervening sheet. Both the top sheet and intervening sheet should be sufficiently large as to be able to be tucked in under the mattress, thus securing the metal sheets in position. Dische (1973) points out that another cause of false alarms may be inadequate laundering of the intervening sheets. Urinary electrolytes previously deposited in a soiled sheet may facilitate conduction by perspiration.

After the child has been dry for two continuous weeks the parent should be told that the chance of later relapse can be reduced by continuing with the bell and pad for a further two weeks, during which time the child is encouraged to drink up to two pints of fluid at night before retiring. In a very few cases this will result in a complete breakdown in continence and the procedure should then be abandoned; however, in most cases continence at night is maintained despite this stress.

Drug Treatment

The bell and pad method can result in a permanent cure in a high proportion of cases and is therefore the treatment of choice. Nevertheless, there are a number of situations in which treatment with imipramine or other TCA is appropriate as, for example, when (1) it is important to obtain an immediate short term effect, as when a child is first seen just before going away on vacation. (2) The wetting has become the focus of aggressive and hostile behavior on the part of parents or siblings. A rapidly effective treatment may serve to reduce the stresses in the family until such a time as the bell and pad can be used. (3) Conditions for the use of the buzzer are likely to improve in the near future; for example, a family living in overcrowded conditions anticipates relocating. (4) The bell and pad have not worked. This should be a conclusion based on experience rather than anticipation. Some apparently disorganized and inadequate families seem able to use the bell and pad successfully under the most difficult circumstances even, for example, when the enuretic child is sharing the bed with a sibling.

Tricyclics are potent pharmacological agents that have a spectrum of anticholinergic and cardiovascular side effects. Since these agents have a significant influence on cardiac electrical conductivity, it is advisable to obtain a baseline EKG and standing and supine blood pressure readings. The length of the PR interval, QRS width, and heart rate must be recorded because these parameters will be the first indices to change indicating cardiotoxicity. If the baseline EKG is beyond normal limits, pharmacotherapy should not be used.

All TCAs are equally effective in enuresis; therefore, the choice of one particular agent is based on the relative frequency of its known side effects. For example, the tertiary amines, imipramine, amytriptyline, doxepin, are more sedating and have greater anticholinergic properties than the secondary amines such as desipramine, nortriptyline, and protriptyline. Anticholinergic side effects include dry mouth and constipation and less commonly nausea, epigastric pain, blurred vision, headaches, and diaphoresis.

Particularly bothersome reactions to TCAs may be orthostatic hypotension (Koehl & Wenzel, 1972) or hypertension (Werry et al., 1975). The systolic–diastolic pressures (standing and supine) should be kept below 145/95. If symptoms of orthostatic hypotension occur, the tricyclic dose should be lowered. Occasionally, chest pains, tremors, and a rare syndrome of cognitive impairment are also noticed. These symptoms are relatively uncommon at the dosages required for enuresis control. The incidence of side effects is dose dependent, and it is greater with higher plasma levels of tricyclics (Rapoport et al., 1980). If treatment is started with a tertiary amine and anticholinergic side effects, blood pressure disturbances, or sedation becomes excessive, changing to a secondary amine or decreasing the dose may alleviate the problem.

Cardiotoxicity is of major concern and this is usually the most serious aspect of tricyclic overdose. Because the effective dose range for tricyclics in enuresis is considerably lower than that needed for its antidepressant action, cardiac electrical conductivity is marginally affected during treatment for bedwetting. It is recommended that EKG parameters be followed if the oral dose is raised to 3 mg/kg/day. It is uncommon that an enuretic child will need such a high dose. The EKG parameters should not exceed the following guidelines: PR interval greater than .21 msec., QRS width greater than 130 percent of baseline, rate greater than 130/minute. If these parameters are exceeded, medication must be lowered. Despramine and nortriptyline tend to induce fewer cardiac conduction abnormalities.

Effective oral doses of tricyclics in enuresis range from 10–125 mg/day; most reports note response in the 10–75 mg/day range. A child can be started on 10–25 mg nightly, the dose being increased every three or four days by 10–25 mg until maximal dryness is obtained. Some enuretic children who are transient responders may exhibit a renewed response if their medication is increased to 125 mg/day but even then might relapse (Rapport et al., 1980). Dose response relationships, nonetheless, are observed when dosages are adjusted to maximize benefit (Rapoport et al., 1980; Jorgensen et al., 1980; Dugas et al., 1980). When using imipramine, a 60 percent or greater decrease in wetting frequency occurs when the combined plasma level of imipramine and desipramine is above 50–60 ng/ml (Rapoport et al., 1980; Jorgensen et al., 1980). Imipramine is metabolized to desipramine so that both tricyclics are in the plasma after an oral dose. One report that used chlorimipramine noted a therapeutic window where maximal benefit occurred between 20–60 ng/ml (Dugas et al., 1980). Monitoring TCA plasma levels does not ensure greater therapeutic efficacy; therefore, the child's response to TCAs can be followed on an empirical basis.

Bed wetting is a self-limiting disorder, although there is no way to predict when dryness will occur. Pharmacotherapy, therefore, should be terminated every three to four months in order to reassess the need for continued treatment. Since wetting returns quite rapidly once medication has stopped, this drug holiday need only last two weeks. Acute discontinuation of a tricyclic, however, can provoke withdrawal emergent symptoms that include vomiting, abdominal cramps, drowsiness, decreased appetite, tearfulness, apathy/withdrawal, headache, and agitation (Law et al., 1980). A flulike illness with gastrointestinal symptoms may also appear. These symptoms will generally abate within one hour after 25 mg of tricyclic by mouth. Withdrawal emergent symptoms are more noticeable if the child is on larger dosages, so tapering withdrawal over one to two weeks in these subjects is desirable.

Overdose of tricyclics is a very serious medical emergency (Callahan, 1979) because of a low therapeutic toxicity ratio. Tricyclic toxicity produces cardiac arrhythmias, seizures, coma, and death. Management should include (1) Ipecac or gastric lavage up to 18 hours after ingestion, and using large volumes for lavage since a significant percentage of the circulating drug is secreted in gastric juices; (2) activated charcoal 50–100 mg in eight ounces of water administered every two hours by mouth or through a nasal gastric tube (use lower amounts for children less than 40 kilograms); (3) EKG monitoring, the width of the QRS complex being the best gauge of cardiotoxicity; (4) intravenous fluids to maintain volume; (5) sodium bicarbonate (1–3 mEq/kg) is recommended to treat tachycardia; (6) seizure precautions; (7) admission to an intensive care unit for a minimum of 24 hours for observation. The following are not helpful: dialysis, since most of the drug is protein bound; induced diuresis; acidification of urine (which increases the risk of cardiac arrhythmias). It needs to be emphasied that intraveneous physostigmine is not an antidote for tricyclic overdose. It may clear the sensorium if anticholinergic blockage is present but will have no effect on cardiotoxicity or seizure propensity.

Management of Day-Time Wetting

It is especially important that the urine of children who wet during the day be examined bacteriologically to exclude the presence of an occult urinary infection.

In some cases daytime wetting is situation specific. The patient is a young, timid child who has started to wet only since starting school, wets only at school and never during weekends or holidays. In these children school anxiety may be the most important factor, the child being reluctant to use the school lavatories or leave the classroom during lessons. In such cases a suggestion to the teacher that she tactfully encourage the child to use the toilet at regular intervals may be all that is needed.

More systematic approaches to treatment include "habit training" and operant reinforcement of appropriate elimination. Habit training requires the child to go regularly and frequently to the toilet at predetermined times. This approach has been widely used with retarded adults and children and the results of various treatment studies are reviewed by Rentfrow and Rentfrow (1969).

Rather than relying on prescheduled toileting, Azrin and Foxx (1971) and Foxx and Azrin (1973) have given their treatment subjects an increased fluid intake and have reinforced appropriate toileting when the urge to pass urine was felt spontaneously by their subjects. By increasing fluid intake they increased the number of responses available for reinforcement and obtained good results with very young and retarded children after short but extremely intensive treatment sessions.

THE TREATMENT OF OTHER SLEEP DISORDERS

DSM-III classifies sleep disorders into four major groups. These are disorders of (1) initiating and maintaining sleep (insomnias), (2) disorders of excess somnolence (hypersomnias), (3) sleep-wake schedule disorders, and (4) dysfunctions associated with sleep, sleep stages, or partial arousals (parasomnias). The syndromes associated with this classification scheme should be separated from sleep-related behavior such as fears of the dark, going to sleep, sleeping alone, and other bedtime rituals. A careful history will clarify diagnosis and indicate the appropriate therapeutic intervention.

Insomnia

It is unusual that a child will present with a primary insomnia, but some adult insomniacs report childhood onset of sleep difficulty (ASDC, 1979). There have been reports that symptoms of insomnia are more frequent in child psychiatric patients (Dixon et al., 1981). In child patients with depression and with Attention Deficit Disorder (ADD), clinical reports of sleep difficulty often correlate poorly with actual polysomnographic evidence of sleep architecture disturbances (Puig-Antich et al., 1982; Greenhill et al., 1983). If a child does present with insomnia as a chief complaint, it is necessary to assess whether the child is ingesting excessive dietary and/or pharmacological stimulants, is experiencing acute anxiety from psychosocial stressors, or has a phobic or separation anxiety disorder or a major depressive disorder (Puig-Antich et al., 1982).

Drug Treatment.   When identifiable stress appears to be the cause of the insomnia, and where this cannot be modified, a low dose of a benzodiazepine such as diazepam (2–15 mg) can be given before bedtime. Other medication includes hydroxyzine (10–50 mg), chloral hydrate (10–20 mg/kg; single dose not to exceed 2 gm) or diphenydramine (1 mg/kg) all of which may be effective in initiating sleep. Sedatives used in these situations should be employed only as temporary aides for the child and parent.

Parasomnias

These include nightmares, sleepwalking, and sleep terrors (pavor nocturnus). Simmonds and Parraga (1982) have recently reported the prevalence of a comprehensive group of sleep disorders and behaviors in school-aged children.

Nightmares are "dream anxiety attacks" and should be distinguished from pavor nocturnus. In the former disorder, the child is woken from sleep by a remembered disturbing dream; however, in the latter condition, the child awakens in an agitated state seemingly confused and disoriented. Additionally, the child with night terrors may exhibit perseverative motor movements and signs of autonomic arousal (e.g., tachycardia, mydriasis, diaphoresis, piloerection). The child is usually unresponsive to calming efforts until the agitation and confusion subside. There is frequently no recall of a frightening dream, and morning amnesia is common. Polysomnographic differences will distinguish nightmares from night terrors. Pavor nocturnus characteristically occurs in deep sleep during stage three and four (non-REM sleep) prior to the transition to REM sleep; nightmares are associated with REM sleep stages (Jacobson, 1968). Individuals are more difficult to arouse from deep sleep stages and if awakened, appear disoriented and confused. Sleep walking also occurs during these deep sleep phases (Guilleminault & Anders, 1976).

The parasomnias can be *treated* with pharmacological agents if the child is endangering himself and/or if the sleep dysfunction is producing excessive anxiety in either parent or child. The treatment of choice for night terrors and sleep walking are the benzodiazapines, which shorten the time spent in stage three and four sleep (Fisher et al., 1973; Harvey, 1980). A 5–15 mg dose of diazepam or its equivalent given before bed should be sufficient. Tricyclics should not be used since these agents may induce nightmares. The parasomnias decrease in frequency with increasing age (Simmonds & Parraga, 1982). The need for continued pharmacotherapy should therefore be reassessed periodically.

Other Syndromes

Other syndromes associated with insomnia or subsequent daytime hypersomnia are sleep apnea, alveolar hypoventilation, nocturnal myoclonus, and "restless legs" syndrome. The prevalence of these disorders has not been ascertained in children, however, some are serious medical problems, are genetically linked (Strohl et al., 1978), and require polysomnographic confirmation in the sleep laboratory (Guilliminaut et al., 1976).

Hypersomnias that are associated with Klein-Levine and Pickwickian syndromes are generally readily identified because of their association with bulimia (Gilbert, 1964) and obesity with respiratory insufficiency (Burwell et al., 1956) respectively. Narcolepsy is a disorder of excessive daytime sleepiness with sleep attacks characteristically beginning with REM period sleep, cateplexy, sleep paralysis, and hypnogogic, and/or hypnopompic hallucinations. The prevalence in the general population is less than .1% and the symptoms are unusual before adolescence (Karacan et al., 1979). Pharmacotherapy is with stimulant medication although tricyclics may also be helpful since they will suppress REM sleep.

Sleep-wake schedule disorders (i.e., circadian shifts) in children are not common although irregular sleep-wake patterns do occur in some infants. This pattern may be reported by the parent as difficulties in settling to bed or as night waking. There is evidence suggesting a positive correlation of these sleep disturbances with environmental stressors, neonatal, and perinatal complications; however, few of these infants have been adequately studied in detail (Anders, 1982). In these clinical situations, therefore, the consulting psychiatrist should obtain a thorough neurodevelopmental and family history before administering any soporiphic medication. In the grade schooler and in the older adolescent, circadian shifts in sleep may be an early sign of an incipient affective or psychotic process.

REFERENCES

Aladjem, M., Wohl, R., Boichis, H., Orda, S., Lotan, D., & Freedman S. (1982). Desmopressin in nocturnal enuresis. *Archives of Disease in Childhood, 57,* 137–140.

Ambrosini, P. J., Fried, J. E. (1983). Pilot study: Amantadine hydrocloride in childhood enuresis. Presented at the American Academy of Child Psychiatry, San Francisco.

American Academy of Pediatrics. (1980). Excretory urography for evaluation of enuresis. *Pediatrics. 65,* 644–645.

Anders, T. F. (1982). Neurophysiological studies of sleep in infants. *Journal of Child Psychology and Psychiatry, 23,* 75–83.

Angel, A. (1935). From the analysis of a bedwetter. *Psychoanalytic Quarterly,* 120–134.

Association of Sleep Disorders Center (ASDC). (1979). Diagnostic Classifications of sleep and arousal disorders (1st ed.) prepared by the Sleep Disorders Classification Committee, H. P. Roffwarg, Chairman. *Sleep, 2,* 50–51.

Azrin, N. H., & Foxx, R. M. (1971). A rapid method of toilet training the institutionalized retarded. *Journal of Applied Behavior Analysis,* 4, 89–99.

Azrin, N. H., Sneed, T. J., & Foxx, R. M. (1974). Dry bed: A rapid method of eliminating bed-wetting (enuresis) of the retarded. *Behavior Research and Therapy, 11,* 427–434.

Azrin, N. H., & Thienes, P. M. (1978). Rapid elimination of enuresis by intensive learning without a conditioning apparatus. *Behavior Research and Therapy, 9,* 342–54.

Bakwin, H. (1961). Enuresis in children. *Journal of Pediatrics, 58,* 806–819.

Bakwin H. (1973). The genetics of bed-wetting. In I. Kolvin, I., R. MacKeith, & R. S. Meadow, (Eds.), *Bladder control and enuresis.* London: Heinemann/SIMP Clinics in Developmental Medicine. Nos. 48–49, pp. 73–77.

Baldessarini, R. J. (1980). Drugs and the treatment of psychiatric disorders. In A. G. Gilman, L. S. Goodman, A. Gilman (Eds.), *The pharmacological basis of therapeutics* (pp. 391–446). New York: Macmillan.

Bindeglas, P. M., Dee, G. H., & Enos, F. A. (1968). Medical and psychosocial factors in enuretic children treated with imipramine hydrochloride. *American Journal of Psychiatry, 124,* 1107–1112.

Blackwell, B., & Currah, J. (1973). The psychopharmacology of nocturnal enuresis. In I. Kolvin, R. MacKeith, & S. R. Meadow (Eds.), *Bladder control and enuresis.* London: Heinemann/SIMP Clinics in *Developmental* Medicine, Nos. 48/49, pp. 231–257.

Burwell, C. S., Robin, E. G., Whaley, R. D., & Bickelmann, H. G. (1956). Extreme obesity associated with alveolar hypoventilation—A Pickwickian syndrome. *American Journal of Medicine, 21,* 811–818.

Boon, F. (1981). Nocturnal enuresis and psychotropic drugs. Letter to the *American Journal of Psychiatry, 138,* 538.

Buttarazzi, P. J. (1977). Oxybutynin chloride (Ditropan) in enuresis. *Journal of Urology, 118,* 46.

Callahan, M. (1979). Tricyclic antidepressant overdose. *JACEP, 8,* 413–425.

DeLeon G., & Mandell W. (1966). A comparison of conditioning and psychotherapy in the treatment of enuresis. *Journal of Clinical Psychology, 22,* 326–330.

Diokno, A. C., Hyndman, C. W., Hardy, D. A., & Lapides, J. (1972). Comparison of action of imipramine (Tofranil) and propantheline (Probanthine) on detrussor contraction. *Journal of Urology, 107,* 42–43.

Dische, S. (1973). Treatment of enuresis with an enuresis alarm. In I. Kolvin, R. MacKeith, & S. R. Meadow, (Eds.), *Bladder control and enuresis.* London: Heinemann/SIMP Clinics in Developmental Medicine, Nos. 48/49, pp. 211–230.

Dische, S., Yule, W., Corbett, J. & Hand, D. (1983). Childhood nocturnal enuresis: Factors associated with outcome of treatment with an enuresis alarm. *Developmental Medicine and Child Neurology, 25,* 67–81.

Dixon, K. N., Monroe, L. J., & Jakim, S. (1981). Insomniac children, *Sleep, 4,* 313–318.

Dodge, W. F., West, E. F., Bridgforth, M. S., & Travis, L. B. (1970). Nocturnal enuresis in 6–10-year-old children. *American Journal of Disability in Children, 120,* 32–35.

Douglas, J. W. B. (1973). Early disturbing events and later enuresis. In I. Kolvin, R. Mac-Keith, & S. R. Meadow. (Eds.), *Bladder control and enuresis.* London: Heinemann/SIMP Clinics in Developmental Medicine Nos. 48/49, 109–117.

Dugas, M., Zarifian, E., Leheuzey, M. F., Rovei, V., Duran, G., Morselli, P. (1980). Preliminary observations of the significance of monitoring tricyclic antidepressant plasma levels in the pediatric patient. *Therapeutic Drug Monitoring,* 307–314.

Essen, J., & Peckham, C. (1976). Noctural Enuresis in childhood. *Developmental Medicine and Child Neurogy, 18,* 577–89.

Felthous, A.R., & Bernhard H. (1978). Enuresis, firesetting, and cruelty to animals: The significance of two thirds of this triad. *Journal of Forensic Sciences, 45,* 240–246.

Fielding, D. (1980). The response of day and night wetting children and children who wet only at night to retention control training and the enuresis alarm. *Behavior Research and Therapy, 18,* 305–317.

Finley, W. W., Besserman, R. L., Clapp, R. K., & Finley P. (1973). The effect of continuous, intermittent and placebo reinforcement on the effectiveness of the conditioning treatment for enuresis nocturna. *Behavior Research and Therapy, 11,* 289–297.

Finley, W. W., & Wansley, R. A. (1977). Auditory intensity as a variable in the conditioning treatment of enuresis nocturna. *Behavior Research and Therapy, 15,* 181–185.

Fischer, C., Kahn, E., Edwards, A., & David, D. M. (1973). A psychophysiological study of nightmares and night terrors: The suppression of stage 4 night terrors with diazepama. *Archives of General Psychiatry, 28,* 252–259.

Forsythe, W. I., & Merrett, J. D. (1969). A controlled trial of imipramine (Tofranil) and nortriptyline (Allergon) in the treatment of enuresis. *British Journal of Clinical Practice, 23,* 210–215.

Forsythe, W. I., & Redmond, A. (1974). Enuresis and spontaneous cure rate. A stydy of 1129 enuretics. *Archives of Diseases in Childhood, 49,* 259–263.

Foxx, R. M., & Azrin, N. H. (1973). Dry pants. A rapid method of toilet training children. *Behavior Research and Therapy, 11,* 435–442.

Fritz, G. K., & Anders, T. F. (1979). Enuresis: The clinical application of an etiologically-based classification system. *Child Psychiatry and Human Development, 10,* 103–113.

Gilbert, G. J. (1964). Periodic hypersomnia and bulimia. The Klein-Levine syndrome. *Neurology, 14,* 844–850.

Greenhill, L., Puig-Antich, J., Goetz, R., Hanlon, C., & Davies, M. (1983). Sleep architecture and REM sleep measures in prepubertal children with attention deficit disorder with hyperactivity. *Sleep, 6,* 91–101.

Guilleminault, C., & Anders, T. (1976). Sleep disorders in children. In I. Schulman (Ed.). *Advances in pediatrics,* Vol. 22. Chicago: Yearbook Medical Publishers, pp. 151–174.

Guilleminault, C., Eldridge, F. L., Simmon, S., Dement, W. C. J. (1976). Sleep apnea in eight children. *Pediatrics, 58,* 23–31.

Hagglund, T. B. (1965). Enuretic children treated on fluid restriction or forced drinks. A clinical and cystometric study. *Annales Paediatriae Fenniae, 11,* 84–90.

Hallgren, B. (1956). Enuresis. A study with reference to certain physical, mental and social factors possibly associated with enuresis. *Acta Psychiatrica et Neurologica Scandinavica, 31,* 405–436.

Hallgren, B. (1960). Nocturnal enuresis in twins. *Acta Psychiatrica et Neurologica Scandinavica, 35,* 73–90.

Hansen, G. D. (1979). Enuresis control through fading, escape, and avoidance training. *Journal of Applied Behavior Analysis, 12,* 303–307.

Harris, L. S. (1977). Bladder training and enuresis. *Behavior Research and Therapy, 15,* 485–490.

Harvey, S. C. (1980). Hypnotices and sedatives. In A. G. Gilman, L. S. Goodman, & A. Gilman (Eds.), *The pharmacological basis of therapeutics* (pp. 339–375). New York: Macmillan.

Jacobson, A., & Kaler, J. D. (1968). Clinical and electrophysiological correlation or sleep disorders in children. In A. Kales (Ed.), *Sleep physiology and pathology* (pp. 109–118). Philadelphia: J. B. Lippincott.

Janknegt, R. A., Moonen, W. A., & Schrienemechars, L. M. H. (1979). Transsection of the bladder as a method of treatment in adult enuresis nocturna. *British Journal of Urology, 51,* 275–277.

Johnston, J. H., Koff, S. A., & Glassberg, K. I. (1978). The pseudo-obstructed bladder in enuretic children. *British Journal of Urology, 550,* 505–510.

Jones, B., Gerrard, J. W., Shokeir, M. K., & Houston, C. S. (1972). Recurrent urinary infection in girls: Relation to enuresis. *Canadian Medical Association Journal, 106,* 127–130.

Jorgensen, O. S., Lober, M., Christiansen, J., & Gram, L. F. (1980). *Clinical Pharmacokinetics, 5,* 386–393.

Kaffman, M., & Elizur, E. (1977). Infants who become enuretics. A longitudinal study of 161 kibbutz children. *Monogr. Soc. Res. in Child. Dev., 42,* (2), 170.

Karacan, I., Moore C. A., & Williams, R. L. (1979). The narcoleptic syndrome. *Psychiatric Annals, 9,* 377–381.

Koehl, G. W., & Wenzel, J. E. (1972). Severe postural hypotension due to imipramine therapy. *Pediatrics, 47,* 132–134.

Koff, S. A., Lapides, J., & Piazza, D. H. (1978). Uninhibited bladder in children: Causes for urinary obstruction infection and reflux. In (J. Hodson & P. Kinkaid-Smith (Eds.), *Reflux nephropathy* (pp. 161–170), New York: Masson.

Kolvin, I., Taunch, J., Currah, J., Garside, M. F., Nolan, J., & Shaw, W. B. (1972). Enuresis: A descriptive analysis and a controlled trial. *Developmental Medicine and Child Neurology, 14,* 715–726.

Korczyn, A. D., & Kish, I. (1979). The mechanism of imipramine in enuresis nocturna. *J. Clinical and Experimental Pharmacology and Physiology, 6,* 31–35.

Kunin, C. M., Zacha, E., & Paquin, A. J., Jr. (1962). Urinary tract infections in school children: An epidemiologic, clinical and laboratory study. *New England Journal of Medicine, 266,* 1287–1296.

Kunin, S. A., Limbert, D. J., Platzker, A. C., & McGinley, J. (1970). The efficacy of imipramine in the management of enuresis. *Journal of Urology, 104,* 621–625.

Kvarstein, B., & Mathison, W. (1981). Sigmoidocystoplasty in adults with enuresis. *Surgery, Gynecology and Obstetrics, 153,* 65–66.

Law, W., Petti, T. A., Kazdin, A. E. (1981). Withdrawal symptoms after graduation cessartion of imipramine in children. *American Journal of Psychiatry, 138*, 647–650.

Leiderman, P. C., Wasserman, D. H., Leiderman, V. R. (1969). Desipramine in the treatment of enuresis. *Journal of Urology, 101*, 314–316.

Lickorish, J. R. (1964). One hundred enuretics. *Journal of Psychosomatic Research, 7*, 263–267.

Lovibond, S. H. (1964). *Conditioning and enuresis.* Oxford: Pergamon.

McKendry, J. B. J., & Stuart, D. A. (1974). Enuresis. *Pediatric Clinics of North America, 21*, 1019–1028.

Mahoney, D. T. (1971). Studies of enuresis: I. Incidence of obstructive lesions and pathophysiology and enuresis. *Journal of Urology, 106*, 951–958.

Mattsson, J. L., & Ollendick, T. H. (1977). Issues in training normal children. *Behavior Therapy, 8*, 549–553.

Meadow, S. R., White R. H. R., & Johnson, N. M. (1969). Prevalence of symptomless urinary tract disease in Birmingham school children. *British Medical Journal, 3*, 81–84.

Michaels, J. J. (1961). Enuresis in murderous aggressive children and adolescents. *Archives of General Psychiatry, 5*, 490–493.

Mikkelson, E. J., Rapoport, J. L., and Nee, L., Gruenau, C., Mendelson, W., & Gillin, J. C. (1980). Childhood enuresis I. Sleep patterns and psychopathology. *Archives of General Psychiatry, 37*, 1139–1145.

Miller, F. J. W., Court, S. D. M., Walton, W. S., & Knox, E. G. (1960). *Growing up in Newcastle-upon-Tyne.* London: Oxford, University Press.

Miller, P. M. (1973). An experimental analysis in retention control training in the treatment of nocturnal enuresis in two institutionalized adolescents. *Behavior Therapy, 4*, 288–294.

Milner, G., & Hills, N. F. (1968). A double-blind assessment of antidepressants in the treatment of 212 enuretic patients. *Medical Journal of Australia, 1*, 943–947.

Mowrer O. H., & Mowrer, W. M. (1938). Enuresis: A method for its study and treatment. *American Journal of Othropsychiatry, 8*, 436–459.

Nettelbeck, T., & Langeluddecke, P. (1979). *Behavior Research and Therapy, 17*, 403–404.

Noark, C. H. (1964). Enuresis nocturna: A long term study of 44 children treated with imipramine hydrochlorid (Tofranil) and other drugs. *Medical Journal of Australia, 1*, 191–192.

Nurnberg, H. G., & Ambrosini, P. J. (1979). Urinary incontenence in patients receiving neuroleptics. *Journal of Clinical Psychiatry, 40*, 271–274.

Oppel, W. C., Harper, P. A., & Rider, R. V. (1968). Social, psychological and neurological factors associated with enuresis. *Pediatrics, 42*, 627–641.

Paschalis, A. P., Kimmel, H. D., & Kimmel, E. (1972). Further study of diurnal instrumental conditioning in the treatment of enuresis nocturna. *Journal of Behavior Therapy and Experimental Psychiatry, 3*, 253–256.

Petersen, K. E., Anderson, O. O., & Hansen, T. (1973). The mode of action of imipramine and related drugs and their value in the treatment of different categories of enuresis nocturna. *Acta Paed. Scand.*, Supplement, *236*, 63–64.

Petersen, K. E., Anderson, O. O., Hansen, T. (1974). Mode of action and relative value of imipramine and similar drugs in the treatment of nocturnal enuresis. *European Journal of Clinical Pharmacology, 7*, 187–194.

Pfaundler, M. (1904). Demonstration eines Apparetes zur selbstatig Signalisierung statt-gehabter Bettnassung. *Verhandlungen der Gesellschuft Kinde. Heilkd. 21*, 219–220.

Poussaint, A. F., Koegler, R. R., & Riehl, J. L. (1967). Enuresis, epilepsy, and the EEG. *American Journal of Psychiatry, 123*, 1294–1295.

Puig-Antich, J., Goetz, R., Hanlon, C., Davies, M., Thompson, J., Chambers, W. J., Tabraizi, M. A., Weitzman, E. D. (1982). Sleep architecture and REM sleep measures in prepubertal children with major depression. *Archives of General Psychiatry, 39*, 932–939.

Rapoport, J. L., Mikkelsen, E. J., Zavardil, A., et al. (1980) Childhood enuresis II. Psychopathology, tricylic concentration in plasma, and anti-enuretic effect. *Archives of General Psychiatry, 37*, 1146–1152.

Redman, J. E., & Seibert, J. J. (1979). Urographic evaluation of the enuretic child. *Journal of Urology, 122*, 699–801.

Rentfrow, R. K., & Rentfrow, D. K. (1969). Studies related to toilet training of the mentally retarded. *American Journal of Occupational Therapy, 23*, 425–430.

Roberts, K. E., & Schoellkopf, J. A. (1951). Eating, sleeping, and elimination practices in a group of 2-1/2 year olds. *American Journal of Diseases of Children, 82*, 144–152.

Rutter, M. L., Yule, W., & Graham, P. J. (1973). Enuresis and behavioral deviance: Some epidemiological considerations. In I. Kolvin, R. MacKeith, & S. R. Meadow (Eds.), *Bladder control and enuresis*. London: SIMP/Heinemann Clinics in Developmental Medicine, Nos. 48/49, pp. 137–147.

Salmon, M. A. (1973). The concept of day-time treatment for primary nocturnal enuresis. In I. Kolvin, R. MacKeith, & S. R. Meadow (Eds.), *Bladder control and enuresis* Philadelphia: J. B. Lippincott. Pp. 189–194.

Shaffer D. (1973). The association between enuresis and psychiatric disorder in childhood. (pp. 118–136). S.I.M.P. Heinemann, London. In I. Kolvin, R. MacKeith, & S. R. Meadow (Eds.), *Bladder control and enuresis*. London: SIMP/Heinemann Clinics in Developmental Medicine, No. 1, pp. 48–49.

Shaffer, D. (1985) Enuresis. In M. Rutter & L. Hersov (Eds.), *Child psychiatry: Modern approaches* (2nd ed.) Oxford: Blackwell.

Shaffer, D., Costello, A. J., & Hill, J. D. (1968). Control of enuresis with imipramine. *Archives of Diseases in Childhood, 43*, 665–671.

Shaffer, D., Gardner, A., & Hedge, B. (1985). Behavior and bladder disturbance in enuretics: The rational classification of a common disorder. *Developmental Medicine and Child Neurology.*

Shaffer, D., Hedge, B., & Stephenson, J. D. (1978). Trial of an alpha-adrenolytic drug (Indoramin) for noctural enuresis. *Developmental Medicine and Child Neurology, 20*, 183–188.

Shenoy, R. S. (1980). Nocturnal enuresis caused by psychotropic drugs. American Journal of Psychiatry, 137, 739–740.

Simmonds, J. F., & Parraga, H. (1982). Prevalence of sleep disorders and sleep behaviors in children and adolescents. *Journal of the American Academy of Child Psychiatry, 21*, 383–388.

Smith, E. H., & Gonzalez, R. (1967). Nortriptyline hydrochloride in the treatment of enuresis in mentally retarded boys. *American Journal of Mental Deficiency, 71*, 825–827.

Smith, D. R. (1969). Critique of the concept of vesical neck obstruction in children. *Journal of the American Medical Association, 207*, 1686–1692.

Strohl, K. P., Saunders, N. A., Feldman, N. T., & Hallett, M. (1978). Obstructive sleep apnea in family members. *New England Journal of Medicine, 299,* 969–973.

Smith, L. J. (1981). Training severely and profoundly mentally handicap nocturnal in family members. *New England Journal of Medicine, 299,* 969–973.

Starfield, S. B. (1967). Functional bladder capacity in enuretic and non-enuretic children. *Journal of Pediatrics, 70,* 777–781.

Stedman, J. M. (1972). The extension of the Kimmel treatment method for enuresis to an adolescent: A case report. *Journal of Behavior Therapy and Experimental Psychiatry, 3,* 307–309.

Strohl, K. P., Saunders, N. A., Feldman, N. T., & Hallett, M. (1978). Obstructive sleep apnea in family members. *New England Journal of Medicine, 299,* 969–973.

Thompson, I. M., & Lauvetz, R. (1976). Oxybutynin in bladder spasm, neurogenic bladder and enuresis, *Urology, 8,* 452–454.

Torrens, M., & Hald, T. (1979). Bladder denevation procedures. *Urological Clinics of North America, 6,* 283–293.

Troup, C. W., & Hodgson, N. B. (1971). Nocturnal functional bladder capacity in enuretic children. *Journal of Urology, 105,* 129–130.

Turner, R. K. (1973). Conditioning, treatment of nocturnal enuresis: Present studies. In I. Kolvin, R. MacKeith, & S. R. Meadow (Eds.), *Bladder control and enuresis.* London: Heinemann/SIMP Clinics in Developmental Medicine, Nos. 48/49, pp. 195–210.

VanPutten, T., Malkin, M. D., & Weiss, M. S. (1972). Phenothiozine induced stress incontinence. *Journal of Urology, 109,* 625–626.

Wallace, I. R., & Forsythe, W. I. (1969). The treatment of enuresis. A controlled clinical trial of propoantheline, propantheline and phenobarbitone, and placebo. *British Journal of Clinical Practice, 23,* 207–210.

Werry, J. S., Aman, M. G., Dowrick, M. A., & Lampen, E. L. (1977). Imipramine and chlordiazepoxide inenuresis. *Psychopharmacology Bulletin, 13,* 38–39.

Werry, J. S., Dowrick, P. W., Lampen, E. L., & Vamos, M. J. (1975). Imipramine in enuresis—psychological and physiological effects. *Journal of Child Psychology and Psychiatry, 16,* 289–300.

Young, G. C., & Morgan, R. T. T. (1972). Overlearning in the conditioning treatment of enuresis. *Behavior Research and Therapy, 10,* 147–151.

Young, G. C., & Morgan, R. T. T. (1973). Rapidity of response to the treatment of enuresis. *Developmental Medicine and Child Neurology, 15,* 488–496.

Young, G. C., & Turner, R. K. (1965). C. N. S. stimulant drugs and conditioning treatment of nocturnal enuresis. *Behavior Research and Therapy, 3,* 93–101.

Conclusion

Summary and Prospect

JERRY M. WIENER, M.D.

As reflected in this textbook on the psychopharmacology of childhood disorders and by the research and clinical issues presented in these chapters, the field of child psychiatry is fully participant in the so-called biological revolution that has dominated psychiatry since the 1950s. Although the use of stimulants in heterogeneous groups of childhood disorders began with Bradley's work in the 1930s, it was the discovery of phenothiazine efficacy for psychosis just over 30 years ago that marks the beginnings of a scientific study of the neurobiology of psychiatric disorders. For the first several years drugs were tried first in adult-diagnosed disorders and then applied to children, either with similar symptoms (and therefore presumably or hopefully with the same illness) or with the same diagnosis even if the illness itself seemed quite different (e.g., DSM-II adult and childhood schizophrenia). With a few exceptions—the study and treatment of "hyperactivity" and the application of antidepressants for enuresis—child psychiatry psychopharmacology research lurched in the wake of its adult conterpart with, if anything, greater methodological limitations and a more limited diagnostic classification.

How much this scenario has changed is exemplified in this volume, and indeed many of the most important changes are a reflection of the contributions made by several of the chapter authors, who represent a combination of the first and second generations of child psychiatry research in psychopharmacology.

This volume is organized into two major sections: first, one dealing with basic and broader issues of historical development (Chapter 1), the ever-important consideration of the interaction of drugs with the developmental process itself (Chapter 2), and a comprehensively scholarly presentation of methodological issues (and pitfalls), and assessment instruments useful in research and clinical practice (Chapter 3); and second, the section on clinical psychopharmacology, organized according to DSM-III diagnostic categories rather than (as a pharmacology text) by type of drug. While these chapters contain a true wealth of material related to theoretical and research issues, they are intended more than anything for the clinician treating childhood psychiatric disorders, and focus on issues of diagnosis and clinical usage relevant to clinical practice.

Several themes recur in these chapters.

1. Both the significant advantages and serious clinical limitations represented by the development during the 1970s and adoption in 1980 of DSM-III. For the first time more homogeneous groupings of children could be reliably identified and studied under carefully controlled conditions. This is necessary to establish drug efficacy and at the same time

test the validity and refine the diagnostic assessment. Assessment is repeatedly emphasized, with rigid adherence to DSM-III criteria for research studies, and a more flexible application for clinical usage.

2. With few exceptions, a conservative approach is still indicated for the use of drugs in most categories of childhood disorders. It is worth noting that in no category of childhood disorder for which drugs are effective is etiology yet established. Much more is now known about the neurobiology of the brain, and information is rapidly accumulating about genetic, neurotransmitter, neuroendocrine, and neurophysiologic aspects of many disorders. But little is yet known about long term effects on development of drug use begun in childhood; there is reason for concern about the serious adverse effets of many medications, again both of themselves and on the developmental process, and little is known, for example, about how drugs may influence or alter important ego-developmental tasks related to mastery, cognition, drive and affect states. It should be mentioned that a conservative approach refers to the decision to use medication, the expectations and cost–benefit ratio of medication and the duration of use, but not to the use of therapeutically ineffective low doses and/or for too brief a period for a valid trial. These latter usages reflect inexperience rather than conservative management.

3. Related to the above is an emphasis on the importance of known adverse effects in determining the benefit–risk ratio and the duration of treatment. There is a reemphasis on both the direct observation and subjective experience of the child in monitoring potentially serious effects and/or those which compromise compliance.

4. Other time-tested, nonbiological interventions are consistently emphasized, often as the initial treatment approach. These include traditional psychotherapies, family interventions, special educational and remedial programs, and behavioral therapies. This perspective respects the larger totality of the child's overall developmental needs within the family and school, and views medication as only part of a comprehensive treatment plan.

SUMMARY OF CHAPTERS

Historical Overview

From its beginnings with the use of Benzedrine sulfate in the 1930s, research and usage for each class of drugs is reviewed decade by decade, with special emphasis on the period 1970–1984. One can trace the gradual definition of the condition now classified in DSM-III as Attention Deficit Disorder (ADD), with and (still controversial) without hyperactivity, as a function of its clinical response first to stimulant medication and then to the tricyclic antidepressants (TCAs). Each category of drugs —antipsychotics, stimulants, antidepressants, and antimanic—is presented from the year of its introduction and reviewed according to the accumulation of studies establishing rationale, indications, clinical usage, adverse affects, and degrees of efficacy. The period from 1970–1984 is given particular emphasis because it marks: (1) the introduction of reasonably reliable diagnostic criteria, allowing for more homogeneous groupings of carefully diagnosed subject groups; (2) a growing critical number of research scientists in childhood psychopharmacology, increasingly able to apply acceptable methodologies and sophisticated statistical analysis; (3) the development of standardized assessment instruments and observational techniques; (4) an increasing concern for and attention to the short and long term adverse affects of drugs.

It is during this period from 1970 that one can identify the emergence of a more mature and truly scientific psychopharmacology for childhood and adolescent disorders, with extensive studies of: (1) affective disorders and their treatment with TCAs, lithium, and newer drugs such as carbamazapine; (2) the indications, effects, and dosage rationale for the stimulant medications; (3) the use of antipsychotics in autism, schizophrenia in children, Tourette's Syndrome and more recently in conduct-disordered children; and (4) the use of lithium in bipolar disorders and conduct disorders.

Developmental Considerations

This chapter is largely theoretical and conceptual, raising many important questions to which complete answers are not available, but that must be considered in any decision to use medication in a still growing and developing child. Here the child psychiatrist will find a discussion of medication usage in relationship to developmental theory as the framework for the clinician's role, goals, and professional identity. It is a particularly balanced presentation of the importance of combining knowledge and theory about biological, intrapsychic, and sociocultural influences in reaching a sophisticated clinical judgment about the use of drugs in a given individual child.

Methodologic and Assessment Issues

This chapter is a thorough and systematic review of research study design, emphasizing the importance of fitting method to the nature of the question, the type of data best gathered, and the characteristics of the study population. Here the reader will find a definition and discussion of the number and types of variables that must be considered, and a review of assessment instruments and measurements available for both research and clinical usage. An understanding of the issues discussed in this chapter is necessary certainly to do research, more broadly to be able to evaluate the research literature, and finally for effective and informed clinical practice.

Schizophrenic Disorders and Pervasive Developmental Disorders: Infantile Autism

This chapter initiates the clinical usage section. It begins with a thorough discussion of the concept of these disorders and their definition by current diagnostic criteria, followed by a thorough review of the pertinent literature and clinical usage according to the most recent available studies. Particular attention is given to the description of and concerns about both short and long term effects of antipsychotic (dopaminergic blocking) agents, especially the withdrawal-emergence syndrome (WES), and the risks for tardive dyskinesia in children. The author emphasizes the overall limitations of any medication yet available in altering the major deficits of pervasive early-onset disorders such as infantile autism, and the directions in which research is moving. The specific benefits of a drug such as haloperidol, both alone and in combination with behavioral approaches, are identified in the treatment of infantile autism. In addition the current status of fenfluramine as a possibly more effective treatment for infantile autism is presented.

Affective Disorders

Perhaps no issue in child psychiatry in the past 10–15 years has been so extensively debated and carefully studied as that of affective disorders in childhood. From an initial period in which the condition itself was considered for theoretical reasons not to exist in children, there is now a concensus (although not unanimous agreement) that major depressive disorder, analogous to that in adults as diagnosed by DSM-III criteria, does indeed afflict children. Furthermore, there has been much study given to a genetically related broader concept of depression that explores relationships with such diverse conditions as ADD, conduct disorders, anorexia nervosa, and separation anxiety disorders. While the diagnosis of major depression in childhood is generally accepted, the indications for and efficacy of different treatments is currently uncertain and controversial. A large number of older studies with various methodological limitations report efficacy for TCAs (imipramine) and monoamine oxidase inhibitors. More recent and methodologically sound studies either fail to document the superiority of TCAs over placebo or report mixed results. Answers for these surprising findings may be found in more careful studies of the relationship between total TCA plasma levels and antidepressant response. Furthermore, current studies also suggest that to the degree effective for the vegetative, mood, and cognitive symptoms, medication is limited in effecting important relationship, self-concept, and self-esteem issues. It is clear that a strong research base exists that has explored assessment, diagnostic, biological, genetic and treatment issues, and from which much further research must be done.

Attention Deficit Disorders (ADD)

Drug treatment of the diagnostic antecedants of this disorder began in the 1930s and still continues. There has been a progressive evolution of diagnostic terms related to etiologic and/or descriptive concepts—brain damage, brain dysfunction, hyperactivity, focusing on the attentional disorder as central. Both stimulant and TCA medication are unquestionably effective in modifying many of the core symptoms of this disorder, and a concensus has emerged for the use of stimulants. Short term effects are well known; the longer term benefits and adverse effects are still uncertain. Initially simply prescribed on an empirical basis, dosage is now on a mg/kg/dose regimen, and much more is known about the pharmacokinetics for accurate prescribing. At the same time uncertainty remains about the relationships among dosage, plasma level, and response, and there are still questions about the specificity of different symptom responses at different dosage levels.

Pharmacological treatment of ADD (with hyperactivity) is the best described and most extensively studied treatment among child psychiatric disorders. It is safe and effective. Clinical experience and sophistication is required for its proper use within an overall treatment program. Drugs alone always are insufficient.

Anxiety Disorders

In contrast to many other areas, the issue of anxiety disorders has received relatively little attention. Among the most common of childhood symptoms and disorders, it is perhaps the least studied and understood, especially from a biological and pharmacological point of view. Anxiety itself is ubiquitous, not pathological. Anxiety related to the normal pressures of developmental conflicts and stage transitions must be differentiated from pathological anxiety. Despite the impression of wide usage, it is surprising if not amazing that we have few if any methodologically acceptable studies of medication effects in anxiety disorders. The lone exception may be studies done in the early 1970s on the use of TCAs in separation anxiety disorders with school phobia presentation. No controlled studies exist on the efficacy of the benzodiazepines in anxiety disorders in children. Much basic work remains to be done.

Stereotyped Movement Disorders and Tourette's Syndrome

For several reasons this topic has received increasing attention in the past several years. First, it is in itself an intriguing and often very serious disorder. Second, effective drug treatment with haloperidol, pimozide, and clonidine is available, albeit with concern about the adverse effects of long term treatment. Third, Tourette's Syndrome has been tentatively linked to a variety of other disorders—simple and complex chronic tic syndromes and Attention Deficit Disorder—both broadening the concept of the disorder and raising further interesting and important questions about pathophysiology and mechanisms of drug action.

Tourette's Syndrome and related disorders are discussed within a comprehensive, holistic, biopsychosocial framework. The diagnostic criteria and varieties of clinical presentations and clinical course are described in detail, along with theories of etiology and approaches to treatment. While the use of medication is thoroughly covered, the discussion emphasizes the importance of developmental, educational, and psychosocial considerations as critical elements in every treatment plan.

Conduct Disorders

That this topic remains largely terra incognita in child psychiatry is reflected in the careful review and presentation of the many theoretical, diagnostic, and treatment perspectives applied by the field. This category (with particular emphasis on the aggressive and unsocialized subtypes) is perhaps the least satisfactory and/or least helpful major diagnostic category for childhood disorders. Likewise, its treatment by any method—pharmacological, psychotherapeutic, milieu, and behavioral—remains controversial, with little established on the basis of acceptable data.

What is known and what is conjectured are reviewed. The relationship of conduct disorders to a variety of etiological possibilities and other

342 Summary and Prospect

disorders is examined, including genetic, familial, and constitutional factors, developmental disturbances, early deprivation, maladaptive learning, socioeconomic factors, and the overlap between conduct disorders and such conditions as seizure disorders, depression, attention deficit disorder, and other neurological impairment.

The literature is reviewed on each class of drugs used in the treatment of conduct disorders—including neuroleptics, lithium, anticonvulsants, and miscellaneous others, particularly the antidepressants. Their possible range of efficacy or lack thereof, and their adverse effects are considered. Overall, the point is made that these children and their families will require behavioral and psychosocial treatments no matter how helpful medication may be.

Eating Disorders

Anorexia nervosa, bulimia, and combinations of the two are increasing in incidence, perhaps related to a sociocultural idealization of thinness, especially for women. The perplexing nature of these disorders, their association with a variety of DSM-III Axis I and Axis II diagnoses, and their often chronic course, along with uncertainty about etiology, have all combined to lead to the use of a number of different medications for treatment. Antipsychotic, anticonvulsant, antihistaminic, antimanic, and antianxiety agents have all been tried without significant documented success. More recently attention has been focused on the relationship (familial and clinical) between eating disorders and depression. This has led to studies on the use of antidepressants, both tricyclics and monoamine oxidase inhibitors. So far antidepressant medication holds more promise for bulimia than for anorexia nervosa.

Enuresis and Sleep Disorders

The characteristics, prevalence, and natural history of bed wetting lead into questions about etiological factors and treatment approaches. The authors review the range of etiological possibilities—genetic, obstructive (organic), developmental, learned behavior, drug-induced, and relationship to psychiatric disorder—recognizing that there is no one disorder or cause. The use and limitations of TCA medication are presented, as well as studies of a vasopressin compound, antispasmodics, benzodiazepines, and dopamine agonists. Although TCA medication is well established as an effective treatment, albeit with long term limitations, a conservative conditioning-type regimen is recommended for most cases before medication is indicated. As to other sleep disorders, primary insomnia is rare in children. The parasomnias of night terrors and sleep walking can be identified and usually, when indicated, effectively treated with benzodiazepines.

PROSPECTS FOR THE FUTURE

At the risk of redundancy, it is clear that significant advances have been made and that much opportunity exists for further research.

1.   While DSM-III has allowed for a greater cohesion and consistency in the diagnosis and study of more reliable and homogeneous subject groups, it is limited in its usefulness for childhood disorders. The prospect is for an improvement in DSM-IV, leading to further reciprocal advances between diagnosis and medication specificity and efficacy.

2.   Certainly much more remains to be learned about the relationship between mechanism and site of action of drugs and aspects of etiology. The two are surely not the same, but will continue to inform each other in future research.

3.   Badly needed is a better understanding of the relationship between biological and psychotherapeutic/psychosocial treatment approaches, as well as their comparative and combined efficacies. This type of study is only in its early stages with adult disorders, and/methodologically acceptable designs to answer these questions are even more difficult to come by in studying childhood disorders. Yet the work must be done.

4.   Medication is increasingly established on a scientific basis as a treatment for many important childhood disorders and as a possibility for several others. Hopefully all child psychiatrists will become increasingly knowledgeable and clinically comptetent in the targeted use of medication and, as important, in the consideration and management of acute and longer term adverse effects.

The dangers are overusage and underdosage. The promise is that increasingly children will be prescribed specifically indicated medication in appropriate doses for a sufficient time to achieve their maximum developmental potential, and that to do this it will be understood that almost without exception medication will be only one component of a more comprehensive treatment plan.

Author Index

Subject Index

365

Benadryl, 11, 15. *See also*
Diphenhydramine
Benzedrine, 4–8, 12, 36
Benzodiazepines, 189
ADDH, 189
anorexia nervosa, 299
anxiety disorders, 210–211
Benztropine, 231
Bipolar affective disorders, 154–155
lithium, 33
Brief Psychiatric Rating Scale, 118
Bulimia, 290–300
and affective disorders, 291–293
anticonvulsants, 297–298
antidepressants, 293–295
chlorpromazine, 298–299
diagnosis, 290–291
drug treatment, 293–300
imipramine, 294
phenelzine, 294
phenothiazines, 298–299
tranylcypromine, 294
Bulimia nervosa, 292, 294
Mianserin, 294

Caffeine, in ADDH, 182–183
Captodiamine, 12
Carbamazepine, 36, 171
anorexia nervosa, 297–298
conduct disorders, 272–274
Cerebral palsy, 10–11
Chloral hydrate, 324
Chlordiazepoxide, 21, 158, 210, 231, 317
separation anxiety disorder, 208
Chlorpromazine, 9–12, 15, 17, 18–20, 26,
29, 58, 141
anorexia nervosa, 298–299
bulimia, 298–299
cerebral palsy, 10–11
combination with methylphenidate,
135
emotional disturbances, 10
infantile autism, 130
mental retardation, 10
plasma levels, 98
primary behavior disorder, 11
schizophrenic disorders, childhood,
134–135
Chlorprothixene, 19
Clinical Global Impressions scale, 118

Clomipramine:
anorexia nervosa, 293–294
obsessive-compulsive disorder, 206
Clonidine, 28, 238–239
Tourette's syndrome, 220, 223–224
Compazine, *see* Prochlorperazine
Compliance, 94–95
Conduct disorders, 28, 250–280, 341–342
and ADD, 276–277
anticonvulsants, 269–275
antidepressants, 277–278
delinquency, predictors, 259–260
diagnostic systems, 253–256
diphenylhydantoin, 270–272
etiology, 256–259
genetics, 258–259
haloperidol, 261–262
imipramine, 278
lithium, 261–269
medications, 261–279
methylphenidate, 276
natural history, 250–253
neuroleptics, 261–262
predictive factors, 259–260
propranolol, 278–279
socialized, aggressive, 255
socialized, non-aggressive, 255–256
stimulants, 275–277
undersocialized:
aggressive, 254
nonaggressive, 254–255
Connors Parent Symptom Questionnaire,
14, 87
Connors Rating Scales, and ADDH, 190
Connors Teacher Rating Scale, 14, 87
Coprolalia, 219
Cortisol hypersecretion, in depression, 31
Cyproheptadine, anorexia nervosa, 296–
297

Data analysis, 101–103
Daytime wetting, 322–323
Deanol, 17
ADDH, 182–184
Delinquency, predictors of, 259–260
Delta-9-tetrahydrocannabinol, 299
Delusions, depressive, 154
Dependent variables, 100–101
Depression, 30–32
childhood, biological correlates, 31